Pediatric Firearm Injuries and Fatalities

Lois K. Lee • Eric W. Fleegler
Editors

Pediatric Firearm Injuries and Fatalities

The Clinician's Guide to Policies
and Approaches to Firearm Harm Prevention

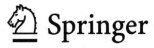

Editors
Lois K. Lee
Department of Pediatrics
Division of Emergency Medicine
Boston Children's Hospital
Harvard Medical School
Boston, MA
USA

Eric W. Fleegler
Department of Pediatrics
Division of Emergency Medicine
Boston Children's Hospital
Harvard Medical School
Boston, MA
USA

ISBN 978-3-030-62247-3   ISBN 978-3-030-62245-9   (eBook)
https://doi.org/10.1007/978-3-030-62245-9

This Springer imprint is published by the registered company Springer Nature Switzerland AG
The registered company address is: Gewerbestrasse 11, 6330 Cham, Switzerland

To my mother and father, Sue and Henry Lee, who showed me what is possible through hard work and helping others.

To my husband, Young-Jo, who supports and sustains me through everything, and my children, Alex and Lauren, who inspire me every day.

~Lois K. Lee

To my mom and dad, Kathy and Earl Fleegler, and my brother, Michael Fleegler, you always believed in and supported me, and you will remain in my heart always.

To Marisa, the best wife, partner, and friend I could ever ask for, and to Joshua, Naomi, and Sonia, my passionate children who will each carry their own torches forward to light up the night.

~Eric W. Fleegler

And finally, to our patients, especially those affected by gun violence,

who motivate us to work to make this world safer.

Foreword

As I write this in early spring 2020, the globe is in the midst of confronting the pandemic caused by SARS-CoV-2. Our world has dramatically changed in ways few could have imagined and the future over the next months is uncertain.

Children have been the population group with the lowest proportion of severe illness and extremely rare mortality from COVID-19. The jobs of pediatric healthcare workers have been less directly affected by the virus than those of our adult medicine colleagues, but all have been indirectly affected by the changes the pandemic has brought on the healthcare system and our communities.

Contrast the risk to our children from SARS-CoV-2 to that from firearms. According to the Centers for Disease Control and Prevention (CDC), as of December 10, 2020, there were 162 deaths among children in the United States with COVID-19 disease. In contrast, 22 children and adolescents were killed *per day* in 2018 from firearms. A silver lining of stay-at-home orders is that the nation has been spared from the horrible specter of children being shepherded from schools by SWAT teams in response to a mass shooting in their classrooms. Shelter-in-place now has more hopeful implications as children stay home from school and parents work from home, rather than the use of the term in association with school shootings.

However, firearm sales have skyrocketed as people rush to buy handguns and rifles in response to the fear generated by the pandemic. The FBI reports that the week of March 16–23, 2020 had the highest number of firearm background checks – 1,197,788 – conducted by the National Instant Criminal Background Check system for purchases of firearms since the system was set up in 1998. In short, firearms appear to be a more immediate threat to our nation's children than SARS-CoV-2.

This book is important reading for healthcare workers for many reasons. Firearm injuries and the policies governing firearm access are complicated. The issues can't be summarized on a bumper sticker or a tweet – regardless of where a person stands on the political spectrum. The descriptive data on firearm deaths is straightforward but the causes that result in those numbers and the methods to reduce them are not. The chapters in this book lay out the science as we know it in 2020, information that is not as robust as it should be because of the 24-year hiatus in funding by the CDC for firearm research. That hiatus has now ended with requests for proposals on firearm research issued this year by the CDC, National Institutes of Health (NIH), National Institute of Justice (NIJ), and private organizations such as the National Collaborative on Gun Violence Research. One of the lessons of the COVID-19 pandemic is that science *is* important and should drive policy when the health of the public is threatened. The same is true for policies related to firearms. Healthcare professionals need to educate themselves about the issues and know the science behind firearm injuries and policies. This book provides the science to make all of us better informed.

As the data in these pages show, some groups of children are much more affected by firearms than are others. Children living in urban areas are more at risk of firearm-related assaults and death than their counterparts in rural sections of the country. On the other hand, youth in rural communities have seen an increase in firearm-related suicide. African American young males have rates of firearm homicide that are an order of magnitude greater than that for young white males. American Indian and Native Alaskan youth have unconscionably high rates of firearm suicide. An astounding proportion of children in inner cities hear gunshots every year, and many have had firearm murders in their neighborhoods. The reasons for these high rates of firearm injuries and deaths in certain groups all ultimately stem from poverty and systemic racism. These same issues are responsible for the high rate of COVID-19 deaths in these communities. Solutions to reducing these rates must be found.

Another important COVID-19 lesson for the country has been that healthcare workers – physicians, nurses, emergency medical service providers – are critical professionals in the community who are dedicated to saving lives. The respect that members of this profession have earned in the last few months is probably greater than it has ever been in most of the lifetimes of the readers of this book. That new-found respect can give us a meaningful voice whether it be talking with patients and families or engaging our local, state, and national policy makers about the risks to our children related to unfettered access to firearms.

The critical role that public health plays in the lives of communities has never been more clear. Firearms do affect the health of the community, and the role of public health is critical to better understand the scope of the firearm injury problem and its consequences to the community. We do not have adequate surveillance for non-fatal firearm injuries. NORC at the University of Chicago published a report in October 2019 that outlined the serious data limitations the nation currently has on firearms and firearm-related injuries and crimes. Health professionals will need to team with the public health community to obtain those data to better inform our policy makers as well as those on the front lines of caring for victims, families, and communities affected by firearms.

Crises create the realization that we are all dependent on one another and that threats to the health, safety, and welfare of any of us affect us all and require a response from us together. As the nation and the world slowly recovers from the immediate threat of the pandemic, we have a chance to create new paradigms for our children. In the US, individual firearm ownership is protected by the Second Amendment to the Constitution, and the reasons why firearms are owned are highly varied. We must all respect those rights as we work together to develop better solutions to reducing the toll of firearms. It will not be a new drug or vaccine. It will require us to learn the facts put forth in this book and use this information to help our children. It is their right and our duty.

Seattle, WA, USA   Frederick P. Rivara
April 2020

Preface

The world is a dangerous place, not because of those who do evil, but because of those who look on and do nothing. (Albert Einstein (1879–1955))

Philadelphia, 1995: 140 children and young adults died due to firearm homicide; 80% were black and almost all lived in poor neighborhoods. Caring for children in Philadelphia in the 1990s, our careers in academic medicine were profoundly influenced by the poverty and gun violence affecting our patients and their families. These experiences continue to shape our clinical, research, and advocacy work as pediatric emergency medicine physicians today. Our injury prevention and health policy research focuses not only on understanding who is at risk for traumatic injuries, but more importantly, on what are the policies that could prevent these injuries and deaths in the first place.

Over 7000 children and young adults die by firearms each year in the United States, and rates of homicides and suicides have been increasing. Isolated and shocking events such as the 1999 shooting at Columbine High School in Colorado have tragically become commonplace today. If we look around the world, we know gun violence need not be a constant in our daily lives. Yes – the United States is an extreme outlier in rates of gun-related injuries and deaths compared to other nations, but we know that thoughtful interventions and appropriate legislation decrease gun violence.

Change does not come easily. After decades of effort, a multi-pronged approach to reduce motor vehicle collisions now has children and youth dying at less than half the rate of just 20 years ago. Gun violence must follow the same trajectory. To accomplish this requires a willingness to rethink the role of guns in our society, the implementation of meaningful legislation, and the support of our government to fund the research that will guide us.

This book will inform you about the scope of the gun violence epidemic in the United States, focusing on our children and youth. We hope it will inspire you to affect change. We believe that we can work together and make the world a safer place for all our children.

Boston, MA, USA   Eric W. Fleegler
Boston, MA, USA   Lois K. Lee

Contents

List of Contributors

Deborah Azrael, PhD Harvard School of Public Health, Harvard Injury Control Research Center, Boston, MA, USA

Patrick M. Carter, MD Department of Emergency Medicine, Injury Prevention Center, University of Michigan, Ann Arbor, MI, USA

Andrew Conner, BS Frank H. Netter MD School of Medicine at Quinnipiac University, North Haven, CT, USA

Rebecca M. Cunningham, MD Department of Emergency Medicine, Injury Prevention Center, University of Michigan, Ann Arbor, MI, USA

James Dodington, MD Department of Pediatrics, Yale University School of Medicine, New Haven, CT, USA

Elizabeth Dugan, LICSW Department of Emergency Medicine, Boston Medical Center, Boston, MA, USA

Joel A. Fein, MD, MPH Department of Pediatrics, Children's Hospital of Philadelphia at the University of Pennsylvania School of Medicine, Philadelphia, PA, USA

Eric W. Fleegler, MD, MPH Department of Pediatrics, Division of Emergency Medicine, Boston Children's Hospital, Harvard Medical School, Boston, MA, USA

Francesca Fontin, MPH Department of Emergency Medicine, Boston Medical Center, Boston, MA, USA

Erin Grinshteyn, PhD Health Professions Department, School of Nursing and Health Professions, University of San Francisco, San Francisco, CA, USA

David Hemenway, PhD Department of Health Policy and Management, Harvard T.H. Chan School of Public Health, Boston, MA, USA

Michael P. Hirsh, MD Department of Surgery, University of Massachusetts Medical School, Worcester, MA, USA

David M. Jaffe, MD Formerly Department of Emergency Medicine, University of California, San Francisco, San Francisco, CA, USA

Lois K. Lee, MD, MPH Department of Pediatrics, Division of Emergency Medicine, Boston Children's Hospital, Harvard Medical School, Boston, MA, USA

Jody Lyneé Madeira, MS, JD, PhD Maurer School of Law, Center for Law, Society, & Culture, Indiana University, Bloomington, IN, USA

Rebekah Mannix, MD, MPH Department of Pediatricis, Division of Emergency Medicine, Boston Children's Hospital, Harvard Medical School, Boston, MA, USA

Peter T. Masiakos, MD Department of Pediatric Surgery, Massachusetts General Hospital, Harvard Medical School, Boston, MA, USA

Matthew Miller, MD, MPH, ScD Bouve College of Health Sciences, Northeastern University, Boston, MA, USA

Harvard Injury Control Research Center, Harvard T.H. Chan School of Public Health, Boston, MA, USA

Michael C. Monuteaux, ScD Department of Pediatrics, Division of Emergency Medicine, Boston Children's Hospital, Boston, MA, USA

Elizabeth C. Pino, PhD Department of Emergency Medicine, Boston Medical Center, Boston, MA, USA

Zheala Qayyum, MBBS, MD Department of Psychiatry & Behavioral Sciences, Boston Children's Hospital, Harvard Medical School, Boston, MA, USA

Department of Psychiatry, Yale University School of Medicine, New Haven, CT, USA

Chris A. Rees, MD, MPH Department of Pediatrics, Division of Emergency Medicine, Boston Children's Hospital, Harvard Medical School, Boston, MA, USA

Naveen F. Sangji, MD, MPH Department of Acute Care Surgery, University of Michigan, Ann Arbor, MI, USA

Judy Schaechter, MD, MBA Department of Pediatrics, University of Miami, Miller School of Medicine, Miami, FL, USA

Cynthia Wilson, MD Department of Psychiatry, Yale University, New Haven, CT, USA

Chapter 1
Children and Firearms: Inevitable Interactions or Needless Calamities?

Lois K. Lee and Eric W. Fleegler

Jacksonville school officials urge parents to lock up their weapons after boy packs gun

By The Times-Union
February 19, 2019. *The Florida Times-Union*

1.1 The US Firearm Experience

By 2013, two-thirds of US public school students participated in firearm drills, often three to four times per year. The days of tornado and hurricane drills have been supplemented or supplanted with frequently intense "active shooter drills" designed to teach children to hide in closets, black out windows, and throw school supplies at a shooter. Children sometimes do not know whether the event was a drill or someone was actually trying to kill them until it is over, 7–10 minutes into their concealment. The emergence of this new type of school safety drill has occurred as a result of recent, seminal school shootings in the US, including at Sandy Hook Elementary School in Connecticut in 2012, Marjory Stoneman Douglas High School in Florida in 2018, and then again 3 months later at the Santa Fe High School in Texas. While school killings ultimately represent a small percentage of the children who die by guns, a culture of awareness and activism has arisen among US youth and adults to try to curb this epidemic of increasing gun violence.

Although these shootings receive the most press attention related to firearms [1], what should be of greater concern is the increasing rates of firearm suicides, homicides [2], and unintentional deaths as well as the nonfatal firearm injuries inflicted on US children and youth every year. Children and young adults 0–24 years old accounted for 20% of the 39,740 US firearm deaths in 2018. This translates to 22

L. K. Lee (✉) · E. W. Fleegler
Department of Pediatrics, Division of Emergency Medicine, Boston Children's Hospital, Harvard Medical School, Boston, MA, USA
e-mail: Lois.lee@childrens.harvard.edu; eric.fleegler@childrens.harvard.edu

© Springer Nature Switzerland AG 2021   1
L. K. Lee, E. W. Fleegler (eds.), *Pediatric Firearm Injuries and Fatalities*,
https://doi.org/10.1007/978-3-030-62245-9_1

pediatric deaths in the US daily from firearms – the equivalent of an entire school busload of children killed every 4 days. In 2018 there were a total of 7946 deaths due to firearms in children and youth 0–24 years old, of whom there were 3198 suicides (40%), 4358 homicides (55%), and 183 unintentional deaths (2%). When specifically examining the higher-risk group of teenagers 15–19 years old, of the 2807 deaths due to firearms, there were 1094 suicides (39%), 1580 homicides (56%), and 62 unintentional deaths (2%). In the highest-risk group of young adults 20–24 years old, there were 4604 deaths due to firearms including 1901 suicides (41%), 2527 homicides (55%), and 67 unintentional deaths (1%) [3].

The rates and numbers of pediatric firearm deaths have increased over the past two decades (Fig. 1.1). Between 2001 and 2018, significant disparities continued to persist in firearm homicides in the age-adjusted firearm homicide rates among Black, non-Hispanic children (16.6/100,000), American Indian/Alaskan Native (3.4/100,000), and Hispanic children (3.3/100,000) far greater than White, non-Hispanic children (1.1/100,000) and Asian/Pacific Islander children (1.1/100,000) (Fig. 1.2a). Smaller disparities exist in pediatric firearm suicide with American Indian/Alaskan Native children having the highest rates of firearm suicide (4.3/100,000), followed by White, non-Hispanic children (2.6/100,000) versus Black, non-Hispanic children (1.7/100,000), Hispanic children (1.2/100,000), and Asian/Pacific Islander children (0.8/100,000) [3] (Fig. 1.2b).

In addition to fatal injuries, there has been an increase in nonfatal injuries [4]. From 2002 to 2016, pediatric firearm injuries grew from an estimated 27,342 to 48,828, a rate increase of over 65%. For teenagers 15–19 years old, there were an estimated 15,867 nonfatal firearm injuries, and for young adults 20–24 years old, there were an estimated 31,604 nonfatal firearm injuries [3]. These numbers only represent the tip of the iceberg in terms of the magnitude of impact firearm injuries have on the health system. These nonfatal injuries do not account for the continuing care required for those requiring chronic physical rehabilitation, long-term mental

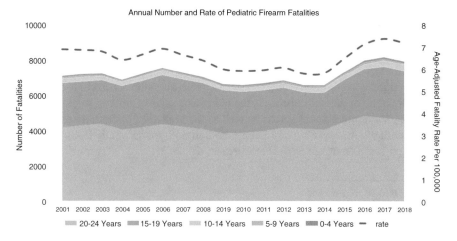

Fig. 1.1 Firearm deaths in the US, 0–24 years old, 2001–2018, by age group

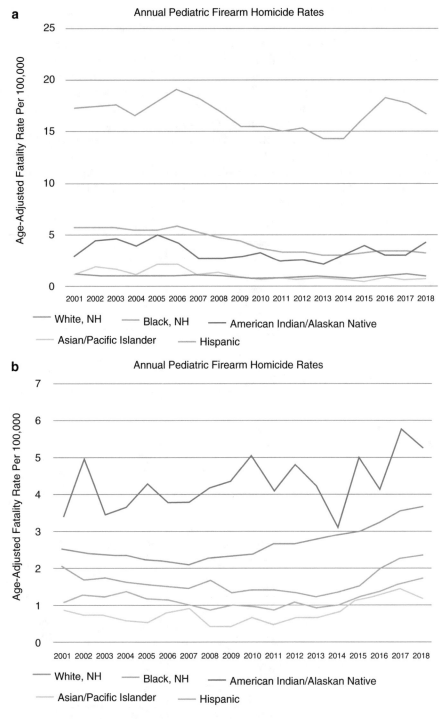

Fig. 1.2 (**a**) Pediatric firearm homicide rates, 2001–2018, by race/ethnicity. (**b**) Anual pediatric firearm suicide rates, 2001–2018, by race/ethnicity

health effects, and years of potential life lost for these young victims. A 2010 estimate put the 1-year medical cost of pediatric firearm injuries and deaths at $424 million and the work loss cost at $13.6 billion [3]. These numbers of course do not speak to the unmeasurable emotional costs to their families and loved ones.

According to national Gallup polls in 2019, about 37% of American households own guns, down from a peak of 51% in 1994 [5]; significant variability exists in state household ownership rates (Table 1.1). Approximately 22.6 million children live in households with firearms. Among them, 4.6 million children, 7% of all US children, are exposed to at least one gun that is loaded and unlocked (the most dangerous storage environment). Another 11.4 million children live in households with the gun loaded and locked, or unloaded and unlocked, each a dangerous storage method into itself [6]. In children with a history of self-harm risk factors, 43.5% live in a household with a firearm present [7].

Table 1.1 Household firearm ownership rates, by state, 2017[a]

State	Ownership rates	Rank
Alabama	50%	44
Alaska	49%	43
Arizona	38%	29
Arkansas	46%	41
California	19%	7
Colorado	32%	17
Connecticut	13%	5
Delaware	25%	10
Florida	30%	12
Georgia	41%	33
Hawaii	5%	1
Idaho	52%	47
Illinois	22%	8
Indiana	34%	22
Iowa	32%	16
Kansas	40%	32
Kentucky	42%	35
Louisiana	43%	38
Maine	43%	37
Maryland	24%	9
Massachusetts	10%	2
Michigan	32%	18
Minnesota	35%	25
Mississippi	48%	42
Missouri	42%	36
Montana	63%	50
Nebraska	34%	21
Nevada	31%	13
New Hampshire	31%	14
New Jersey	12%	4
New Mexico	34%	19

Table 1.1 (continued)

State	Ownership rates	Rank
New York	14%	6
North Carolina	36%	27
North Dakota	53%	48
Ohio	32%	15
Oklahoma	44%	39
Oregon	35%	24
Pennsylvania	34%	20
Rhode Island	12%	3
South Carolina	39%	31
South Dakota	51%	46
Tennessee	45%	40
Texas	35%	26
Utah	36%	28
Vermont	42%	34
Virginia	34%	23
Washington	29%	11
West Virginia	51%	45
Wisconsin	38%	30
Wyoming	59%	49

[a]Ownership rate estimated based on formula using ratio of firearm suicides to total suicides and hunting license rates [3, 20]

Over the last 10 years, support has increased for stricter firearm laws (44% in 2011 versus 64% in 2019). This is consistent with increasing dissatisfaction with US gun policy with 36% very dissatisfied and only 17% very satisfied in 2019. This is compared to 2008 when 21% reported they were very dissatisfied and 14% very satisfied with US gun policy [5]. By 2019, 64% of people felt laws covering firearms should be stricter, versus only 7% who felt they should be less strict. Americans are divided on what type of laws there should be – 29% want to ban the possession of handguns, and 47% want to ban semi-automatic guns ("assault rifles"). The majority of Americans (96%) favor universal background checks for all gun purchases, 75% favor enacting a 30-day waiting period for all gun sales, and 70% favor the requirement that all privately owned guns be registered with the police [5].

Youth in the US in general actually support guns in the home. A national text message survey of US youth reported 66% (506/772 respondents) were "pro" or "conditionally pro" guns in the home. They cite the second amendment, as well as wanting guns for protection and hunting, as reasons for wanting to have a gun [8]. This mirrors a change in mindset across the US – in 2000, 35% of Americans felt guns made a house safer and 51% more dangerous. By 2014 these opinions had completely flipped – 63% felt guns made homes safer, and 30% felt guns made homes more dangerous [9]. This remarkable reversal goes against research over the past 35 years showing that having a gun in home makes it more dangerous as members of the household are far more likely to be killed by a gun in the house than an intruder [10]. This speaks to the powerful messaging of gun rights groups like the National Rifle Association (NRA) and the ineffectiveness of medical and public health organizations in their ability to raise awareness of the potential dangers associated with guns in the home.

To be clear, having a gun in the home increases the risk of firearm injuries in children [11, 12]. The American Academy of Pediatrics (AAP), as well as multiple other medical organizations, recommends that if a gun is to be kept at home, the safest way to store the gun is unloaded, with the ammunition and firearm stored separately and locked and ideally not on the premises of the home [13, 14]. The vast majority (90%) of unintentional shooting deaths occur in a home when children play with an unsecured gun. For suicide attempts and unintentional injuries, more than 75% of the guns used were in the home of the victim, relative, or friend [12]. Firearms are also the most common mechanism of death for victims of intimate partner violence, the majority of whom are female [15, 16]. This is highly relevant to pediatrics since these women are frequently the main caregivers of the children, and children are frequently killed along with their mothers.

One study examining children's knowledge of guns in their home reported 76% of children less than 9 years old knew the location of their parents' firearm and 36% of them had handled the gun. Only 60% of the parents of these children knew their children had handled the gun [17]. In addition to parents' lack of awareness that their children have handled a gun, parents may not realize children as young as 2 years old are strong enough to fire a gun [18]. Thus removal or safe storage of firearms is important to prevent access to guns in the home to decrease unintentional and intentional injuries and deaths, not only by children but also by other individuals at risk for causing harm [11].

1.2   How to Use This Book

Part I, *Epidemiology and Risk Factors*, will dive into the details of pediatric firearm injuries and fatalities in the US. Most data pertain to the children and youth, 0–24 years old. Chapters 2, 3 and 4 take an in-depth look at the most common firearm injury intents – suicide, homicide, and unintentional. Each chapter explores changes over time, risk factors, and disparities. Chapter 5, "School Shootings," takes a close look at this growing American phenomenon, and then Chapter 6 provides an international perspective on pediatric firearm experiences.

Part II, *Interventions*, provides the before, during, and after approach to handling guns and gun violence among children and youth. Chapters 7, 8, 9, 10 and 11 provide the clinician's approach to these potentially challenging conversations, then management of patients in the emergency department and the mental health clinician's office, and care of injured patients both from the medical perspective and the holistic view of violence intervention advocates. Chapter 12 examines the evolving technology of "smart guns." Then Chapters 13 and 14 evaluate the essential role of firearm legislation and how clinicians can and should play a strong advocacy role.

In conclusion, Chapter 15 looks to the future – providing guidance for the interventions, policies, and research that can make the greatest difference in protecting the youth of America.

1.3 Our Philosophy

Pediatric healthcare clinicians have the responsibility to care for not only their pediatric patients but also their patients' families and loved ones. The most important intervention we can provide is the guidance and advice to help families avoid needless – and preventable – tragedies, whether they are deaths from pools, motor vehicle crashes, or firearms. The interventions may take place in primary care offices, emergency departments, operating rooms, trauma services, or intensive care units, as well as the halls of government, departments of public health, and anywhere efforts are made to reduce children's harm from guns. Healthcare clinicians need to play an important role in harm prevention to decrease the risk of unintentional and intentional firearm injuries to children and youth, not only through anticipatory guidance but also through research and advocacy for effective policies designed to save lives.

An open dialog is an important part of informing parents and caregivers of youth about the best way to keep their children safe while being respectful of the family's customs and beliefs. Screening and counseling are effective in increasing safe storage of firearms, and the majority of clinicians and patients find these conversations acceptable and appropriate, though unfortunately they occur infrequently. We should educate and advocate for the promotion of the safe storage of firearms in the home, if a family owns or is considering purchasing a firearm. We can also discuss with parents and caregivers the increased risk of firearm injuries and death in the home when a gun is present and to ask about firearms when their children visit someone else's home. For families where there are substance use or mental health concerns, conversations around firearm means restriction are particularly essential.

On a larger community level, healthcare clinicians and public health advocates need to work towards policy solutions to improve firearm safety in our communities. Community-based efforts to improve the safety of neighborhoods differentially affected by gun violence are critical. The major disparities in firearm fatalities, whether by race or ethnicity, or by poverty concentration, are neither inevitable nor acceptable. Other efforts to decrease firearm injuries and deaths include advocating for the advancement and use of safe gun technology so only an authorized user can fire a gun, as well as effective policies to prevent at-risk individuals from accessing guns must be pursued. Effective policies to promote include universal background checks for firearms and ammunition and extreme risk protection orders to prevent individuals at risk of harming themselves or others from possessing a gun. Our country has a patchwork of firearm legislation that has helped protect citizens of some states while leaving others more vulnerable. For example, only 16 states have enacted strong child access prevention laws [19]. A multipronged strategy is needed to increase the adoption of effective policies to decrease firearm injuries and deaths to children and youth.

As healthcare clinicians and public health advocates for children and youth, we have a responsibility to engage in efforts to keep them safe. Like other public health epidemics, a coordinated approach engaging individuals, communities, corporations, and the government will be critical to address the increasing rates of firearm deaths and injuries in US children and youth. This problem of firearm injuries and death in our youth as well as the effectiveness of certain policies has been well established. We hope this book will engage and educate its readers about the impact firearms have on children and their community, the role of policy in harm reduction, and the importance of advocating for effective policies and robust research. Only by working together can we hope to stem the tide of this firearm epidemic to protect our children and youth.

References

1. Rees CA, Lee LK, Fleegler EW, Mannix R. Mass school shootings in the United States: a novel root cause analysis using lay press reports. Clin Pediatr (Phila). 2019;58(13):1423–8.
2. Lee LK, Mannix R. Increasing fatality rates from preventable deaths in teenagers and young adults. JAMA. 2018;320(6):543–4.
3. Centers for Disease Control and Prevention. Web-based injury statistics query and reporting system [Internet]. [cited 2020 Oct 1]. Available from: https://webappa.cdc.gov/sasweb/ncipc/leadcause.html
4. Gani F, Canner JK. Trends in the incidence of and charges associated with firearm-related injuries among pediatric patients, 2006–2014. JAMA. 2018;172(12):1195–6.
5. Gallup. Guns [Internet]. 2020 [cited 2020 Mar 19]. Available from: https://news.gallup.com/poll/1645/Guns.aspx?g_source=link_newsv9&g_campaign=item_262724&g_medium=copy
6. Azrael D, Cohen J, Salhi C, Miller M. Firearm storage in gun-owning households with children: results of a 2015 national survey. J Urban Health. 2018;95(3):295–304.
7. Scott J, Azrael D, Miller M. Firearm storage in homes with children with self-harm risk factors. Pediatrics. 2018;141(3):e20172600.
8. Van Sparrentak M, Chang T, Miller AL, Nichols LP, Sonneville KR. Youth opinions about guns and gun control in the United States. JAMA Pediatr. 2018;172(9):884–6.
9. Pew Research Center. Views of gun safety and the key responsibilities of gun owners [Internet]. 2017 [cited 2020 Mar 19]. Available from: https://www.pewsocialtrends.org/2017/06/22/views-of-gun-safety-and-the-key-responsibilities-of-gun-owners/
10. Kellermann AL, Reay DT. Protection or peril? An analysis of firearm-related deaths in the house. N Engl J Med. 1986;314(24):1557–60.
11. Grossman DC, Mueller BA, Riedy C, Dowd MD, Villaveces A, Prodzinski J, et al. Gun storage practices and risk of youth suicide and unintentional firearm injuries. J Am Med Assoc. 2005;293(6):707–14.
12. Grossman DC, Reay DT, Baker SA. Self-inflicted and unintentional firearm injuries among children and adolescents: the source of the firearm. Arch Pediatr Adolesc Med. 1999;153(8):875–8.
13. Gardner HG, Quinlan KP, Ewald MB, Ebel BE, Lichenstein R, Melzer-Lange MD, et al. Firearm-related injuries affecting the pediatric population. Pediatrics. 2012;130(5):e1416-23.

14. Pallin R, Spitzer SA, Ranney ML, Betz ME, Wintemute GJ. Preventing firearm-related death and injury. Ann Intern Med. 2019;170(11):ITC81–96.
15. Adhia A, Kernic MA, Hemenway D, Vavilala MS, Rivara FP. Intimate partner homicide of adolescents. JAMA Pediatr. 2019;173(6):571–7.
16. Everytown for Gun Safety. Guns and violence against women [Internet]. 2019. Available from: https://everytownresearch.org/wp-content/uploads/2019/10/IPV-for-WEB-112519B.pdf
17. Baxley F, Miller M. Parental misperceptions about children and firearms. Arch Pediatr Adolesc Med. 2006;160(5):542–7.
18. Naureckas SM, Galanter C, Naureckas ET, Donovan M, Christoffel KK. Children's and women's ability to fire handguns. JAMA Pediatr. 1995;149:1318–1322.
19. Azad HA, Monuteaux MC, Rees CA, Siegel M, Mannix R, Lee LK, et al. Child access prevention firearm laws and firearm fatalities among children aged 0 to 14 years, 1991–2016. JAMA Pediatr. 2020;174(5):463–9.
20. Siegel M, Ross CS, King C 3rd. A new proxy measure for state-level gun ownership in studies of firearm injury prevention. Inj Prev. 2014;20(3):204–7.

Part I
Epidemiology and Risk Factors

Chapter 2
Access to Firearms and Youth Suicide in the US: Implications for Clinical Interventions

Andrew Conner, Deborah Azrael, and Matthew Miller

Despair and guns, a deadly mix for two Rockwall girls who had everything to live for

By Nancy Churnin
June 3, 2013. *The Dallas Morning News*

2.1 Introduction

In 2017, 6774 youth 5–24 years old died by suicide in the US. Of these, almost half (47%) used a firearm. Over the past 10 years, suicide rates in this age group have increased nearly 50%, with the rate in 2017 (8.02 per 100,000) the highest it has been in nearly 40 years [1] (Fig. 2.1). This chapter summarizes the epidemiology of youth suicide and provides an overview of the evidence showing that access to firearms is a risk factor for suicide. It then describes what we know, to date, about counseling parents to prevent their child's access to firearms. The chapter concludes with recommendations for current clinical practice and for future research.

A. Conner
Frank H. Netter MD School of Medicine at Quinnipiac University, North Haven, CT, USA
e-mail: andrew.conner@quinnipiac.edu

D. Azrael
Harvard School of Public Health, Harvard Injury Control Research Center, Boston, MA, USA
e-mail: Azrael@hsph.harvard.edu

M. Miller (✉)
Bouvé College of Health Sciences, Northeastern University, Boston, MA, USA

Harvard Injury Control Research Center, Harvard T.H. Chan School of Public Health, Boston, MA, USA
e-mail: ma.miller@northeastern.edu

© Springer Nature Switzerland AG 2021
L. K. Lee, E. W. Fleegler (eds.), *Pediatric Firearm Injuries and Fatalities*,
https://doi.org/10.1007/978-3-030-62245-9_2

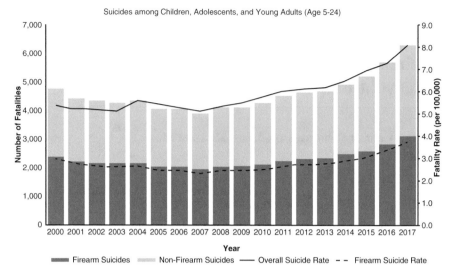

Fig. 2.1 Trends in firearm and non-firearm suicides, as well as overall firearm and non-firearm suicide fatality rates among children, adolescents, and young adults (5–24 years old), United States, 2000–2017. (Adapted from Web-based Injury Statistics Query and Reporting System (WISQARS) [1])

2.2 Epidemiology of Suicide Among Youth

From 2008 to 2017, (the ten most recent years for which mortality data are available), 53,957 youth 5–24 years old died by suicide, making suicide the second leading cause of death in this age group.[1] As is true across all age groups, suicide rates among youth 5–24 years old are three to four times higher among males than among females; higher among White, non-Hispanics than among all other race/ethnicities; and higher in rural, non-metropolitan areas than in urban, metropolitan areas [1].

Firearms are the most common means used in suicides among people of all ages as well as among youth. Of the almost 54,000 suicide deaths among 5–24-year-olds (over the decade 2008 to 2017), 24,226 (45%) were by firearm. The fraction of suicides completed with a firearm varies by age, making up 33% of suicides among 5–14-year-olds, 43% among 15–19-year-olds, and 47% among those aged 20–24 [1].[2] Among youth, as is the case among older age groups as well, firearm suicide rates vary by age and gender. Between 2008 and 2017, for example, rates of firearm suicide ranged from 0.29 per 100,000 among 5–14-year-olds to 6.76 per 100,000 among 20–24-year-olds. Firearm suicide rates among those 5–24 years old are over

---

[1] Motor vehicle crashes killed 81,428 youth aged 5–24 over this time period.

[2] The second most common method of completed suicide among youth overall is suffocation (39.8%), followed by poisoning (7.4%), jumping (2.7%), and drowning (0.9%).

seven times higher for male youth (4.95 per 100,000) than for female youth (0.67 per 100,000) and over two times higher for White, non-Hispanic youth (3.76 per 100,000) than for all other race/ethnicities (1.70 per 100,000), respectively [1].

Firearm (and overall) suicide rates also vary substantially by geography. Across states, for example, rates of youth firearm suicide range from as low as 0.76 deaths per 100,000 in New Jersey to as high as 16.74 deaths per 100,000 in Alaska, and youth firearm suicide rates are higher in non-metropolitan areas compared to metropolitan areas in 2017 [1]. The variation in suicide rates across geography is not explained by demographic differences across place, nor by differences in the prevalence of known behavioral or psychiatric risk factors for suicide. Rather, variation in rates of suicide and firearm suicide are largely explained by variation in household firearm prevalence [2].

2.3 Exposure to Firearms

The US has more firearms in civilian hands than any developed country. Based on survey estimates from 2015, there were an estimated 265 million civilian-owned firearms in the US [3]. By 2019, preliminary data from the 2019 National Firearms Survey suggest that this number has risen to approximately 300 million (unpublished data from authors D.A and M.M.). The US gun stock is distributed across one-third of US households [3]; homes with children are no more or less likely to have firearms than those without children [4]. As such, approximately 13 million households with children less than 18 years old contain at least 1 firearm. Though there has been little research on the characteristics of households with and without children with respect to gun ownership, several studies suggest there are few, if any, differences in the probability that youth with known risk factors for suicide will live in a household with a firearm [4, 5]. Given these observations, it is not surprising that firearms from children's households or the households of family members are often the source of firearms used by youth suicide decedents, with estimates ranging from 80% to 90% [6–8].

The only recent survey to characterize firearm storage in households with children found approximately two in ten such households stored at least one firearm loaded and unlocked (the least safe way with regard to locking and loading), while only three in ten stored all household firearms unloaded and locked up (the safest way) [9]. While fewer gun-owning households with children than households without children stored any firearm loaded and unlocked (20% vs. 30%, respectively), among households with children, those with only older children were more likely to store a firearm unsafely compared with households with younger children (e.g., 17% of households with any child under the age of 5 years and 27% of households with 13–17-year-old children only) [9, 10]. This is *despite* the fact older children are at higher risk than are younger children for firearm injury [1].

2.4   The Relationship Between Firearms and Suicide

2.4.1   Lethality of Suicide Attempts with Firearms Relative to Other Means

Across the US, suicide mortality rates are only modestly correlated with the incidence of suicidal acts (fatal and nonfatal suicide attempts). Rates of suicide attempts (and other strong correlates of suicidal behavior including rates of major psychiatric illness) vary far less across states than do rates of death by suicide and, accordingly, have been found to be weakly, sometimes inconsistently, and occasionally inversely correlated with rates of death by suicide across demographic and geographical groups. Whereas ecologic patterns of suicide mortality are not well explained by patterns of suicide attempt rates, variation in the proportion of suicidal acts that prove fatal – the suicide case fatality rate (CFR) – is strongly correlated with rates of death by suicide [11].

   Variation in overall suicide CFR between sexes and across age groups, regions, and levels of urbanization is largely explained by the distribution of methods used in suicidal acts, which is itself not strongly related to the underlying base rate of suicidal behavior. For example, compared with females, males are less likely to engage in suicidal acts (and only slightly more likely to die by suicide when they use a given method), but three to four times more likely to die in a suicidal act because the methods that males use are, on average, more lethal [12–15]. A similar pattern is observed across age groups. Younger people engage in suicidal acts more often, but older people are far more likely to die in a suicidal act because suicidal acts among older people are more likely to involve the use of highly lethal means [12, 13, 15]. Using data that include only cases of intentional self-inflicted injury that results in either medical evaluation in an emergency department or hospitalization, several studies have found substantial differences in the CFR for various methods used in suicidal acts [12–15]. The most recent of these studies, which used national-level US data from 2007 to 2014, for example, found that 90% of self-inflicted injuries with a firearm and 53% of hangings/suffocations were fatal, whereas only 2% of poisonings with drugs and less than 1% of self-injuries with a sharp instrument resulted in death [15]. In the US, a predominant determinant of the suicide CFR across geographic and demographic subgroups is the proportion of suicidal acts that are completed using firearms.

2.4.2   Evidence from the US that Access to Firearms Is a Risk Factor for Suicide

The strong association between living in a household with a firearm and risk of suicide has been established in a large body of literature, summarized at length elsewhere [11, 16–18]. We provide a brief accounting of the ecologic and individual-level studies that have been conducted, highlighting those that provide estimates of the association for youth.

Firearm suicide rates and overall suicide rates in the US are higher where firearms are more prevalent, a finding that holds across all age groups at the regional, state, and city level [2, 19–27]. By contrast, rates of suicide by methods other than firearms are not significantly correlated with rates of household firearm ownership [2, 19–27].[3] This pattern has been reported in ecologic studies adjusting for several potential confounders, including measures of psychological distress, alcohol and illicit drug use, poverty, education, and unemployment, and even when controlling for underlying suicide attempt rates.[4] For example, using data from the early 2000s, researchers found overall suicide rates among 5–19-year-olds were more than two times higher in high gun prevalence states compared to low gun prevalence states. This finding was driven entirely by a five-and-a-half-fold difference in firearm suicide rates [26].

Household firearm ownership is also a strong and consistent predictor of suicide in studies examining individual-level data. Overall, the pattern observed in ecologic studies – overall suicide rates are higher where firearms are more readily available because firearm suicide rates are higher and non-firearm suicides are not markedly different, compared with places where firearms are less available – has also been observed in individual-level studies with the power to examine suicide by method. This literature was summarized in a 2014 meta-analysis pooling data from 14 observational studies measuring the odds of suicide [28]. This analysis estimated a pooled odds ratio (OR) of 3.24 (95% confidence interval [CI]: 2.41 to 4.40) for suicide among persons *of any age* with access to firearms compared with those without access. A few of the studies included in the meta-analysis focused on adolescents, one of which compared adolescent suicide victims to living population-based community controls. In this study, the odds of suicide were four-fold higher for adolescents who lived in homes with firearms, compared to adolescents who lived in homes without firearms (OR = 4.4, 95% CI: 1.1 to 17.5) [29].

2.4.3   Is the Association Causal?

The association between firearm availability and suicide is not confounded by mental illness or other known suicide risk factors, strengthening the case for a causal effect of guns imposing heightened risk of dying by suicide. Three national surveys

---

[3] Household firearm ownership levels (often the fraction of households in a given geographic area that have one or more guns) are largely derived from surveys such as the General Social Survey or the large Behavioral Risk Factor Surveillance System Survey. Many studies that explore the relationship between firearm prevalence and outcomes such as suicide have also used a validated proxy for household firearm ownership, the fraction of suicides that are committed with a gun (FS/S).

[4] Earlier studies that relied on validated cross-sectional proxies of firearm ownership showed similar relationships.

among adults and one among adolescents found rates of mental illness and suicidality were not higher among those who owned or had access to household guns, compared with those without such access [30–33]. Simonetti et al. used the National Comorbidity Survey – Adolescent Supplement, a nationally representative survey of over 10,000 US adolescents to estimate the prevalence of self-reported in-home firearm access among adolescents with and without mental health-related suicide risk factors [32]. Adolescents with risk factors for suicide were just as likely to report in-home firearm access as those without such risk factors. Sorenson and Vittes analyzed data among adults from the General Social Survey (GSS), which asks about both gun ownership and mental health [33]. No significant associations were detected between personal gun ownership and any measure of mental health. Ilgen et al. analyzed data from the National Comorbidity Survey Replication (NCS-R), which included a question about whether there was a firearm in the respondents' home and several measures of mental health [30]. Here too, no significant difference was found between NCS-R respondents with and without access to firearms in terms of lifetime prevalence of mental illness. Miller et al. also used data from the NCS-R but extended Ilgen *et al.'s* analyses to investigate potential differences in recent (i.e., past year or current) symptoms of mental illness between respondents who lived in homes with firearms and respondents who lived in homes that did not contain firearms [31]. Again, no differences were found among people living in homes with versus without firearms and the odds of a recent diagnosis of mental health conditions.

To explore whether estimates in the peer-reviewed studies linking firearm availability to suicide risk may have been biased to a meaningful extent by failure to account for underlying differences between members of households with and without firearms, Miller, Swanson, and Azrael conducted a bias analysis using estimates of the elevated risk of suicide conferred by firearms from individual-level analyses [34]. This study found any such unmeasured confounder would need to possess an untenable combination of characteristics, including being as potent a suicide risk factor as the psychiatric disorders most strongly linked to suicide (e.g., major depression, major substance use disorders) and an order of magnitude more imbalanced across households with and without firearms than any known risk factor. The authors concluded no such confounder has ever been identified, or even suggested, and consequently, unmeasured confounding alone is unlikely to explain the reported associations between firearm availability and suicide.

Taken as a whole, the literature linking firearms to suicide indicates access to firearms does not serve as a proxy for an unmeasured predisposition to suicide, but instead increases suicide risk by making it more likely that suicidal acts will more often involve firearms, and therefore, will be more likely to result in death.

2.5 Firearm Storage Practices and Access to Firearms

A single case-control study has compared storage practices of household firearms used in suicides (and unintentional injuries) of children and adolescents younger than 20 years of age to storage practices of controls who live in gun-owning households [35]. This study, by Grossman and colleagues, found that firearms used in suicides, compared to firearms from control households, were less likely to be stored unloaded (adjusted odds ratio [aOR] = 0.39, 95% CI: 0.19 to 0.78), stored locked (aOR = 0.27, 95% CI: 0.16 to 0.47), stored separately from ammunition (aOR = 0.56, 95% CI: 0.32 to 0.98), or to have locked ammunition (aOR = 0.40, 95% CI: 0.22 to 0.72). Storage of firearms locked and separate from ammunition resulted in the greatest suicide risk reduction (aOR = 0.22, 95% CI: 0.11 to 0.47). Using the point estimates from Grossman's work, a 2019 study estimated approximately 100 youth suicides (19 years old or younger) could be prevented annually if the proportion of unlocked firearms decreased from 50% (the proportion of unlocked guns among the homes with children and firearms in the 2015 National Firearm Survey) to 30% [36].

Although Grossman and colleagues found that storing household firearms locked, unloaded, and separately from ammunition was associated with reduction in the risk of self-inflicted (and unintentional) firearm injuries among adolescents and children, a non-negligible proportion of case (suicide) firearms were stored in this manner. In other words, several youth who died from self-inflicted firearm injuries (or unintentional firearm injuries) used a firearm that was stored locked, unloaded, and/or separate from ammunition. Of the 106 firearm suicides and unintentional firearm injuries included in the study, 66% involved the use of a firearm stored unloaded, 34% involved a firearm stored locked, 41% involved the use of a firearm stored separate from ammunition, and 17% involved the use of a firearm stored locked with ammunition stored separately. What can be inferred from this is that while safe storage practices may attenuate the risk of suicide among households with firearms, children and adolescents living in a home with a firearm remain at increased risk compared to their counterparts who live in homes without firearms, regardless of storage practices. This is because "safe storage" is only a proxy for making firearms inaccessible to youth to the extent that youth can still access locked (or unloaded) firearms. Consistent with this residual risk, a study including all age groups found that the risk of suicide in the home was two fold higher in homes where all guns were locked compared to homes without any firearms [37].

2.6 Parental and Clinician Perceptions Regarding Risks of Household Gun Ownership

One reason adults in homes with children may store firearms in ways that make household guns accessible to children is that parents and other adults in the household may fail to appreciate the risk these firearms pose, especially with respect to suicide. In fact, many gun owners who store their guns loaded and unlocked may believe that they are keeping their household safe (and not increasing risk) by doing so. A recent study using the 2015 National Firearms Survey found only 3% of gun owners thought that having a gun in the home made the home more dangerous (59%

of gun owners said that guns in the home make it a safer place to be, and 40% said it depends) [38]. Using the same survey, another study found that adults overall, and firearm owners in particular, were unlikely to agree that a gun in the home increases the risk of suicide [39]. For example, only 6% of gun-owning adults agree the presence of a firearm in the home increases the risk for suicide, compared to 9% of adults who do not own a firearm but live with someone who does. This fraction rose only to 10% among gun owners with children. Even among health-care practitioners, only one in three (30.2%, 95% CI: 14.0% to 53.3%) agreed having a household firearm increases suicide risk. Among health-care practitioners who own firearms, 11.8% (95% CI: 4.5% to 27.3%) agreed.

Adults may also believe their household firearm, however stored, is inaccessible to their children. Although there is little research on this topic, one study among younger children (5–14 years old) in a pediatric and family practice clinic in rural Alabama found many parents think their child does not know about and/or cannot access household firearms. On the contrary, the child frequently in fact does know the location and has even accessed the firearm [40].

2.7 Clinical Efforts to Reduce Youth Suicide by Reducing Access to Firearms

Interventions to reduce unauthorized youth access to firearms in the US take, by and large, one of two approaches: (1) legislation imposing penalties on adults if a child could gain or gains access to their guns, especially if access results in fatal or non-fatal injury (Child Access Prevention [CAP] laws) and (2) health practitioner counseling about firearm safety (sometimes referred to as Lethal Means Counseling). Evaluations of these approaches have seldom been conducted, in the case of counseling, or severely limited in their design to permit causal inference, in the case of legislative efforts. We focus here on lethal means counseling, providing a comprehensive review of studies that have sought to evaluate community and clinical interventions to improve firearm storage in households with children.

2.8 Lethal Means Counseling and Safe Firearm Storage

In the US, approaches to preventing suicide by reducing access to firearms and other lethal methods have relied largely on efforts to inform personal decision-making rather than on legislative or public policy levers. For youth, decisions regarding access to firearms and other suicide methods generally rest with parents. Counseling parents to reduce access to potentially lethal suicide methods, an approach known as lethal means counseling (LMC), has been endorsed by several US medical societies, including the American Academy of Pediatrics (AAP), the American College of

Physicians (ACP), the American Medical Association (AMA), and the American College of Emergency Physicians (ACEP) [41–44]. Although parents generally appear to be willing to discuss firearm safety with their child's pediatrician [45–48], to date, few clinicians routinely offer LMC to parents of youth, even of those acutely at risk for suicide [49–64]. One reason LMC may not be routinely offered is that few studies have examined whether, and if so what type and for whom, counseling works. Those studies that have been conducted include evaluations of interventions to reduce youth access to firearms at the community level, in primary care practices, and only recently in acute care settings (i.e., emergency departments).

2.8.1   Community-Based Studies

Several studies have evaluated community-based interventions for safe firearm storage, including firearm storage device giveaway programs and/or community education programs. Studies evaluating storage device giveaway programs have generally found distribution of safe storage devices (such as trigger locks or lock boxes) led to a small increase in self-report of safe firearm storage [65–72]. These studies used different measures of storage to assess changes after intervention and assessed changes as soon as 4 weeks and as long as 18 months after intervention, limiting generalization about the magnitude of any effect. For example, a recent study evaluated changes in firearm storage practices following an intervention that included firearm safety messaging and distribution of a free, participant-selected firearm locking device (firearm trigger lock or lock box). At follow-up, 4–6 weeks after the intervention, 78% of participants reported that all household firearms were stored locked, compared to 64% of participants at baseline [70]. Another study examined if the installation of gun cabinets along with firearm safety messaging improved household firearm storage practices in a rural Alaskan community. At follow-up, 18 months after the intervention, 33% of households reported storing at least one firearm unlocked in the home, compared to 95% of households at baseline [66]. Evaluations of community education initiatives have reported mixed results regarding storage practices, and none have measured removal as a distinct outcome.

2.8.2   Primary Care-Based Studies

In the earliest of the primary care-based studies, a consecutive sample of parents of patients with appointments for routine visits in a single practice received provider-delivered verbal and written firearm safety counseling following the "Steps to Prevent Firearm Injury" (STOP) program of the American Academy of Pediatrics [73]. Among families with matched baseline and follow-up questionnaires (23.6% of families who completed baseline survey), there were no significant difference in household firearm ownership after counseling (at follow-up, 7.0%, vs. baseline,

9.4%, $p = 0.1$) and no significant decrease in the prevalence of storing firearms unlocked (2.7% at follow-up and baseline, $p = 1.0$) or loaded (at follow-up, 0.5%, vs. baseline, 1.6%, $p = 0.3$).

Two quasi-experimental studies examined physician-provided educational messages to parents with children or adolescents in the home around safe firearm storage [74, 75]. In the first study, patients of family medicine physicians received either no counseling, verbal counseling alone, or counseling and a firearm safety brochure from their physician [74]. After adjustment for demographic characteristics and the number and types of firearms owned, patients receiving counseling were three times more likely to make safe changes compared to patients who did not receive any form of counseling (aOR = 3.04, 95% CI: 1.28 to 7.24). Sixty-four percent of the counseling-only group and 58% of the counseling-plus brochure group made at least one or more safe changes between enrollment and follow-up, compared with 33% of the control group. In the second study, gun-owning families presenting to a single pediatric clinic received either firearm safety counseling along with a firearm safety brochure and a free gun lock (the intervention) or usual anticipatory guidance [75]. At 1-month follow-up, families who received counseling were not significantly more likely to have removed all firearms from their homes as compared with families who did not receive counseling. Among the families who received counseling, 61.6% either removed all guns from their homes or improved their firearm storage practices in some manner, whereas 26.9% of the families who received no counseling reported similar types of improvement ($p = 0.001$). Among parents in households continuing to have firearms at follow-up, those who received counseling were four times more likely to report some form of improvement in firearm storage than those who were not counseled (RR = 4.13, 95% CI: 2.06 to 8.30; 38.6% difference between groups).

Three randomized, controlled clinical trials have examined the effect of counseling families on safe storage practices in primary care settings [76–78]. For all three studies, the randomization and intervention were at the level of the clinician [77] or practice [76, 78]. In one study, families seen for a scheduled well-child appointment were given a brief message by their practitioner that depended on the presence of firearms in the home [77]. Families without firearms in the home were informed of the risks associated with household firearm ownership and given a standard information pamphlet. Families with household firearms were given the same information about risks and were told that if they decided to keep firearms in the home, they should be stored locked and unloaded. Families with firearms in the home were also provided with written storage guidelines and discount coupons for firearm storage devices. Over a 3-month follow-up, families receiving counseling were just as likely to acquire new firearms as those who did not (intervention group: 1.3% vs. control group: 0.9%, $p = 0.44$). Among families with household firearms at baseline, there were also no differences between those who received counseling and those who did not in the likelihood of removing firearms from the home at follow-up (intervention group, 6.7%, vs. control group, 5.7%, $p = 0.72$). In another randomized counseling intervention study, providers in pediatric practices were randomized to deliver counseling on either alcohol and tobacco use or firearm safety and bicycle helmet and seatbelt use to families with fifth- and sixth-grade children [78]. All families received brochures, annual newsletters, and reinforcement of messaging at subsequent health-care visits based on the initial counseling they received. Among families with household firearms, those receiving counseling on safe firearm storage were as likely to store all firearms unlocked as those receiving counseling on tobacco and alcohol use (aOR = 1.22, 95% CI: 0.87 to 1.71) (the percentages of firearm storage at follow-up were not reported, nor were unadjusted odds ratios).

The largest primary care intervention study included both counseling and cable lock distribution as its intervention. This study included 137 pediatric practices across the US. These practices were randomly assigned to have their providers either deliver motivational interviewing-based education on a range of safety behaviors (i.e., safe firearm storage, car seat and bicycle helmet use) or deliver no such specific counseling to families with children aged 2–11 years [76]. Families who received counseling and reported having firearms in the home were offered free cable locks. Over a 6-month follow-up, there was an increase in the use of cable locks among families receiving counseling (at 6 months, 68.3%, vs. baseline, 58.6%). These counseled families were significantly more likely to report the use of cable locks compared to those who did not receive the counseling (OR = 2.0, $p < 0.001$; 22% difference between groups).

2.8.3 Emergency Department-Based Studies

Three studies have examined the receipt of LMC in emergency department (ED) settings as it is related to subsequent storage of lethal means, including firearms [79–81]. One study found parents of children who made an ED visit for mental health assessment or treatment and received LMC were nearly four times more likely to take new actions to limit access to lethal means of suicide (i.e., firearms, alcohol, prescription medications, and over-the-counter medications) than parents who did not receive counseling (aOR = 3.6, 95% CI: 1.1 to 12.1) [79]. For example, compared with parents who were not counseled, those who were counseled were more likely to reduce access to prescription drugs (75% vs. 48%) and to firearms (63% vs. 0%). The number of gun-owning households, however, was small: five of eight adults whose households contained firearms at baseline took new action to limit firearm access after LMC (locked or removed all firearms), while none of the seven gun-owning families not counseled took action to limit access. In the other study, psychiatric emergency clinicians were trained to provide LMC, based on the "Counseling on Access to Lethal Means" (CALM) model, to parents of pediatric patients who received care for suicidality in the ED of a children's hospital [80]. A free lock box was provided during counseling. Of the 114 parents who received LMC, 76% reported all medications in the home were locked on the day of the follow-up telephone interview, compared to 9% at the time of the visit. Of the 33 parents who indicated they had firearms in their home at the time of the ED visit (one-third of whom reported unlocked guns at that time), none reported firearms were unlocked at follow-up. Because neither ED-based study had a control group (i.e., ED protocol called for counseling all parents), it is not possible to isolate the treatment effect from other factors that might have motivated parents to store firearms and medications more safely (e.g., routine care provided in the ED or the acute crisis itself).

Only one controlled trial of LMC has been conducted in the acute care setting [81]. This study, a clustered multisite trial in five Colorado EDs, tested whether an ED-based LMC intervention, implemented at the hospital level, led parents or other caregivers to improve household firearm and medication storage following their child's ED visit for a mental health-related concern. The intervention involved training behavioral health clinicians at each ED and providing medication and firearm storage devices for clinicians to offer to parents. During the usual care phase of the study, parents and other caregivers infrequently reported that clinical ED staff spoke with them (or other family members) about firearms (19%) or medications (32%). After hospitals adopted the LMC intervention, however, most caregivers reported having been spoken with about firearms (57%) and medications (71%). Moreover, adopting the intervention resulted in a twofold improvement in medication and firearm storage after returning home from the ED: 45% of caregivers improved medication storage and 22% of caregivers with firearms at home at baseline improved firearm storage during intervention phases, compared with 22% and 11%, respectively, during usual care phases. Findings for medications persisted in analyses that accounted for the staggered rollout of the intervention, but results for improved firearm safety did not, leaving open the possibility that the improvements observed for firearms might have been due to secular changes unrelated to the intervention or, alternatively, to heterogeneity in treatment effect across sites. The authors suggest that attributing improvements in firearm storage to the intervention rather than to external secular changes (i.e., time-varying confounding) is reasonable for several reasons, including that although other suicide prevention interventions occurred in Colorado over our study period, no other contemporary initiative, at study hospitals or elsewhere, had a primary focus on firearm storage.

Considered as a whole, the literature evaluating clinical interventions to reduce access to household firearms has been limited by its reliance on self-reported storage practices and the relatively small sample sizes in specific geographic locations in the studies. None have measured the impact of counseling on firearm injury outcomes. Moreover, significant heterogeneity in the study designs, samples, and interventions makes it difficult to draw strong conclusions regarding the effectiveness of firearm safety counseling as it has been practiced. Nonetheless, as reported by Rowhani-Rahbar, Simonetti, and Rivera in a comprehensive review [82], several studies have found a positive effect of practitioner-delivered counseling on household firearm storage practices, especially when counseling is augmented with firearm storage device provision, a finding supported by the only controlled trial of LMC in an acute care setting that has been conducted. More research is needed in health-care settings to better determine which specific messaging, delivered by whom, and in what setting is most effective at motivating parents to reduce firearm access to the children in their homes.

2.9 Conclusions

The evidence that the presence of a firearm in a child's home substantially increases that child's risk of death by suicide is overwhelming. Evidence that suicide risk is likely moderated by how household firearms are stored when it comes to youth suicide is also compelling, though it is worth emphasizing that no matter how household firearms are stored, the mere presence in the home still places youth at higher risk of death by suicide, compared with having no firearms at home. Indeed, even in homes where all firearms are stored locked, unloaded, and separate from ammunition, youth can sometimes still access these firearms. Important unanswered questions therefore remain about how to effectively reduce youth access to household firearms. For example, while interventions providing parents with firearm storage devices have the strongest evidence for improving in-home storage of firearms, little is known about the extent to which providing such storage devices might work against efforts to remove firearms from the home, arguably the safest way to protect youth. Moving forward, rigorous evaluation of interventions aiming to make good on what we know – that reducing access to firearms will reduce suicide among youth – should be a funding and clinical intervention priority.

Take Home Points
- The presence of a firearm in the home independently increases the risk of death by suicide for all household members, especially young household members.
- Reducing access to household firearms through safe storage practices (i.e., storing all household firearms locked, unloaded, and separate from ammunition) attenuates risk of firearm suicide, particularly among youth.
- Clinical interventions to promote safe storage of household firearms (i.e., lethal means counseling) is endorsed by several professional medical organizations and is widely accepted by pediatricians and parents of children and adolescents living in households with firearms, but is seldom incorporated into routine practice and even anticipatory guidance for youth acutely at-risk of suicide.
- Studies examining the effectiveness of clinician-delivered lethal means counseling on improving household firearm storage practices have yielded mixed results. These studies have been limited by reliance on self-reported outcomes and relatively small sample sizes in specific geographic locations. Although inference from the totality of the literature is hampered by methodological heterogeneity, on balance the evidence suggests that when counselling is accompanied by provision of locking devices, parents move towards safer household firearms storage.
- Future research should include formative qualitative work on what types of messages delivered by whom and in what contexts are most effective at shifting parents towards safer in-home and out-of-home storage.

References

1. Web-based Injury Statistics Query and Reporting System (WISQARS) [Internet]. Centers for disease control and prevention, National Center for Injury Prevention and Control. 2005. Available from: www.cdc.gov/injury/wisqars. Accessed 21 Feb 2020.
2. Miller M, Barber C, White RA, Azrael D. Firearms and suicide in the United States: is risk independent of underlying suicidal behavior? Am J Epidemiol. 2013;178(6):946–55.
3. Azrael D, Hepburn L, Hemenway D, Miller M. The stock and flow of U.S. firearms: results from the 2015 National Firearms Survey. RSF: The Russell Sage Found J Soc Sci. 2017;3(5):38–57.
4. Scott J, Azrael D, Miller M. Firearm storage in homes with children with self-harm risk factors. Pediatrics. 2018;141(3):e20172600.
5. Simonetti JA, Theis MK, Rowhani-Rahbar A, Ludman EJ, Grossman DC. Firearm storage practices in households of adolescents with and without mental illness. J Adolesc Health. 2017;61(5):583–90.
6. Grossman DC, Reay DT, Baker SA. Self-inflicted and unintentional firearm injuries among children and adolescents: the source of the firearm. Arch Pediatr Adolesc Med. 1999;153(8):875–8.
7. Johnson RM, Barber C, Azrael D, Clark DE, Hemenway D. Who are the owners of firearms used in adolescent suicides? Suicide Life Threat Behav. 2010;40(6):609–11.
8. Schnitzer PG, Dykstra HK, Trigylidas TE, Lichenstein R. Firearm suicide among youth in the United States, 2004–2015. J Behav Med. 2019;42(4):584–90.
9. Azrael D, Cohen J, Salhi C, Miller M. Firearm storage in gun-owning households with children: results of a 2015 national survey. J Urban Health. 2018;95(3):295–304.
10. Berrigan J, Azrael D, Hemenway D, Miller M. Firearms training and storage practices among US gun owners: a nationally representative study. Inj Prev. 2019;25(Suppl 1):31–8.
11. Miller M, Azrael D, Barber C. Suicide mortality in the United States: the importance of attending to method in understanding population-level disparities in the burden of suicide. Annu Rev Public Health. 2012;33(1):393–408.
12. Spicer RS, Miller TR. Suicide acts in 8 states: incidence and case fatality rates by demographics and method. Am J Public Health. 2000;90(12):1885–91.
13. Miller M, Azrael D, Hemenway D. The epidemiology of case fatality rates for suicide in the Northeast. Ann Emerg Med. 2004;43(6):723–30.
14. Vyrostek SB, Annest JL, Ryan GW. Surveillance for fatal and nonfatal injuries—United States, 2001. MMWR Surveill Summ. 2004;53(7):1–57.
15. Conner A, Azrael D, Miller M. Suicide case-fatality rates in the United States, 2007 to 2014: a nationwide population-based study. Ann Intern Med. 2019;171(12):885–95.
16. Azrael D, Miller M. Reducing suicide without affecting underlying mental health: theoretical underpinnings and a review of the evidence base linking the availability of lethal means and suicide. In: O'Connor RC, Pirkis J, editors. The international handbook of suicide prevention. 2nd ed. West Sussex: John Wiley & Sons, Ltd; 2016. p. 637–62.
17. Barber CW, Miller MJ. Reducing a suicidal person's access to lethal means of suicide: a research agenda. Am J Prev Med. 2014;47(3 Suppl 2):264–72.
18. Miller M, Hemenway D. The relationship between firearms and suicide: a review of the literature. Aggress Violent Behav. 1999;4(1):59–75.
19. Birckmayer J, Hemenway D. Suicide and firearm prevalence: are youth disproportionately affected? Suicide Life Threat Behav. 2001;31(3):303–10.
20. Hemenway D, Miller M. Association of rates of household handgun ownership, lifetime major depression, and serious suicidal thoughts with rates of suicide across US census regions. Inj Prev. 2002;8(4):313–6.
21. Kposowa A, Hamilton D, Wang K. Impact of firearm availability and gun regulation on state suicide rates. Suicide Life Threat Behav. 2016;46(6):678–96.
22. Miller M, Azrael D, Hemenway D. Firearm availability and unintentional firearm deaths, suicide, and homicide among 5–14 year olds. J Trauma. 2002;52(2):267–75.

23. Miller M, Azrael D, Hemenway D. Firearm availability and suicide, homicide, and unintentional firearm deaths among women. J Urban Health. 2002;79:26–38.
24. Miller M, Azrael D, Hemenway D. Household firearm ownership and suicide rates in the United States. Epidemiology. 2002;13(5):517–24.
25. Miller M, Hemenway D, Azrael D. Firearms and suicide in the Northeast. J Trauma. 2004;57(3):626–32.
26. Miller M, Lippmann SJ, Azrael D, Hemenway D. Household firearm ownership and rates of suicide across the 50 United States. J Trauma. 2007;62(4):1029–35.
27. Miller M, Warren M, Hemenway D, Azrael D. Firearms and suicide in US cities. Inj Prev. 2015;21(E1):e116–9.
28. Anglemyer A, Horvath T, Rutherford G. The accessibility of firearms and risk for suicide and homicide victimization among household members: a systematic review and meta-analysis. Ann Intern Med. 2014;160(2):101–10.
29. Brent DA, Perper JA, Moritz G, Baugher M, Schweers J, Roth C. Firearms and adolescent suicide: a community case-control study. Am J Dis Child. 1993;147(10):1066–71.
30. Ilgen MA, Zivin K, McCammon RJ, Valenstein M. Mental illness, previous suicidality, and access to guns in the United States. Psychiatr Serv. 2008;59(2):198–200.
31. Miller M, Barber C, Azrael D, Hemenway D, Molnar BE. Recent psychopathology, suicidal thoughts and suicide attempts in households with and without firearms: findings from the National Comorbidity Study Replication. Inj Prev. 2009;15(3):183–7.
32. Simonetti JA, Mackelprang JL, Rowhani-Rahbar A, Zatzick D, Rivara FP. Psychiatric comorbidity, suicidality, and in-home firearm access among a nationally representative sample of adolescents. JAMA Psychiat. 2015;72(2):152–9.
33. Sorenson SB, Vittes KA. Mental health and firearms in community-based surveys: implications for suicide prevention. Eval Rev. 2008;32(3):239–56.
34. Miller M, Swanson SA, Azrael D. Are we missing something pertinent? A bias analysis of unmeasured confounding in the firearm-suicide literature. Epidemiol Rev. 2016;38(1):62–9.
35. Grossman DC, Mueller BA, Riedy C, Dowd MD, Villaveces A, Prodzinski J, et al. Gun storage practices and risk of youth suicide and unintentional firearm injuries. JAMA. 2005;293(6):707–14.
36. Monuteaux MC, Azrael D, Miller M. Association of increased safe household firearm storage with firearm suicide and unintentional death among US youths. JAMA Pediatr. 2019;173(7):657–62.
37. Kellermann AL, Rivara FP, Somes G, Francisco J, Banton JG, Prodzinski J, et al. Suicide in the home in relation to gun ownership. N Engl J Med. 199;327(7):467–72.
38. Mauri A, Wolfson JA, Azrael D, Miller M. Firearm storage practices and risk perceptions. Am J Prev Med. 2019;57(6):830–5.
39. Conner A, Azrael D, Miller M. Public opinion about the relationship between firearm availability and suicide: results from a national survey. Ann Intern Med. 2018;168(2):153–5.
40. Baxley F, Miller M. Parental misperceptions about children and firearms. Arch Pediatr Adolesc Med. 2006;160(5):542–7.
41. American Academy of Pediatrics. Firearm-related injuries affecting the pediatric population. Committee on injury and poison prevention. Pediatrics. 2000;105(4):888–95.
42. American College of Emergency Physicians. Firearm safety and injury prevention. Revised 2019. https://www.acep.org/patient-care/policy-statements/firearm-safety-and-injury-prevention. Accessed 21 Feb 2020.
43. American College of Physicians, Ginsburg JA. Firearm injury prevention. Ann Intern Med. 1998;128(3):236–41.
44. Knox LM, Lomonaco C, Elster A. American Medical Association's youth violence prevention training and outreach guide. Am J Prev Med. 2005;29(5 Suppl 2):226–9.
45. Forbis SG, McAllister TR, Monk SM, Schlorman CA, Stolfi A, Pascoe JM. Children and firearms in the home: a Southwestern Ohio Ambulatory Research Network (SOAR-Net) study. J Am Board Fam Med. 2007;20(4):385–91.

46. Garbutt JM, Bobenhouse N, Dodd S, Sterkel R, Strunk RC. What are parents willing to discuss with their pediatrician about firearm safety? A parental survey. J Pediatr. 2016;179:166–71.
47. Haught K, Grossman D, Connell F. Parents' attitudes toward firearm injury prevention counseling in urban pediatric clinics. Pediatrics. 1995;96(4):649–53.
48. Webster DW, Wilson MEH, Duggan AK, Pakula LC. Parents' beliefs about preventing gun injuries to children. Pediatrics. 1992;89(5):908–14.
49. Barkin S, Duan N, Fink A, Brook RH, Gelberg L. Do clinicians follow guidelines on firearm safety counseling? Arch Pediatr Adolesc Med. 1998;152(8):749–56.
50. Barkin S, Fink A, Gelberg L. Predicting clinician injury prevention counseling for young children. Arch Pediatr Adolesc Med. 1999;153(12):1226–31.
51. Becher EC, Christakis NA. Firearm injury prevention counseling: are we missing the mark? Pediatrics. 1999;104(3):530–5.
52. Beidas RS, Jager-Hyman S, Becker-Haimes EM, Wolk CB, Ahmedani BK, Zeber JE, et al. Acceptability and use of evidence-based practices for firearm storage in pediatric primary care. Acad Pediatr. 2019;19(6):670–6.
53. Cheng TL, DeWitt TG, Savageau JA, O'Connor KG. Determinants of counseling in primary care pediatric practice: physician attitudes about time, money, and health issues. Arch Pediatr Adolesc Med. 1999;153(6):629–35.
54. Cohen LR, Runyan CW, Bowling M. Social determinants of pediatric residents' injury prevention counseling. Arch Pediatr Adolesc Med. 1998;152(2):169–75.
55. Fargason CA, Johnston C. Gun ownership and counseling of Alabama pediatricians. Arch Pediatr Adolesc Med. 1995;149(4):442–6.
56. Finch SA, Weiley V, Ip EH, Barkin S. Impact of pediatricians' perceived self-efficacy and confidence on violence prevention counseling: a national study. Matern Child Health J. 2008;12(1):75–82.
57. Giggie MA, Olvera RL, Joshi MN. Screening for risk factors associated with violence in pediatric patients presenting to a psychiatric emergency department. J Psychiatr Pract. 2007;13(4):246–52.
58. Grossman DC, Mang K, Rivara FP. Firearm injury prevention counseling by pediatricians and family physicians: practices and beliefs. Arch Pediatr Adolesc Med. 1995;149(9):973–7.
59. Hoops K, Crifasi C. Pediatric resident firearm-related anticipatory guidance: why are we still not talking about guns? Prev Med. 2019;124:29–32.
60. Naureckas Li C, Sacks CA, McGregor KA, Masiakos PT, Flaherty MR. Screening for access to firearms by pediatric trainees in high-risk patients. Acad Pediatr. 2019;19(6):659–64.
61. Olson LM, Christoffel KK, O'Connor KG. Pediatricians' involvement in gun injury prevention. Inj Prev. 2007;13(2):99–104.
62. Olson LM, Christoffel KK, O'Connor KG. Pediatricians' experience with and attitudes toward firearms: results of a national survey. Arch Pediatr Adolesc Med. 1997;151(4):352–9.
63. Solomon BS, Duggan AK, Webster D, Serwint JR. Pediatric residents' attitudes and behaviors related to counseling adolescents and their parents about firearm safety. Arch Pediatr Adolesc Med. 2002;156(8):769–75.
64. Webster DW, Wilson MEH, Duggan AK, Pakula LC. Firearm injury prevention counseling: a study of pediatricians' beliefs and practices. Pediatrics. 1992;89(5):902–7.
65. Coyne-Beasley T, Schoenbach VJ, Johnson RM. "Love our kids, lock your guns": a community-based firearm safety counseling and gun lock distribution program. Arch Pediatr Adolesc Med. 2001;155(6):659–64.
66. Grossman DC, Stafford HA, Koepsell TD, Hill R, Retzer KD, Jones W. Improving firearm storage in Alaska native villages: a randomized trial of household gun cabinets. Am J Public Health. 2012;102(Suppl 2):291–7.
67. Horn A, Grossman DC, Jones W, Berger LR. Community based program to improve firearm storage practices in rural Alaska. Inj Prev. 2003;9(3):231–4.

68. Roberto A, Meyer G, Johnson AJ, Atkin C, Smith P. Promoting gun trigger-lock use: insights and implications from a radio-based health communication intervention. J Appl Commun Res. 2002;30(3):210–30.
69. Sidman EA, Grossman DC, Koepsell TD, D'Ambrosio L, Britt J, Simpson ES, et al. Evaluation of a community-based handgun safe-storage campaign. Pediatrics. 2005;115(6):654–61.
70. Simonetti JA, Rowhani-Rahbar A, King C, Bennett E, Rivara FP. Evaluation of a community-based safe firearm and ammunition storage intervention. Inj Prev. 2018;24(3):218–23.
71. Wafer MS, Carruth A. "Locks for life": a gun lock distribution community health intervention program. J Emerg Nurs. 2003;29(4):349–51.
72. Wargo C, Erdman DA, Smith JG, Widom K, Reardon J. Community gun safety in Central Pennsylvania. J Trauma Nurs. 2013;20(1):67–73.
73. Oatis PJ, Fenn Buderer NM, Cummings P, Fleitz R. Pediatric practice based evaluation of the steps to prevent firearm injury program. Inj Prev. 1999;5(1):48–52.
74. Albright TL, Burge SK. Improving firearm storage habits: impact of brief office counseling by family physicians. J Am Board Fam Pract. 2003;16(1):40–6.
75. Carbone PS, Clemens CJ, Ball TM. Effectiveness of gun-safety counseling and a gun lock giveaway in a Hispanic community. Arch Pediatr Adolesc Med. 2005;159(11):1049–54.
76. Barkin SL, Finch SA, Ip EH, Scheindlin B, Craig JA, Steffes J, et al. Is office-based counseling about media use, timeouts, and firearm storage effective? Results from a cluster-randomized, controlled trial. Pediatrics. 2008;122(1):15–25.
77. Grossman DC, Cummings P, Koepsell TD, Marshall J, D'Ambrosio L, Thompson RS, Mack C. Firearm safety counseling in primary care pediatrics: a randomized, controlled trial. Pediatrics. 2000;106(1):22–6.
78. Stevens MM, Olson AL, Gaffney CA, Tosteson TD, Mott LA, Starr P. A pediatric, practice-based, randomized trial of drinking and smoking prevention and bicycle helmet, gun, and seatbelt safety promotion. Pediatrics. 2002;109(3):490–7.
79. Kruesi MJP, Grossman J, Pennington JM, Woodward PJ, Duda D, Hirsch JG. Suicide and violence prevention: parent education in the emergency department. J Am Acad Child Adolesc Psychiatry. 1999;38(3):250–5.
80. Runyan CW, Becker A, Brandspigel S, Barber C, Trudeau A, Novins D. Lethal means counseling for parents of youth seeking emergency care for suicidality. West J Emerg Med. 2016;17(1):8–14.
81. Miller M, Salhi C, Barber C, et al. Changes in firearm and medication storage practices in homes of youths at risk for suicide: results of the SAFETY Study, a clustered, emergency department-based, multisite, stepped-wedge trial. Ann Emerg Med. 2020;76(2):194–205.
82. Rowhani-Rahbar A, Simonetti JA, Rivara FP. Effectiveness of interventions to promote safe firearm storage. Epidemiol Rev. 2016;38(1):111–24.

Chapter 3
Firearm Homicide and Assaults

Patrick M. Carter and Rebecca M. Cunningham

A Dire Weekly Total for the U.S.: 25 Children Killed by Guns

By Nicholas Bakalar
June 19, 2017. *The New York Times*

3.1 Introduction

Among US children and adolescents (age 1–19 years), firearm injuries are the second leading cause of death, with homicides responsible for nearly 60% of firearm deaths among this population [1, 2]. In addition to the nearly 2000 firearm youth homicides, there are approximately 12,500 non-fatal firearm assault injuries requiring emergency department (ED) treatment every year among US children and adolescents [1]. Pediatric patients suffering violent injuries are at high risk for repeat injury related to interpersonal violence, with 59% reporting subsequent involvement in firearm violence [3] and 37% having another violent injury within the next 2 years [4]. In addition to subsequent violence-related outcomes (e.g., repeat fatal and non-fatal violent injuries) [3–5], these children and adolescents are at risk for a range of additional health and social consequences related to experiencing injuries from interpersonal firearm assault. Some of these consequences include developing substance use disorders [6], mental health disorders (e.g., post-traumatic stress disorder, anxiety, depression) [7], and long-term disabilities due to physical injury [8]. In addition these youth are at increased risk for experiencing negative criminal justice outcomes (e.g., arrest, incarceration) [5, 9].

The CDC 2010 cost estimates for all firearm fatalities for ages 0–19 years are $26.9 million for medical costs and $4.8 billion for work lost costs. There are no data for injuries (hospitalizations or ED visits) because of the instability of these estimates.

P. M. Carter (✉) · R. M. Cunningham
Department of Emergency Medicine, Injury Prevention Center, University of Michigan,
Ann Arbor, MI, USA
e-mail: cartpatr@med.umich.edu; stroh@umich.edu

© Springer Nature Switzerland AG 2021
L. K. Lee, E. W. Fleegler (eds.), *Pediatric Firearm Injuries and Fatalities*,
https://doi.org/10.1007/978-3-030-62245-9_3

Given the substantial human and economic costs resulting from such violence [10–12], leading medical and health policy organizations [13–18], including the American Academy of Pediatrics (AAP) [16] and the National Academy of Medicine (NAM, formerly the Institute of Medicine) [18], have highlighted a need for a renewed focus on the prevention of firearm homicide and assaults among pediatric populations. Research groups such as the Firearm Safety Among Children and Teens (FACTS) Consortium have also recently outlined both the current state of the science [19–24] and a set of research priorities to better understand the science of the problem and the necessary research essential to preventing future firearm homicide deaths and assault-related injuries among pediatric populations [25]. In the present chapter, we review the current state of our knowledge about the epidemiology of firearm homicide and non-fatal firearm assaults, trends in such injuries over time, and risk and protective factors associated with interpersonal firearm violence and outline a pathway forward for the prevention of interpersonal firearm violence among children and adolescents.

3.2 Epidemiology

3.2.1 Pediatric Firearm Homicide

In 2017, homicides resulted in 2470 fatalities (3.2 fatalities per 100,000) in the United States (Fig. 3.1) among children and adolescents (1–19 years old) [26]. Firearms were the underlying mechanism responsible in the majority (78%; 1915) of these homicides [26]. There were an additional 34 homicides in 2017 resulting

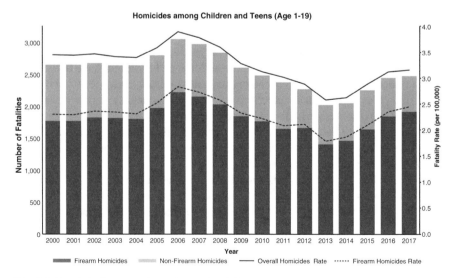

Fig. 3.1 Trends in firearm and non-firearm homicides, as well as overall firearm and non-firearm homicide fatality rates among children and adolescents (1–19 years old), United States, 2000–2017 [1]

from legal intervention by law enforcement, with nearly all of these (97%) resulting from firearm-related injuries [26]. Examining trends over time, while overall homicide rates remain lower than the peak rates observed in 1993 (6.6 homicides per 100,000), rates of homicide during the past 4 years have steadily increased 22.2%, rising from a rate of 2.6 fatalities per 100,000 in 2013 to 3.2 fatalities per 100,000 children and adolescents in 2017 [26]. This increase is exclusively the result of increases in firearm-related homicides, which have risen 37.0% since 2013, while non-firearm-related homicides have actually decreased nearly 11.0% during the corresponding time period [26]. While overall rates for fatal firearm homicide due to legal intervention are relatively low by comparison to general rates of firearm homicide, they have remained stable without improvement during the past decade [26].

3.2.2 Health Disparities: Age, Sex, Urbanicity, and Race/Ethnicity

Across the pediatric and adolescent age spectrum (1–19 years), firearm homicides disproportionately impact children during the developmental period of adolescence, with 93.7% of firearm homicides during the past decade (2008–2017) occurring among adolescents between 10 and 19 years old [26]. Among younger children (1–9 years old), firearm homicide rates during the past decade have remained comparable between male and female children [26]. However, after 10 years of age, disparities by sex become more pronounced, with evidence of a widening gap between male and female adolescents for each additional year of life [26]. Overall, rates of male adolescent deaths due to firearm homicide (10–19 years old) are seven times higher than those for female adolescents [26]. Such sex-related disparities, especially those observed among older adolescent populations, likely reflect differential socialization and normative constraints leading to higher levels of risk-taking behavior among male adolescents [27].

While firearm fatality rates for children and adolescents are similar across urban, suburban, and rural communities throughout the United States [2], injury-related intent varies for firearm deaths by urbanicity [26]. Firearm homicide disproportionately impacts urban communities, with rates (2.7 per 100,000) over the past decade nearly 2.5 times higher than those observed for rural communities (1.1 per 100,000) and 1.5 times higher than suburban communities (1.8 per 100,000) [26]. Observed sex disparities for firearm homicide also vary by urbanicity and are more pronounced in urban settings [26]. Male adolescents in urban settings are six times more likely to suffer a fatal firearm homicide than females. This is in comparison to either suburban or rural communities where males are five times and three times more likely than female adolescents to succumb to firearm homicide [26]. These disparities are almost exclusively the result of differences among older age adolescents, as rates for younger children (0–9 years old) are similar between males and females regardless of urbanicity [26].

With regard to race and ethnicity, disparities for firearm homicide rates are most pronounced among Black children and adolescents, among whom firearm homicide has been the leading cause of death for well over the past two decades [26]. In fact, firearm homicide fatality rates during the past 10 years of available data (2008–2017) for Black children and adolescents (8.2 per 100,000) are more than eight times higher than those observed for other racial groups, including Whites (1.0 per 100,000), Asian/Pacific Islanders (0.4 per 100,000), and American Indian/Alaska Natives (0.4 per 100,000) [26]. While this is primarily the result of higher rates of firearm homicide fatalities among older Black adolescents (10–19 years old), such disparities are also apparent among younger children (1–9 years old). Firearm homicide fatality rates are three times higher for young Black children compared to other racial groups [26]. Disparities among younger Black children also do not differ by sex [26]. Among adolescents (10–19 years old), firearm fatality rates are nine times higher for Black youth than other racial groups, with the highest fatality rates occurring among Black male adolescents (26.1 per 100,000).

With regard to ethnicity, non-Hispanic (2.2 per 100,000) and Hispanic/Latino (2.0 per 100,000) children and adolescents are noted to have comparable rates of death due to firearm homicide during the past decade [26]. However, it is important to note that CDC WONDER fatality data may underestimate rates of deaths among Hispanic populations [26]. Other analyses examining Hispanic youth (15–24 years old) populations have identified homicide as the second leading cause of death, with 82% of homicide deaths resulting from firearms [28, 29]. It is important to note these disparities persist regardless of neighborhood income. This suggests racial/ethnic differences in firearm homicide risk do not result solely from socioeconomic differences and likely also stem from a legacy of structural racism and segregation (e.g., redlining) of ethnic minority communities [30–32].

3.2.3   Global Comparisons

Rates of homicide (all mechanisms) among US children and adolescents are significantly higher compared to other high-income countries. This finding primarily results from markedly higher firearm homicide rates [2, 33, 34]. Based on World Health Organization (WHO) mortality data from 2010, rates of homicide by all mechanisms were 6, 3, and 14 times higher for US children and youth in all pediatric age groups (0–4; 5–14; 15–24 years old, respectively) than homicide rates in the next 23 high-income countries combined [33]. This disparity is mainly driven by firearm homicide rates that are 22, 19, and 49 times higher in the United States than these countries by corresponding age category. In fact, when comparing all deaths due to firearm homicide in the United States to this set of similar high-income countries, 93% of all firearm deaths in high-income countries occur within the United States for youth less than 25 years old [33]. While not disaggregated by firearm injury intent (e.g., homicide vs. suicide), similar results have been reported from the 2016 WHO mortality data comparing rates of overall firearm deaths among children and adolescents in the United States and both high-income and low-income countries [2].

3.2.4 Non-fatal Firearm Assault Injuries

For every firearm homicide among children and adolescents, there are more than seven non-fatal firearm assault injuries [35]. Although national ED data regarding non-fatal firearm injuries are incomplete due to the use of probability sampling strategies to create a weighted national sample [35], best estimates available report 12,500 ED visits for pediatric firearm assaults annually between 2008 and 2017 [35]. This may be a substantial underestimate, but no other robust national data source for non-fatal firearm injuries currently exists outside of administrative billing datasets. Firearm assault injuries represent nearly 4% of all intentional violence injuries (estimated at 365,000/year) seen and treated in EDs across the United States for children and adolescents [35]. Over 93.8% of these firearm assaults are among older adolescents (15–19 years old). Males are nearly eight times more likely than female children and adolescents to require ED treatment for a non-fatal firearm injury. Black children and adolescents represent nearly 50% of ED patients seeking care for a firearm assault. The vast majority (95%) of assault injuries (all mechanisms) occurring among children and adolescents do not require hospital admission. In contrast, 47.1% of firearm assaults require hospital admission. This is an indication of the higher severity of firearm injuries compared to other mechanisms causing violent injuries but also speaks to the need for prevention-based programs to start in the ED to engage with the high percentage of patients discharged home and not admitted to the hospital (see Chaps. 8 and 11) [35].

Among body areas injured in pediatric firearm assaults, nearly 80% involved upper and/or lower extremity injuries, while over 20% are thoracoabdominal injuries; over 20% are head, neck, or spinal cord injuries; and 20% are poly-trauma injuries [36]. In addition to the considerations for the acute injuries, the long-term morbidity resulting from firearm injuries is substantial. Nearly 50% of all children hospitalized after a firearm injury sustain long-term disabilities requiring rehabilitative care (see Chap. 10). This equals ~3200 children annually who are unable to independently perform age-specific activities of daily living (ADLs) [8].

3.2.5 Contextual Factors Related to Pediatric Homicide and Firearm Assaults

Police-reported incident data highlight characteristics of homicides occurring among pediatric populations (1–17 years old) [37]. The FBI's supplementary homicide report (SHR) of 2015 data indicates the relationship between the perpetrating offender and pediatric victim varies substantially by age of the victim (Fig. 3.2). Over two-thirds of all child homicide victims less than 6 years old are from homicide by a family member (e.g., mother, father, brother, sister) in cases where the perpetrator-victim relationship was known [37]. In two-thirds of cases among younger children (0–11 years old), the perpetrator was an older adult male family member (18–49 years old) [37]. Among adolescents (12–17 years old), in cases

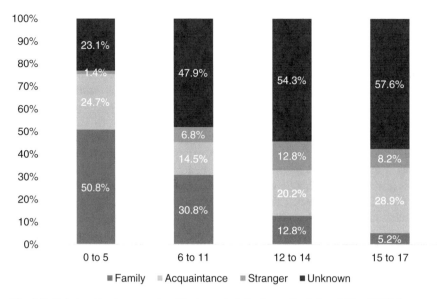

Fig. 3.2 Relationships between the offender and victim for pediatric homicides (2015) by age of the pediatric victim (0–17 years old) [37]. *FBI Supplemental Homicide Report (SHR) definition of victim-offender relationships: family,* husband, wife, common-law husband, common-law wife, mother, father, son, daughter, brother, sister, in-law, stepfather, stepmother, stepson, stepdaughter, and other family members; *acquaintance,* acquaintance, boyfriend, girlfriend, ex-husband, ex-wife, employee, employer, friend, homosexual relation, neighbor, and other known individuals; *stranger,* stranger; *unknown,* relationship unknown

where the perpetrator-victim relationship was known, the perpetrator was most likely to be either an acquaintance (e.g., friend, neighbor, boyfriend/girlfriend, employer) or stranger [37]. For adolescents, the relationship between the perpetrator and victim was more likely to be a similar-aged aggressor, with over 70% of perpetrators from a similar (12–17 years old) or slightly older (18–24 years old) age group [37]. Perpetrator-victim relationships have remained unchanged over the past decade among police incident data [37].

Data from the National Violent Death Reporting System (NVDRS) yields similar findings, highlighting firearm homicides among younger children (≤ 12 years old) are most often the result of intimate partner violence. This is typically the result of conflicts between intimate partners (e.g., parents) in which the child victim is a bystander or is related to recent family crises and/or relationship problems [38]. The overwhelming majority of homicides among younger children occur at home (85%) and result from handguns (75%) rather than long guns (25%) (e.g., rifle or shotgun) [38]. Firearm homicides occurring among older adolescents (13–17 years old) were more likely related to peer fighting/arguments (40%) or more likely precipitated by a crime (31%), gang activity (21%), drug involvement (13%), and/or weapon use by the victim (6%) [38]. Firearm homicides among older adolescents most likely occur either on the street or another public location (53%) and less likely occur within the home setting (39%) [38]. As with firearm homicides among younger children, adolescent firearm homicide was most likely the result of handguns (85%) as compared to long guns (15%) [38].

Similar data have been found when examining non-fatal firearm assaults among youth (14–24 years old). In one study comparing firearm assaults among youth to non-firearm assaults [39], violent encounters involving firearms were noted to involve less reciprocal violence (i.e., both aggression and victimization behaviors) than non-firearm assaults. They were also more likely to occur with a stranger or peer, than with a known family member/acquaintance [39]. Further, firearm assaults were overwhelmingly motivated by issues of retaliatory violence, the need to establish power or respect within the surrounding neighborhood, and retrieval of personal belongings [39]. This is in contrast to non-firearm violent encounters, which are motivated most often by issues of jealousy and rumors between known combatants (e.g., boyfriend/girlfriend, friends) [39]. Further, it is important to note that while adolescent violence encounters are overwhelmingly related to substance use before a violent conflict, the type of substance varies by the underlying mechanism of violence. Conflicts involving firearms are more likely to be preceded by either marijuana use and/or prescription drug use than non-firearm conflicts, which are more likely preceded by alcohol use. Such differences likely relate to the underlying motivation for conflict, with non-firearm encounters often involving low-level altercations escalating to a violent conflict in the presence of alcohol use (e.g., at a social event or party). In contrast, more planned firearm violence encounters are likely occurring among adolescents with more severe persistent substance use and/or substance use disorders (i.e., dependence). Additionally, prior literature also indicates these adolescents may self-medicate for underlying anxiety or other mental health issues (e.g., PTSD) by using drugs, such as marijuana, in an attempt to decrease aggressive impulses before a violent encounter. It is notable, that while alcohol preceded firearm assaults less often than non-firearm assaults, among those who were engaged in firearm assaults, alcohol was utilized more often on a day of firearm violence than on days not involving firearm violence [39].

3.2.6   School-Associated Homicides and Active Shooter Incidents

School-associated homicides include those occurring while a student is on the way to school, is returning from school, or is attending school or a school-sponsored event [40]. In the most recent year of available FBI data (2015 to 2016 school year), there were 18 school-associated homicide deaths among children and adolescents (5–18 years old) in the U.S. [40]. Media attention to these tragic events may magnify the public's expectation about numbers of school fatalities. This represents 1.2% of the total number of all homicides occurring among all similar-aged children and adolescents during the same time period [40]. Examining trends over time, since 2000, there have been a total of 311 school-associated homicides, averaging nearly 20 deaths annually every school year [40]. This includes those homicides resulting from active shooter events (described below). While the absolute number of school-associated homicides has fluctuated greatly during the past two decades, the percentage of overall homicides occurring *related to school activities* has remained stable at 1.3% of all homicides for school-aged children during the same time period [40].

In contrast, active shooter incidents are defined by the FBI to include those where one or more individuals are actively engaged in killing or attempting to kill people in a populated area such as a school setting (see Chap. 5) [40]. Between 2000 and 2017, there were 52 school-associated active shooter incidents (i.e., shooting events) occurring at elementary, secondary, and post-secondary educational institutions, with the majority (71.2%) occurring within elementary and secondary school settings [40]. The 37 active shooter incidents occurring in elementary and secondary school settings between 2000 and 2017 resulted in 153 casualties, including 67 firearm fatalities and 86 non-fatal firearm-related injuries [40]. Of these, the shooter used a single firearm in nearly two-thirds of incidents [40]. Among the 58 total firearms used in 37 active shooter incidents at elementary or secondary schools, 60.3% were handguns [40]. When long guns were used in active shooter incidents, the majority were rifles and not shotguns [40]. Among perpetrators responsible for active shooter incidents, the majority were current or former students at the same elementary or secondary school as the shooting incident, and 70% were adolescents of similar age (12–18 years old) [40]. All of the perpetrators involved in active shooter incidents were male, and each incident involved a single perpetrator [40]. Perpetrators were apprehended in 59.5% of the cases, with the shooter either committing suicide (37.8%) or being killed by law enforcement (2.7%) in the remainder of situations [40].

3.2.7 Firearm Carriage Among Adolescent Populations

Carrying a firearm is a key risk factor for interpersonal firearm violence, as well as for less lethal forms of upstream adolescent violence-related behaviors, including bullying, physical fighting, and non-firearm violence (please see "Risk and Protective Factors" section below) [41–49]. Firearm carriage poses a significant risk of both serious injury and death to the adolescents who carry the firearm, as well as the peer groups surrounding them [42, 44–46, 50–55]. Studies examining firearm carriage among adolescent populations have found between 5% and 10% of adolescents nationwide report having recently carried a firearm in any setting (e.g., in studies with timeframes ranging between past 12 months, past 6 months, and past 30 days) [41, 56–71], with lifetime carriage rates averaging between 15% and 20% for adolescents [63, 72–80]. Rates of adolescent firearm carriage only while traveling to and from school or while in the school setting in multiple studies range between 1% and 3% of youth sampled [65, 78, 79, 81–84]. Mean age of initiating firearm carriage for adolescents is 18 years old. Other studies have reported adolescents as young as 10 years old start to carry firearms, with linear increases in carriage for each additional year of adolescence [73, 75].

In general, studies report adolescent youth carry intermittently, rather than continuously, throughout the adolescent developmental period [73–76, 85]. In one study examining firearm carriage across the lifespan, researchers identified approximately 4–6% of adolescents report carrying a firearm during any single study wave (~12-month period of time). These youth report they carry firearms on average for slightly less than 3 years in duration during the adolescent developmental period with peak initiation of carriage at 15 years old [73].

Motives for firearm carriage among adolescents mostly relate to perceived needs for protection and/or self-defense [41, 78, 79, 86–92]. One study among rural youth identified the primary motive for carrying a firearm to school was the intention to use the weapon in an aggressive act [84]. Qualitative studies have identified similar results regarding protection as a primary motive, highlighting that among urban youth, carrying a firearm (a) provides a "sense of security" in risky places/situations; (b) serves as a means of protection against specific retaliatory threats and is a way to "prove to others" they aren't afraid to defend themselves; and (c) is a way of establishing "respect" among likely aggressors [93]. Other studies conducted among male youth in the criminal justice system for violence-related offenses have reported firearm carriage is a method of protection used by these youth and their peer group as they travel through dangerous neighborhoods. Firearms also provide a mechanism for retaliation or safety after they have been involved in a physical fight [88]. Notably, multiple studies have identified youth rarely carry firearms solely to achieve "status," as a means to impress others, or to gain social recognition [41, 87, 88, 93]. Among youth with access to firearms who do not regularly carry them, reasons for avoiding daily carriage include a fear of arrest or the perception that a firearm is not needed due to a lower risk of victimization (e.g., not carrying when they are traveling through safer neighborhoods during daytime hours) [94].

3.3 Risk and Protective Factors for Interpersonal Firearm Violence

Reducing interpersonal firearm violence among children and adolescents is a key national objective outlined in the Healthy People 2020 initiative [95]. Further, the National Academy of Medicine (NAM), the American Academy of Pediatrics (AAP), and organizations such as the Firearm Safety among Children and Teens (FACTS) have identified firearm violence prevention among pediatric populations as a key research priority [16, 18, 25]. Fundamental to developing, testing, and implementing effective tailored prevention efforts is understanding the range of risk and protective factors contributing to interpersonal firearm violence [96–98]. Risk factors are those factors, which increase the possibility of becoming a victim or perpetrator of firearm violence. Protective factors are those that lower the possibility of firearm violence involvement or reduce the negative impact of risk factors, which increase the likelihood of engagement in firearm violence [99]. Limitations in conducting firearm prevention research during the past two decades, strongly effected by Congress' elimination of funding related to firearm violence [100], have limited our knowledge about the specific subset of risk and protective factors uniquely related to interpersonal firearm violence for children and teens. However, despite this paucity of data, we do have some baseline knowledge from the available research. The remainder of this chapter is dedicated to cataloging the current state of knowledge on risk and protective factors (Table 3.1) influencing pediatric firearm violence involvement.

Table 3.1 Risk and protective factors for interpersonal firearm violence involvement among children and adolescents by level of the ecological model

Risk and protective factors by ecological level	
Risk factors	
Individual level	Prior violence (aggression, victimization, witnessing violence)
	Firearm carriage
	Retaliatory attitudes
	Delinquency/gang membership
	Criminal justice involvement
	Low academic achievement and truancy
	Substance (alcohol, illicit drug, marijuana) use/misuse
	Mental health issues (PTSD, conduct disorder)
Social level	Firearm availability (easy access; firearms in the home)
	Family structure (<2 parents)
	Family relations
	Low parental supervision/monitoring
	Parental substance use
	Parental education/income
	Child welfare involvement
	Peer firearm ownership/carriage
	Peer delinquency/gang membership
	Peer violence exposure/victimization
Community level	Community violence exposure
	Neighborhood disadvantage/disorder
	Alcohol outlets/drug markets
	Violent crime rates
Protective factors	
	Coping strategies/resilience
	Green space coverage

No single risk or protective factor explains why an individual person or group of children or adolescents is at higher or lower risk of engaging in or being a victim of interpersonal firearm violence. Such outcomes are typically the result of complex interactions of many risk and protective factors. Ecological systems theory (EST), as initially described by Bronfenbrenner [101, 102] and adapted for injury and violence research [103–111], characterizes these factors. EST conceptualizes people and their surroundings as nested systems of influence on specific behavioral outcomes (e.g., firearm violence) and implies reciprocal causation between individuals and their environment [101, 102].

Levels of influence within EST include individual, social (e.g., family, peer, school), and community levels [101–103, 112]. Individual-level factors include those corresponding to the person, including his or her attitudes, emotions, cognitive beliefs, and involvement in specific behaviors (e.g., substance use, mental health, academic achievement). Social-level factors include interactions occurring between the individual and the people/places surrounding them. This includes their peers (e.g., peer support, delinquent or pro-social peers), family (family structure, home environment, parental support, family conflict), or school (e.g., school safety, relationships with school personnel) environment. Finally, community-level factors are those including the physical (e.g., neighborhood disadvantage/disorder), social (e.g., social capital), and policy-oriented (e.g., firearm purchase restrictions) characteristics of neighborhoods and communities within which an individual resides and goes about daily life.

Within this socio-ecological model, behaviors such as interpersonal firearm violence are influenced by risk and protective factors at multiple levels and interact with other factors across multiple levels of the individual's environment [113]. For the purposes of this chapter and given that such violence is often bidirectional in nature (e.g., youth are simultaneously at risk for both victimization and aggression), we will discuss risk and protective factors for being involved as either the victim or the perpetrator of firearm violence at each of the relevant EST levels.

At the individual level, research examining interpersonal firearm violence has identified a series of risk factors for involvement in future firearm violence altercations. Prior exposure to interpersonal violence, both directly (e.g., firearm victimization, fighting behaviors, prior violent injury) and indirectly (e.g., witnessing violence/shootings among peers/within neighborhoods), is a particularly salient risk factor for future engagement in firearm violence, including risk for future firearm victimization and aggression [3, 4, 114–116]. Among these, personally being threatened or victimized with a firearm emerges as one of the most robust risk factors for future aggression with a firearm [3, 4, 115, 116]. This likely stems from altercations motivated by retaliatory violence. In fact, prior literature has also identified adolescent youth with positive attitudes favoring retaliation (i.e., retaliatory attitudes) have an increased likelihood of engaging in or being the victim of firearm violence [3, 39, 88]. This is consistent with research highlighting retaliation as a key motivation underlying all forms of interpersonal violence among adolescents [3, 39, 117]. It is also consistent with broader theoretical constructs (i.e., code of the street theory) [117, 118] proposing adolescent youth perceive retaliatory violence is necessary to correct perceived injustices, to restore and maintain peer respect after being victimized, and to deter future victimization risk [117–119]. The widespread availability and carriage of firearms by previously assaulted adolescent youth, often justified as a means of protecting themselves against repeat victimization [41], increases the lethality of such retaliatory incidents.

Substance use, including marijuana, alcohol, illicit drug, and prescription drug use and misuse have been widely identified in the literature as individual-level risk factors for firearm violence involvement, including firearm perpetration and victimization [3, 39, 41, 114]. In addition, alcohol and other drugs have been identified in prior literature as risk factors for adolescent firearm carriage. Multiple studies identify the initiation of substance use at an earlier age and higher severity use as a higher risk for both carriage and perpetration than occasional substance use [3, 39, 58, 62, 65, 66, 68, 78, 80, 82, 120–123]. The relationship between substance use and interpersonal violence is explained by several factors, including the pharmacological effects of alcohol and drug (e.g., cocaine, prescription stimulants) use [124–126], shared risk/promotive factors between drugs (e.g., marijuana) and firearms/violence [127], and the association of violence and firearms with the illicit drug trade [128]. Pharmacologically, alcohol increases aggression by impairing cognitive processing/impulse control, which increases the risk for escalation of low-level conflict to lethal violence, particularly in the presence of firearms [124, 125]. Acute impairment may also increase victimization risk by impairing cognitive and physical functioning, as well as decreasing risk perception in violent situations [129, 130]. While marijuana may increase anxiety, arousal, confusion, and perceptual distortion in some individuals [131–134], potentially escalating violent conflict [135], most studies suggest the association between marijuana and violence reflects either the impact of withdrawal symptoms among chronic or dependent users or the co-occurrence of socio-contextual factors increasing violence risk (e.g., engaging in buying/selling drugs or attending social events with co-occurring drug use and violence risk) [128]. Drug use prior to a violent conflict may also be an attempt, as noted above, to self-regulate aggressive impulses, while drug and alcohol use following a violent conflict may be an attempt by adolescents to cope with negative effects or to self-medicate for pain or injuries resulting from violence [39, 136, 137].

Behavioral and mental health disorders have also been identified as individual-level risk factors for firearm violence involvement. Attention and learning problems (e.g., low academic achievement), anti-social beliefs/attitudes (e.g., conduct disorder), and delinquency behaviors (e.g., truancy, gang membership, firearm carriage, criminal justice involvement) have been associated in prior cross-sectional and longitudinal studies with adolescent firearm victimization and aggression [3, 9, 39, 41, 116, 138–141]. Such factors likely relate to clustering of co-occurring problem behaviors (e.g., substance use, firearm carriage, low school achievement) among high-risk adolescent youth during this developmental period (i.e., Jessor's problem behavior theory) [127]. Such behaviors are compounded, as noted above, by the widespread availability and carriage/possession of firearms, which remain one of the most potent risk factors for firearm homicide and non-fatal firearm assault in national case-control studies and/or ED samples [3, 39, 41, 42, 142–145]. In fact, in one analysis, researchers found adolescent firearm carriage increased firearm victimization risk by an estimated 150% [146].

Mental health disorders, including anxiety and post-traumatic stress disorder (PTSD), have also emerged as salient risk factors for interpersonal firearm violence, most often owing to previous neighborhood violence exposure or interpersonal violence victimization [3, 4, 147–149]. Among assault-injured youth, a significant portion experience symptoms of acute stress disorder (ASD), including nightmares, hypervigilance, and emotional numbing at the time of the violent injury [148]. Further, compared to adolescents hospitalized for non-violence reasons, violently injured youth have been demonstrated to have elevated rates of anxiety, depression, and PTSD.

PTSD has also been identified as an independent risk factor for both repeat violent injury and subsequent negative firearm outcomes among such youth in the subsequent 2 years after they experience an initial violent injury [3, 4, 147–149]. Underlying mechanisms explaining this association are thought to relate to the constellation of PTSD symptoms experienced by youth. Hyperarousal symptoms are thought to increase the likelihood of aggressive impulses, while hypervigilance and impaired processing are thought to decrease the potential for youth to recognize potentially dangerous situations, increasing their risk for victimization. Risks for aggression and victimization are especially high when combined with elevated substance use rates among youth attempting to self-treat PTSD symptoms [150, 151]. It is important to note that while not studied specifically among adolescent populations, serious mental illnesses (e.g., schizophrenia) have *not* been found to be a significant risk factor for firearm aggression. These mental health issues are more likely to increase an individual's risk of victimization [152].

Risk factors beyond the individual level have generally been understudied within the context of their relationship to interpersonal firearm violence, particularly the influence of school context (e.g., school support) [22]. By contrast, social factors, including family and peer-related factors, have been examined more in depth in prior literature. The most significant family-related factor to emerge in prior literature for both firearm victimization and aggression is the accessibility of firearms within the home [139, 143, 145, 153, 154]. Three separate nationally representative samples have identified the presence of a firearm within the home environment increases the risk for pediatric firearm homicide, including for both younger children and older adolescent populations [143, 145, 154]. Further, two prior studies identified household firearm access as a risk factor for subsequent adolescent firearm perpetration/aggression [140, 154].

Other identified family-level risk factors for firearm victimization include parental substance use, family structure (i.e., households with less than two parents), low levels of parental supervision, and a lack of family closeness or connectedness [138, 139, 153, 155, 156]. Family risk factors associated with firearm aggression include family environments where child welfare services were involved [116].

The most salient peer-related factors include peer firearm ownership and carriage, peer delinquency, and peer violence exposure [88, 115, 140, 141, 157, 158]. Research has identified as many as 95% of youth who are involved in interpersonal violence reported their peers/friends possessed or routinely carry firearms, and nearly 80% report having peers that had used a firearm in a criminal act or violent encounter [88]. This is consistent with other research reporting firearm violence is often concentrated within discrete social networks (i.e., contagion effect), with an increased risk of firearm assaults for adolescent youth who associate with other adolescents injured by firearms and/or those who are part of co-offending social/peer groups (e.g., gang membership) [157, 158]. Such delinquent peer associations also increase the likelihood of youth using firearms aggressively. Research has identified having peers in their social network who have either been victimized by firearms or have used firearms aggressively in the past is associated with an increased risk of other youth peers engaging in aggressive firearm behaviors, likely by normalizing the use of firearms as a means for solving conflicts [115, 140, 141].

It is important to note in terms of the burden of firearm injury that firearm deaths occur at the same rate in urban, rural, and suburban communities. However, in rural communities the intent is more often suicide than homicide/assault [2]. At the community level, firearm assaults and homicides among children and adolescents are more likely to occur within neighborhoods characterized by lower socioeconomic status (SES) indicators, fewer resources, and higher levels of neighborhood disadvantage and disorder [36, 139, 145, 155, 159]. Further, high concentrations of firearm availability, alcohol outlets, illegal drug markets, and gangs have also been associated with an increased risk for firearm victimization for children and adolescents [145, 156, 159, 160]. Higher prevalence of violent crime within a community, including robberies and aggravated assault, has also been shown to increase the risk of adolescent firearm homicide [145]. In addition to objective markers (e.g., violent crime rates), youth perceptions of community violence (e.g., hearing gunshots, seeing gangs, personal robbery) have also been associated with youth engaging in high-risk firearm behaviors (e.g., firing firearms, carrying in risky situations), as well as engaging in firearm violence (i.e., threats/use of a firearm) [114, 161].

Few studies have explored protective individual- or community-level factors specifically associated with firearm violence outcomes among children and adolescents (Table 3.1). At the individual level, coping skills and resiliency have been associated with lower likelihood of engaging in risky firearm behaviors, including firearm aggression [161]. At the community level, urban green spaces have been found to be protective against firearm victimization, with one study finding that tree coverage reduced the risk of firearm assault among urban youth, especially those in low-income areas [162].

3.4 Reducing Firearm Homicide and Assaults in Children and Adolescents

The significant morbidity and mortality resulting from firearm homicide and assaults among children and adolescents are overwhelming preventable [2, 100]. However, achieving progress toward reducing firearm homicide as a leading cause of death will require a renewed focus on this increasing public health problem [24]. Research funding, and as a result publications and evidence-based interventions to decrease interpersonal firearm violence, have lagged substantially behind funding for diseases or other mechanisms of injury and death among pediatric populations over the past 20 years [163]. Recent increased rates of pediatric firearm homicide deaths, including the increased frequency of mass school shootings, have both raised public awareness of this problem and propelled an increasing number of scientists to renew their focus on addressing the critical need for more prevention-based research [24]. If a substantial federal investment in research and prevention follows, the data needed to understand the epidemiology, risk and protective factors, and prevention-based solutions will emerge from this research. These data will provide key information for use by researchers and policy makers to guide communities, law enforcement, and schools on best practices to decrease this leading cause of death. The sound application of rigorous scientific public health methods in other areas of injury prevention science (e.g., motor vehicle crashes, drowning, residential fires) has resulted in considerable success preventing fatal and non-fatal injury outcomes [2, 100]. Expanding on this success by applying similar standards to the public health problem of interpersonal firearm violence could lead to substantial parallel success addressing this leading cause of death, as well as the substantial health disparities resulting from firearm homicide.

Take Home Points
- Among firearm deaths occurring in the US pediatric population (1–19 years old), approximately 60% are due to homicide.
- There are significant disparities in pediatric firearm homicide with rates nine times higher in Black adolescents (10–19 years old) and three times higher for younger Black children (0–9 years old), compared to other racial groups by age.
- For every firearm homicide among US children and youth, there are more than seven non-fatal injuries due to firearm assault.
- Children and youth who are involved in firearm violence are at risk for repeat injury and longer-term health and social consequences related to interpersonal violence.
- Identifying risk and protective factors for interpersonal firearm violence among children and adolescents using ecological systems theory, including factors at the individual, social, and community level, are fundamental for implementing effective firearm violence injury prevention.
- Investment in research and prevention are necessary to guide communities, law enforcement, and schools on best practices to decrease firearm homicides and assault injuries to US children and youth.

References

1. Centers for Disease Control and Prevention, National Center for Health Statistics. Compressed mortality file 1999–2016 on CDC WONDER online database [Internet]. 2017; https://wonder.cdc.gov/cmf-icd10.html. Accessed 6 May 2018.
2. Cunningham RM, Walton MA, Carter PM. The major causes of death in children and adolescents in the United States. N Engl J Med. 2018;379(25):2468–75.
3. Carter PM, Walton MA, Roehler DR, et al. Firearm violence among high-risk emergency department youth after an assault injury. Pediatrics. 2015;135(5):805–15.
4. Cunningham RM, Carter PM, Ranney M, et al. Violent reinjury and mortality among youth seeking emergency department care for assault-related injury. JAMA Pediatr. 2015;169(1):63.
5. Rowhani-Rahbar A, Zatzick D, Wang J, et al. Firearm-related hospitalization and risk for subsequent violent injury, death, or crime perpetration: a cohort study. Ann Intern Med. 2015;162(7):492–500.
6. Walton M, Epstein-Ngo Q, Carter P, et al. Marijuana use trajectories among drug-using youth presenting to an urban emergency department: violence and social influences. Drug Alcohol Depend. 2017;173:117–25.
7. Garbarino J, Bradshaw CP, Vorrasi JA. Mitigating the effects of gun violence on children and youth. Future Child. 2002;12(2):73–86.
8. DiScala C, Sege R. Outcomes in children and young adults who are hospitalized for firearms-related injuries. Pediatrics. 2004;113(5):1306–12.
9. Carter PM, Dora-Laskey AD, Goldstick JE, et al. Arrests among high-risk youth following emergency department treatment for an assault injury. Am J Prev Med. 2018;55(6):812–21.

10. Corso PS, Mercy JA, Simon TR, Finkelstein EA, Miller TR. Medical costs and productivity losses due to interpersonal and self-directed violence in the United States. Am J Prev Med. 2007;32(6):474–82.
11. Howell EM, Abraham P. The hospital costs firearm assaults. Washington, DC: The Urban Institute; 2013.
12. Peek-Asa C, Butcher B, Cavanaugh JE. Cost of hospitalization for firearm injuries by firearm type, intent, and payer in the United States. Inj Epidemiol. 2017;4(1):20.
13. Butkus R, Doherty R, Bornstein SS. Reducing firearm injuries and deaths in the United States: a position paper from the American College of Physicians. Ann Intern Med. 2018;169(10):704–7.
14. Ranney ML, Fletcher J, Alter H, et al. A consensus-driven agenda for emergency medicine firearm injury prevention research. Ann Emerg Med. 2017;69(2):227–40.
15. Bauchner H, Rivara FP, Bonow RO, et al. Death by gun violence—a public health crisis. JAMA Psychiat. 2017;74(12):1195–6.
16. Dowd M, Sege R. Council on injury, violence, and poison prevention executive committee; American Academy of Pediatrics. Firearm-related injuries affecting the pediatric population. Pediatrics. 2012;130(5):e1416–23.
17. Wintemute GJ. Responding to the crisis of firearm violence in the United States: comment on "Firearm legislation and firearm-related fatalities in the United States". JAMA Intern Med. 2013;173(9):740.
18. Leshner AI, Altevogt BM, Lee AF, McCoy MA, Kelley PW. Institute of Medicine. Priorities for research to reduce the threat of firearm-related violence. Washington, DC: National Academies Press; 2013.
19. Ngo QM, Sigel E, Moon A, et al. State of the science: a scoping review of primary prevention of firearm injuries among children and adolescents. J Behav Med. 2019;42(4):811–29.
20. Oliphant SN, Mouch CA, Rowhani-Rahbar A, et al. A scoping review of patterns, motives, and risk and protective factors for adolescent firearm carriage. J Behav Med. 2019;42(4):763–810.
21. Ranney M, Karb R, Ehrlich P, et al. What are the long-term consequences of youth exposure to firearm injury, and how do we prevent them? A scoping review. J Behav Med. 2019;42(4):724–40.
22. Schmidt CJ, Rupp L, Pizarro JM, Lee DB, Branas CC, Zimmerman MA. Risk and protective factors related to youth firearm violence: a scoping review and directions for future research. J Behav Med. 2019;42(4):706–23.
23. Zeoli AM, Goldstick J, Mauri A, et al. The association of firearm laws with firearm outcomes among children and adolescents: a scoping review. J Behav Med. 2019;42(4):741–62.
24. Cunningham RM, Carter PM, Zimmerman M. The firearm safety among children and teens (FACTS) consortium: defining the current state of the science on pediatric firearm injury prevention. J Behav Med. 2019;42(4):702–5.
25. Cunningham R, Carter P, Ranney M, et al. Prevention of firearm injuries among children and adolescents: consensus-driven research agenda from the firearm safety among children and teens (FACTS) consortium. JAMA Pediatr. 2019;173(8):780–9.
26. Centers for Disease Control and Prevention. National Center for Health Statistics. Underlying cause of death 1999–2017 on CDC WONDER online database [Internet]. https://wonder.cdc.gov/ucd-icd10.html. Accessed 19 Aug 2019, Online Database, released December, 2018.
27. Byrnes JP, Miller DC, Schafer WD. Gender differences in risk taking: a meta-analysis. Psychol Bull. 1999;125(3):367.
28. Violence Policy Center. Hispanic victims of lethal firearm violence in the United States [Internet]. 2018; www.vpc.org. Accessed 21 Sept 2019.
29. Walker GN, McLone S, Mason M, Sheehan K. Rates of firearm homicide by Chicago region, age, sex, and race/ethnicity, 2005–2010. J Trauma Acute Care Surg. 2016;81(4):S48–53.
30. Kalesan B, Vyliparambil MA, Bogue E, et al. Race and ethnicity, neighborhood poverty and pediatric firearm hospitalizations in the United States. Ann Epidemiol. 2016;26(1):1–6. e2.
31. Beard JH, Morrison CN, Jacoby SF, et al. Quantifying disparities in urban firearm violence by race and place in Philadelphia, Pennsylvania: a cartographic study. Am J Public Health. 2017;107(3):371–3.

32. Slopen N, Shonkoff JP, Albert MA, et al. Racial disparities in child adversity in the US: interactions with family immigration history and income. Am J Prev Med. 2016;50(1):47–56.
33. Grinshteyn E, Hemenway D. Violent death rates: the United States compared to other high-income OECD countries, 2010. Am J Med. 2016;129(3):266–73.
34. Hemenway D, Miller M. Firearm availability and homicide rates across 26 high-income countries. J Trauma Acute Care Surg. 2000;49(6):985–8.
35. WISQARS (Web-based injury statistics query and reporting system). National Center for Injury Prevention and Control [Internet]. 2019. www.cdc.gov/injury/wisqars/index.html. Accessed 9 Sept 2019.
36. Carter PM, Cook LJ, Macy ML, et al. Individual and neighborhood characteristics of children seeking emergency department care for firearm injuries within the PECARN network. Acad Emerg Med. 2017;24(7):803–13.
37. Puzzanchera C, Chamberlin G, Kang W. Easy access to the FBI's supplementary homicide reports: 1980–2016 [Internet]. 2018; https://www.ojjdp.gov/ojstatbb/ezashr/. Accessed 9 Sept 2019.
38. Fowler KA, Dahlberg LL, Haileyesus T, Gutierrez C, Bacon S. Childhood firearm injuries in the United States. Pediatrics. 2017;140(1):e20163486.
39. Carter PM, Walton MA, Goldstick J, et al. Violent firearm-related conflicts among high-risk youth: an event-level and daily calendar analysis. Prev Med. 2017;102:112–9.
40. Musu L, Zhang A, Wang K, Zhang J, Oudekerk B. Indicators of school crime and safety: 2018 National Center for Education Statistics: U.S. Department of Education, and Bureau of Justice Statistics, Office of Justice Programs, U.S. Department of Justice. Washington, DC; 2019.
41. Carter PM, Walton MA, Newton MF, et al. Firearm possession among adolescents presenting to an urban emergency department for assault. Pediatrics. 2013;132(2):213–21.
42. Branas CC, Richmond TS, Culhane DP, Ten Have TR, Wiebe DJ. Investigating the link between gun possession and gun assault. Am J Public Health. 2009;99(11):2034–40.
43. van Geel M, Vedder P, Tanilon J. Bullying and weapon carrying: a meta-analysis. JAMA Pediatr. 2014;168(8):714–20.
44. Pickett W, Craig W, Harel Y, et al. Cross-national study of fighting and weapon carrying as determinants of adolescent injury. Pediatrics. 2005;116(6):e855–63.
45. DuRant RH, Kahn J, Beckford PH, Woods ER. The association of weapon carrying and fighting on school property and other health risk and problem behaviors among high school students. Arch Pediatr Adolesc Med. 1997;151(4):360–6.
46. Lowry R, Powell K, Kann L, Collins J, Kolbe L. Weapon-carrying, physical fighting, and fight-related injury among U.S. adolescents. Am J Prev Med. 1998;14(2):122–9.
47. Borowsky IW, Mozayeny S, Stuenkel K, Ireland M. Effects of a primary care-based intervention on violent behavior and injury in children. Pediatrics. 2004;114(4):e392–9.
48. Dukarm CP, Byrd RS, Auinger P, Weitzman M. Illicit substance use, gender, and the risk of violent behavior among adolescents. Arch Pediatr Adolesc Med. 1996;150:797–801.
49. Forrest CB, Tambor E, Riley AW, Ensminger ME, Starfield B. The health profile of incarcerated male youths. Pediatrics. 2000;105(1 Pt 3):286–91.
50. Durant RH, Getts AG, Cadenhead C, Woods ER. The association between weapon carrying and the use of violence among adolescents living in and around public housing. J Adolesc Health. 1995;17(6):376–80.
51. Cheng TL, Johnson S, Wright JL, et al. Assault-injured adolescents presenting to the emergency department: causes and circumstances. Acad Emerg Med. 2006;13(6):610–6.
52. Felson RB, Steadman HJ. Situational factors in disputes leading to criminal violence. Criminology. 1983;21(1):59–74.
53. McDowall D, Loftin C, Wiersema B. The incidence of civilian defensive firearm use. Unpublished manuscript. University of Maryland-College Park, Inst Criminal Justice; 1992.
54. Cook PJ. The effect of gun availability on violent crime patterns. Ann Am Acad Pol Soc Sci. 1981;455(1):63–79.
55. Loughran TA, Reid JA, Collins ME, Mulvey EP. Effect of gun carrying on perceptions of risk among adolescent offenders. Am J Public Health. 2016;106(2):350–2.

56. Arria AM, Wood NP, Anthony JC. Prevalence of carrying a weapon and related behaviors in urban schoolchildren, 1989 to 1993. Arch Pediatr Adolesc Med. 1995;149(12):1345–50.
57. Apel R, Burrow JD. Adolescent victimization and violent self-help. Youth Violence Juvenile Justice. 2011;9(2):112–33.
58. Cunningham RM, Resko SM, Harrison SR, et al. Screening adolescents in the emergency department for weapon carriage. Acad Emerg Med. 2010;17(2):168–76.
59. Cook PJ, Ludwig J. Does gun prevalence affect teen gun carrying after all? Criminology. 2004;42(1):27–54.
60. Hayes DN, Hemenway D. Age-within-school-class and adolescent gun-carrying. Pediatrics. 1999;103(5):e64.
61. Hemenway D, Vriniotis M, Johnson RM, Miller M, Azrael D. Gun carrying by high school students in Boston, MA: does overestimation of peer gun carrying matter? J Adolesc. 2011;34(5):997–1003.
62. Lizotte AJ, Krohn MD, Howell JC, Tobin K, Howard GJ. Factors influencing gun carrying among young urban males over the adolescent-young adult life course. Criminology. 2000;38(3):811–34.
63. Luster T, Oh SM. Correlates of male adolescents carrying handguns among their peers. J Marriage Fam. 2001;63(3):714–26.
64. Orpinas P, Murray N, Kelder S. Parental influences on students' aggressive behaviors and weapon carrying. Health Educ Behav. 1999;26(6):774–87.
65. Peleg-Oren N, Saint-Jean G, Cardenas GA, Tammara H, Pierre C. Drinking alcohol before age 13 and negative outcomes in late adolescence. Alcohol Clin Exp Res. 2009;33(11):1966–72.
66. Ruggles KV, Rajan S. Gun possession among American youth: a discovery-based approach to understand gun violence. PLoS One. 2014;9(11):e111893.
67. Tigri HB, Reid S, Turner MG, Devinney JM. Investigating the relationship between gang membership and carrying a firearm: results from a national sample. Am J Crim Justice. 2016;41(2):168–84.
68. Vaughn MG, Perron BE, Abdon A, Olate R, Groom R, Wu L-T. Correlates of handgun carrying among adolescents in the United States. J Interpers Violence. 2012;27(10):2003–21.
69. Vaughn MG, Nelson EJ, Salas-Wright CP, DeLisi M, Qian Z. Handgun carrying among white youth increasing in the United States: new evidence from the National Survey on drug use and health 2002–2013. Prev Med. 2016;88:127–33.
70. Williams SS, Mulhall PF, Reis JS, De Ville JO. Adolescents carrying handguns and taking them to school: psychosocial correlates among public school students in Illinois. J Adolesc. 2002;25(5):551–67.
71. Xuan Z, Hemenway D. State gun law environment and youth gun carrying in the United States. JAMA Pediatr. 2015;169(11):1024–31.
72. Beardslee J, Docherty M, Mulvey E, Schubert C, Pardini D. Childhood risk factors associated with adolescent gun carrying among Black and White males: an examination of self-protection, social influence, and antisocial propensity explanations. Law Hum Behav. 2018;42(2):110.
73. Dong B, Wiebe DJ. Violence and beyond: life-course features of handgun carrying in the urban United States and the associated long-term life consequences. J Crim Just. 2018;54:1–11.
74. Lizotte AJ, Howard GJ, Krohn MD, Thronberry TP. Patterns of illegal gun carrying among young urban males. [Internet] Val UL Rev. 1996;31:375-93. Available from: https://scholar.valpo.edu/vulr/vol31/iss2/4.
75. Loeber R, Burke JD, Mutchka J, Lahey BB. Gun carrying and conduct disorder: a highly combustible combination?: implications for juvenile justice and mental and public health. Arch Pediatr Adolesc Med. 2004;158(2):138–45.
76. Steinman KJ, Zimmerman MA. Episodic and persistent gun-carrying among urban African-American adolescents. J Adolesc Health. 2003;32(5):356–64.
77. Webster DW, Gainer PS, Champion HR. Weapon-carrying among inner-city junior high school students: defensive behavior vs. aggressive delinquency. Am J Public Health. 1993;83:1604–8.

78. Hemenway D, Prothrow-Stith D, Bergstein JM, Ander R, Kennedy BP. Gun carrying among adolescents. Law Contemp Probl. 1996;59(1):39–53.
79. Bergstein JM, Hemenway D, Kennedy B, Quaday S, Ander R. Guns in young hands: a survey of urban teenagers' attitudes and behaviors related to handgun violence. J Trauma Acute Care Surg. 1996;41(5):794–8.
80. Simon TR, Richardson JL, Dent CW, Chou C-P, Flay BR. Prospective psychosocial, inter-personal, and behavioral predictors of handgun carrying among adolescents. Am J Public Health. 1998;88(6):960–3.
81. Cao L, Zhang Y, He N. Carrying weapons to school for protection: an analysis of the 2001 school crime supplement data. J Crim Just. 2008;36(2):154–64.
82. DuRant RH, Krowchuk DP, Kreiter S, Sinal SH, Woods CR. Weapon carrying on school property among middle school students. Arch Pediatr Adolesc Med. 1999;153(1):21–6.
83. May DC. Scared kids, unattached kids, or peer pressure: why do students carry firearms to school? Youth Soc. 1999;31(1):100–27.
84. Kingery P, Pruitt B, Heuberger G. A profile of rural Texas adolescents who carry handguns to school. J Sch Health. 1996;66(1):18–22.
85. Reid JA, Richards TN, Loughran TA, Mulvey EP. The relationships among exposure to vio-lence, psychological distress, and gun carrying among male adolescents found guilty of seri-ous legal offenses: a longitudinal cohort study. Ann Intern Med. 2017;166(6):412–8.
86. McNabb SJ, Farley TA, Powell KE, Rolka HR, Horan JM. Correlates of gun-carrying among adolescents in South Louisiana. Am J Prev Med. 1996;12(2):96–102.
87. Sheley JF, Wright JD. Motivations for gun possession and carrying among serious juvenile offenders. Behav Sci Law. 1993;11(4):375–88.
88. Wilkinson DL, McBryde MS, Williams B, Bloom S, Bell K. Peers and gun use among urban adolescent males: an examination of social embeddedness. J Contemp Crim Justice. 2009;25(1):20–44.
89. Ash P, Kellermann AL, Fuqua-Whitley D, Johnson A. Gun acquisition and use by juvenile offenders. JAMA. 1996;275(22):1754–8.
90. Black S, Hausman A. Adolescents' views of guns in a high-violence community. J Adolesc Res. 2008;23(5):592–610.
91. Lane MA, Cunningham SD, Ellen JM. The intention of adolescents to carry a knife or a gun: a study of low-income African-American adolescents. J Adolesc Health. 2004;34(1):72–8.
92. Wilkinson DL, Fagan J. The role of firearms in violence 'scripts': the dynamics of gun events among adolescent males. Law Contemp Probl. 1996;59(1):55–89.
93. Mateu-Gelabert P. Dreams, gangs, and guns: the interplay between adolescent violence and immigration in a New York City neighborhood. New York: Vera Institute of Justice; 2002;1–41. Available from: https://www.vera.org/downloads/Publications/dreams-gangs-and-guns-the-interplay-between-adolescent-violence-and-immigration-in-a-new-york-city-neighborhood/legacy_downloads/Dreams_gangs_and_guns.pdf.
94. Freed LH, Webster DW, Longwell JJ, Carrese J, Wilson MH. Factors preventing gun acqui-sition and carrying among incarcerated adolescent males. Arch Pediatr Adolesc Med. 2001;155(3):335–41.
95. HealthyPeople. 2020 Topics and objectives: injury and violence prevention [Internet]. Available from: https://www.healthypeople.gov/2020/topics-objectives/topic/injury-and-violence-prevention, 2018.
96. Hawkins JD, Catalano RF, Arthur MW. Promoting science-based prevention in communities. Addict Behav. 2002;27(6):951–76.
97. Herrenkohl TI, Maguin E, Hill KG, Hawkins JD, Abbott RD, Catalano RF. Developmental risk factors for youth violence. J Adolesc Health. 2000;26(3):176–86.
98. Pollard JA, Hawkins JD, Arthur MW. Risk and protection: are both necessary to understand diverse behavioral outcomes in adolescence? Soc Work Res. 1999;23(3):145–58.
99. Kim BE, Gloppen KM, Rhew IC, Oesterle S, Hawkins JD. Effects of the communities that care prevention system on youth reports of protective factors. Prev Sci. 2015;16(5):652–62.

100. Carter PM, Cunningham RM. Adequate funding for injury prevention research is the next critical step to reduce morbidity and mortality from firearm injuries. Acad Emerg Med. 2016;23(8):952–5.
101. Bronfenbrenner U. Toward an experimental ecology of human development. Am Psychol. 1977;32(7):513–31.
102. Bronfenbrenner U. The ecology of human development: experiments by design and nature. Cambridge, MA: Harvard University Press; 1979;1–349.
103. Dahlberg LL, Butchart A. State of the science: violence prevention efforts in developing and developed countries. Int J Inj Control Saf Promot. 2005;12(2):93–104.
104. Garbarino J, Abramowitz R, Asp E, et al. Adolescent development. An ecological perspective. Columbus: Charles Merrill; 1985;1–665.
105. Tolan P, Guerra N. What works in reducing adolescent violence. Center for the Study and Prevention of Violence Institute of Behavioral Science University of Colorado, Boulder; 1994;1–70.
106. Garbarino J, Crouter A. Defining the community context for parent-child relations: the correlates of child maltreatment. Child Dev. 1978;49:604–16.
107. Chalk R, King PA, editors. Institute of Medicine and National Research Council. Violence in families: assessing prevention and treatment programs. Washington, DC: National Academic Press; 1998.
108. Heise LL. Violence against women: an integrated, ecological framework. Violence Against Women. 1998;4(3):262–90.
109. Schiamberg LB, Gans D. An ecological framework for contextual risk factors in elder abuse by adult children. J Elder Abuse Negl. 1999;11(1):79–103.
110. Schiamberg LB, Gans D. Elder abuse by adult children: an applied ecological framework for understanding contextual risk factors and the intergenerational character of quality of life. Int J Aging Hum Dev. 2000;50(4):329–59.
111. Carp FM. Elder abuse in the family: an interdisciplinary model for research. New York: Springer Publishing Company; 2000.
112. Dahlberg L, Krug E. Violence: a global public health problem. Geneva: World Health Organization. In: Krug E, Dahlberg LL, Mercy JA, Zwi AB, Lozano R, editors. World report on violence and health. Geneva: World Health Organization; 2002. p. 1–21.
113. Sallis JF, Owen N, Fisher EB. Ecological models of health behavior. In: Glanz K, Rimer BK, Viswanath K, (Eds.). Health behavior and health education: theory, research, and practice. Jossey-Bass; 2008. p. 465–86.
114. Goldstick JE, Carter PM, Walton MA, et al. Development of the SaFETy score: a clinical screening tool for predicting future firearm violence risk development of the SaFETy score. Ann Intern Med. 2017;166(10):707–14.
115. McGee ZT, Logan K, Samuel J, Nunn T. A multivariate analysis of gun violence among urban youth: the impact of direct victimization, indirect victimization, and victimization among peers. Cogent Soc Sci. 2017;3(1):1328772.
116. Sumner SA, Maenner MJ, Socias CM, et al. Sentinel events preceding youth firearm violence: an investigation of administrative data in Delaware. Am J Prev Med. 2016;51(5):647–55.
117. Copeland-Linder N, Jones VC, Haynie DL, Simons-Morton BG, Wright JL, Cheng TL. Factors associated with retaliatory attitudes among African American adolescents who have been assaulted. J Pediatr Psychol. 2007;32(7):760–70.
118. Anderson E. Code of the street: decency, violence, and the moral life of the inner city. New York: W.W. Norton; 1999.
119. Cota-McKinley AL, Woody WD, Bell PA. Vengeance: effects of gender, age, and religious background. Aggress Behav. 2001;27(5):343–50.
120. Orpinas PK, Basen-Engquist K, Grunbaum JA, Parcel GS. The co-morbidity of violence-related behaviors with health-risk behaviors in a population of high school students. J Adolesc Health. 1995;16(3):216–25.
121. Sheley JF. Drugs and guns among inner-city high school students. J Drug Educ. 1994;24(4):303–21.

122. Sheley JF, Brewer VE. Possession and carrying of firearms among suburban youth. Public Health Rep. 1995;110(1):18–26.
123. Vaughn MG, Salas-Wright CP, Boutwell BB, DeLisi M, Curtis MP. Handgun carrying among youth in the United States: an analysis of subtypes. Youth Violence Juvenile Justice. 2017;15(1):21–37.
124. Chermack ST, Grogan-Kaylor A, Perron BE, Murray RL, De Chavez P, Walton MA. Violence among men and women in substance use disorder treatment: a multi-level event-based analysis. Drug Alcohol Depend. 2010;112(3):194–200.
125. Chermack ST, Giancola PR. The relation between alcohol and aggression: an integrated bio-psychosocial conceptualization. Clin Psychol Rev. 1997;17(6):621–49.
126. Cunningham R, Walton M, Trowbridge M, et al. Correlates of violent behavior among adolescents presenting to an urban emergency department. J Pediatr. 2006;149(6):770–6.
127. Jessor R. Problem-behavior theory, psychosocial development, and adolescent problem drinking. Br J Addict. 1987;82(4):331–42.
128. Goldstein PJ. The drugs/violence nexus: a tripartite conceptual framework. J Drug Issues. 1985;15:493–506.
129. Leonard KE, Quigley BM. Drinking and marital aggression in newlyweds: an event-based analysis of drinking and the occurrence of husband marital aggression. J Stud Alcohol. 1999;60(4):537–45.
130. Cattaneo LB, Bell ME, Goodman LA, Dutton MA. Intimate partner violence victims' accuracy in assessing their risk of re-abuse. J Fam Violence. 2007;22(6):429–40.
131. Green B, Kavanagh D, Young R. Being stoned: a review of self-reported cannabis effects. Drug Alcohol Rev. 2003;22(4):453–60.
132. Hunault CC, Böcker KB, Stellato R, Kenemans JL, de Vries I, Meulenbelt J. Acute subjective effects after smoking joints containing up to 69 mg Δ9-tetrahydrocannabinol in recreational users: a randomized, crossover clinical trial. Psychopharmacology. 2014;231(24):4723–33.
133. Karila L, Roux P, Rolland B, et al. Acute and long-term effects of cannabis use: a review. Curr Pharm Des. 2014;20(25):4112–8.
134. Metrik J, Kahler CW, McGeary JE, Monti PM, Rohsenow DJ. Acute effects of marijuana smoking on negative and positive affect. J Cogn Psychother. 2011;25(1):31–46.
135. Ansell EB, Laws HB, Roche MJ, Sinha R. Effects of marijuana use on impulsivity and hostility in daily life. Drug Alcohol Depend. 2015;148:136–42.
136. Mercado-Crespo MC, Mbah AK. Race and ethnicity, substance use, and physical aggression among US high school students. J Interpers Violence. 2013;28(7):1367–84.
137. Martens K, Gilbert DG. Marijuana and tobacco exposure predict affect-regulation expectancies in dual users. Addict Behav. 2008;33(11):1484–90.
138. Paris C, Edgerton EA, Sifuentes M, Seidel J, Lewis RJ, Gausche M. Risk factors associated with non-fatal adolescent firearm injuries. Inj Prev. 2002;8(2):147–50.
139. Loeber R, DeLamatre M, Tita G, Cohen J, Stouthamer-Loeber M, Farrington DP. Gun injury and mortality: the delinquent backgrounds of juvenile victims. Violence Vict. 1999;14(4):339.
140. Stevens MM, Gaffney CA, Tosteson TD, et al. Children and guns in a well child cohort. Prev Med. 2001;32(3):201–6.
141. Erickson PG, Butters JE, Cousineau MM, Harrison L, Korf D. Girls and weapons: an international study of the perpetration of violence. J Urban Health. 2006;83(5):788–801.
142. Duggan M. More guns, more crime. Cambridge, MA: National Bureau of Economic Research; 2000.
143. Dahlberg LL, Ikeda RM, M-j K. Guns in the home and risk of a violent death in the home: findings from a national study. Am J Epidemiol. 2004;160(10):929–36.
144. Wiebe DJ. Homicide and suicide risks associated with firearms in the home: a national case-control study. Ann Emerg Med. 2003;41(6):771–82.
145. Miller M, Hemenway D, Azrael D. State-level homicide victimization rates in the US in relation to survey measures of household firearm ownership, 2001–2003. Soc Sci Med. 2007;64(3):656–64.

146. Spano R, Freilich JD, Bolland J. Gang membership, gun carrying, and employment: applying routine activities theory to explain violent victimization among Inner City, minority youth living in extreme poverty. Justice Quarterly. 2008;25(2):381–410.
147. Bohnert KM, Walton MA, Ranney M, et al. Understanding the service needs of assault-injured, drug-using youth presenting for care in an urban emergency department. Addict Behav. 2015;41:97–105.
148. Fein JA, Kassam-Adams N, Vu T, Datner EM. Emergency department evaluation of acute stress disorder symptoms in violently injured youths. Ann Emerg Med. 2001;38(4):391–6.
149. Fein JA, Kassam-Adams N, Gavin M, Huang R, Blanchard D, Datner EM. Persistence of posttraumatic stress in violently injured youth seen in the emergency department. Arch Pediatr Adolesc Med. 2002;156(8):836–40.
150. Orcutt HK, Erickson DJ, Wolfe J. A prospective analysis of trauma exposure: the mediating role of PTSD symptomatology. J Trauma Stress. 2002;15(3):259–66.
151. Rich JA, Sullivan LM. Correlates of violent assault among young male primary care patients. J Health Care Poor Underserved. 2001;12(1):103–12.
152. Metzl JM, MacLeish KT. Mental illness, mass shootings, and the politics of American firearms. Am J Public Health. 2015;105(2):240–9.
153. Culyba AJ, Miller E, Ginsburg KR, et al. Adult connection in assault injury prevention among male youth in low-resource urban environments. J Urban Health. 2018;95(3):361–71.
154. Ruback RB, Shaffer JN, Clark VA. Easy access to firearms: juveniles' risks for violent offending and violent victimization. J Interpers Violence. 2011;26(10):2111–38.
155. Dong B, Branas CC, Richmond TS, Morrison CN, Wiebe DJ. Youth's daily activities and situational triggers of gunshot assault in urban environments. J Adolesc Health. 2017;61(6):779–85.
156. Hohl BC, Wiley S, Wiebe DJ, Culyba AJ, Drake R, Branas CC. Association of drug and alcohol use with adolescent firearm homicide at individual, family, and neighborhood levels. JAMA Intern Med. 2017;177(3):317–24.
157. Papachristos AV, Braga AA, Hureau DM. Social networks and the risk of gunshot injury. J Urban Health. 2012;89(6):992–1003.
158. Papachristos AV, Braga AA, Piza E, Grossman LS. The company you keep? The spillover effects of gang membership on individual gunshot victimization in a co-offending network. Criminology. 2015;53(4):624–49.
159. Huebner BM, Martin K, Moule RK Jr, Pyrooz D, Decker SH. Dangerous places: gang members and neighborhood levels of gun assault. Justice Quarterly. 2016;33(5):836–62.
160. Murnan J, Dake JA, Price JH. Association of selected risk factors with variation in child and adolescent firearm mortality by state. J Sch Health. 2004;74(8):335–40.
161. Carter P, Mouch C, Goldstick J, et al. Rates and correlates of risky firearm behaviors among adolescents and young adults treated in an urban emergency department. Prev Med. 2020;130:105891.
162. Kondo MC, South EC, Branas CC, Richmond TS, Wiebe DJ. The association between urban tree cover and gun assault: a case-control and case-crossover study. Am J Epidemiol. 2017;186(3):289–96.
163. Cunningham R, Ranney M, Goldstick J, Kamat S, Roche J, Carter P. Federal funding for research on the leading causes of death among children and adolescents. Health Aff. 2019;38(10):1653–61.

Chapter 4
Unintentional Firearm Injuries in Children

David M. Jaffe

One Week in April Four Toddlers Shot and Killed Themselves

By Jack Healy, Julie Bosman, Alan Blinder and Julie Turkewitz
May 5, 2016. *The New York Times*

Unintentional firearm injuries represent a small fraction of morbidity and mortality due to firearms in the United States, but they disproportionately affect children, especially younger children who are injured by firearms. Most importantly, these deaths are highly preventable. The National Violent Death Reporting System (NVDRS) defines death from unintentional firearm injury as, "A death resulting from a penetrating injury or gunshot wound from a weapon that uses a powder charge to fire a projectile when there was a preponderance of evidence that the shooting was not intentionally directed at the victim." In this chapter we will review the epidemiology and prevention strategies for unintentional firearm injuries and death to children and youth.

4.1 Epidemiology

4.1.1 Fatal Firearm Injuries

As reported in the Centers for Disease Control and Prevention's (CDC) Web-based Injury Statistics Query and Reporting System (WISQARS) in 2018, of the 39,740 firearm-related deaths in the United States (US) (12.2 per 100,000 individuals), 458 (1.2%) were unintentional. Among children and youth 0–17 years old, 1729 children died from firearm-related injury (2.4 per 100,000 children), and 5% were

D. M. Jaffe (✉)
Formerly Department of Emergency Medicine, University of California, San Francisco, San Francisco, CA, USA

unintentional (82 children). However, this number is likely an underestimate. Using the NVDRS, it is estimated that 110 children 0–14 years old die annually from unintentional firearm injuries. There are classification errors regarding intent of firearm injury, particularly in the vital statistics data, with the NVDRS considered to be more accurate. The undercount in vital statistics data is predominantly related to coroner reports, in which medical examiners frequently list as homicide any death in which one person shoots another, regardless of intent. The result of this misclassification is an underestimate of unintentional firearm deaths. The case fatality rate for unintentional firearm injuries is 5%, compared to 19% for assaults with firearms and 85% for self-inflicted firearm injury. From these data it is estimated a child dies of unintentional firearm injury every 3 days. Children 5–14 years old in the United States are 11 times more likely to be killed unintentionally by firearms than in other high-income countries.

Age: The highest rate of fatal firearm injury (all intents) occurs in young adults 25–34 years old and the next highest in youth 15–24 years old. These groups also have the highest rates of unintentional fatal firearm injury at 0.3 and 0.2 per 100,000 respectively. Older children (13–17 years old) have twice the mortality rates as younger children (0–12 years): 0.2 vs. 0.1 /100,000. In most cases, unintentional injuries and fatalities occur when children shoot other children. It is less common for children to be shot unintentionally by unrelated adults, although they can be unintentional victims in drive-by shootings, or shot by unrelated adults unintentionally. Younger children most typically find and play with loaded guns in the home. Older children may fail to realize the guns are loaded as they show them to other children. Most incidents occur in the home, either of the shooter or the victim. In one report 11% of deaths involved hunting, but these included shootings at home before and after the hunt itself. Both younger and older children were more likely to have been killed by another shooter than by themselves. However, the proportion of children shot by another shooter is larger among older children than among younger children (71% vs. 56%).

Sex differences: Males account for 86% of all firearm deaths, and this is 6.5 times that of females (18.1 vs. 2.8 per 100,000). Boys account for 81% of unintentional firearm deaths among children. The shooter in 97% of other-inflicted fatalities is also male.

Urban vs. rural: The overall rates of firearm mortality are similar in rural and urban counties (adjusted rate ratio, aRR 0.91, 95% CI 0.63, 1.3). However, unintentional deaths and suicides are relatively greater in rural counties (aRR for most rural vs. most urban is 2.19, 95% CI 1.27, 3.77). In contrast, firearm homicides are greater in urban counties.

Disparities: Although not as striking as for homicides, there are disparities in unintentional fatal firearm injuries in children. Among reported cases, Black children have twice the rate of unintentional firearm fatalities as White children (0.2/100,000 vs. 0.1/100,000) and four times the rate for Hispanic children (0.05/100,000). This is notable given that surveys of firearm ownership show White household ownership rates of 49%, Black households 32%, and Hispanic households 21%.

Trends: There was an overall decrease in unintentional firearm deaths among children between 2002 and 2014 (annual change = − 2.7%).

To summarize, data from the NVDRS indicate most unintentional firearm deaths occur in the home, about half the victims are younger than 25 years old, and half of all deaths are other-inflicted. Typically, the victim is shot by a friend or family member, often an older brother.

4.1.2 Nonfatal Firearm Injuries

The estimated annual incidence of nonfatal firearm injuries in children 0–19 years old is approximately 19,000 per year (23.9/100,000). This means for every child firearm death, there are nearly 20 nonfatal firearm injuries. It is estimated that 64% of these injuries are unintentional. Approximately 20 children are hospitalized daily for firearm injuries, and for children younger than 10 years old, 75% have an unintentional mechanism. However, as for fatal injuries, there are more nonfatal injuries among older children: nearly five times more among children 10–19 years old, compared to those younger than 10 years old. Ninety percent of pediatric emergency department visits for firearm injuries occur in children 12–19 years old, whereas only 10% are among children younger than 12 years old. Therefore, even though younger children suffer fewer firearm injuries than older children, the proportion of unintentional injuries among those who are shot is greatest in younger children. Boys account for 90% of the ED visits for firearm injury. In one single center study of unintentional firearm injuries, 83% of nonfatal injuries occurred in boys.

There are also significant reported racial disparities for nonfatal unintentional firearm injuries. The hospitalization rate in 2013 for firearm injury among Black children was 7.2/100,000. In contrast, for White children, it was 4.8/100,000; for Hispanic children, it was 2.7 per 100,000; and for other racial categories, it was 2.7/100,000.

Nonfatal firearm injuries also cause significant morbidity. Compared to other injury mechanisms, firearms tend to cause more severe injuries. They cause greater physiologic damage compromise and require more procedure performed by Emergency Medical Services (EMS). Again, compared to other injury mechanisms in children, firearm injuries have the highest injury severity scores (ISS) and the most severe injuries to body systems, including abdominal/pelvic organs and extremities. They also require the greatest proportion of surgical intervention, and almost most half of these children and youth are discharged with a physical or neurological disability. The most common injuries are open wounds (50.2%), fractures (50.4%), and internal injuries of the thorax, abdomen, or pelvis (34.8%). While traumatic brain injury (9.2%) and nerve or spinal cord injury (6.4%) are less common, children younger than 5 years old more commonly have brain injuries (20.8%). In a single center study in Louisiana, extremities were most commonly injured (28%), but the abdomen (15%), head and neck (15%), and thorax (14%) were also commonly injured.

4.1.3 Non-powder Firearm Injuries

Non-powder firearms (such as BB guns, pellet guns, and air rifles) cause an esti-mated 32,000 injuries annually, and more than 75% are to children younger than 15 years old. Half of the injuries in a large single center report were unintentional. These firearms are often treated as toys, and children have relatively easy access to them. Injuries tend to be less severe than with powder firearms, but fatalities have been reported. Body parts injured are the extremities (39%), head and neck (33%), eye (13%), thorax (13%), face (8%), and abdomen (3%).

4.2 Firearm Ownership

Because most unintentional injuries occur in the home and involve children (most often boys) playing with firearms in the household, it is important to understand how these injuries are related to gun ownership and storage in the United States. The US leads the world in per capita gun ownership. Great Britain, for example, has 6.2 firearms per 100 individuals, and Australia has 15 firearms per 100 individuals. Thirty percent of Americans report they own a gun, and 42% of households have at least one firearm. Two-thirds of gun owners report they own more than one gun, and 29% say they own five or more guns. It is estimated there are more than 300 million guns in circulation in the US, with some reports suggesting there are more guns than people in the US.

There are demographic differences in gun ownership. Men are more likely to own guns than women (39% vs. 22%), and 34% of White respondents own a gun compared to 24% of Black residents. Approximately half of adults say they grew up in a household with guns. The proportion of White families with young chil-dren who owned firearms declined from 50% in 1976 to 45% in 2016. Ownership had decreased to 29% in 2002, but it has increased since then. Among Black families with young children, 38% owned firearms in 1976, and this declined to 6% in 2016. There has also been a shift in the type of firearms owned with a decrease in rifles and shotguns and an increase in handguns. Of firearm-owning families, 72% have a handgun in the home. Handguns tend to be more accessible and operable by young children. There are also geographic differences. Whereas 29% of urban households have guns, 41% of suburban and 58% of rural house-holds have them. There are also regional differences with the Northeast having the lowest proportion of households with guns (27%) and approximately 45% of households with guns in other regions of the US. This means in most regions of the US, a child has greater than a 40% chance of living in a household with at least one gun, and similar likelihood that the homes of playmates also have firearms.

4.3 Firearm Storage

The most recent data regarding storage comes from a nationally representative web-based survey conducted in 2015. Approximately one-third of US households in this survey contained at least one gun, and this did not vary by whether there were children in the home. Approximately 21% of households store at least one gun loaded and unlocked, the least safe method of gun storage. An estimated 4.6 million children live in homes with loaded and unlocked guns. Another 50% of households store at least one gun either loaded and locked or unloaded and unlocked, while 30% store the guns unloaded and locked, considered to be the safest method of storage. Fewer households in which there are children younger than 6 years old have loaded and unlocked guns (17%). However, this represents an increase from reports published in the early 2000s in which approximately 10% of households with children younger than 6 years old reported at least one gun loaded and unlocked. More households with handguns compared to long guns (27% vs. 5%) store guns loaded and unlocked. Similarly, more households having guns for protection compared to other uses (e.g., hunting) store guns loaded and unlocked, 29% vs. 3%.

Children often know where the guns are located in the home. When 201 parent-child dyads were questioned separately about guns in their homes, children younger than 10 years old were as likely as older children to know where the guns are stored (73 vs. 79%) – and to have handled a household gun (36% in both age groups). Nearly 40% of parents who thought their children did not know where the gun was stored were contradicted by their children, and 22% of parents who thought their children had never handled a household gun had discordant responses from their children.

Parents and pediatric providers may not realize many young children can pull the trigger of a gun on their own. The one- and two-finger pull strength of children at different ages has been tested using 64 commercially available handguns. Twenty-five percent of children 3–4 years old, 70% of children 5–6 years old, and 90% of children 7–8 years old could pull the triggers. Interestingly, firearms are the only commercial item in the US not regulated for safety by the Consumer Product Safety Commission (CPSC).

We also know young children will play with guns when they find them, even when instructed not to play with them. This was demonstrated in a behavioral study using a convenience sample of boys 8–12 years old. A total of 64 boys were organized into 29 groups of 2 or 3, and each group was sent into a room where 2 obvious toy squirt guns and 1 real disarmed handgun were concealed in drawers. The disarmed handgun was engineered so the study investigators would know if the trigger was pulled by the child. The group of boys were observed through a one-way mirror for up to 15 minutes. The handgun was discovered by 21 of the groups (48 boys): 16 groups handled the gun (30 boys), and 1 or more boys in 10 groups (16 boys) pulled the trigger. Parental estimates of their child's interest in guns did not predict the actual behavior when the boys found the handgun. More than 90% of the boys who handled the gun or pulled the trigger reported they had previously received gun safety instruction – namely, they were instructed, "If you see a gun, don't touch it, and go find an adult."

4.4 Prevention

Strategies for prevention should logically address the epidemiologic evidence that most unintentional firearm injuries occur in the home. This occurs when a child discovers or otherwise obtains a loaded gun and shoots himself or another child. The following cases from the author's emergency department experience are illustrative:

- A 3-year-old boy, son of a policeman, killed himself with his father's loaded pistol found in a dresser drawer.
- A 12-year-old boy was shot in the head by his friend, also 12 years old playing with a loaded pistol kept under the pillow by his grandfather.
- A 4-year-old boy found a handgun in a closet at home, placed the barrel into his mouth, and pulled the trigger as he had often done to get a drink from a similarly designed water pistol.
- A 7-year-old boy was playing "Cops and Robbers" with his 9-year-old cousin who had found a pellet gun. The projectile hit the clavicle, broke a rib, and lodged in the pericardium. The patient lived.

Given the high prevalence of gun ownership and exposure of children to firearms in their homes and the homes of their playmates, it is necessary to employ prevention strategies addressing this reality in the US environment. A 2017 US Government Accountability Office report (GAO 17-665) stated: "Researchers have found that having a firearm in the home is a risk factor for injuries and deaths, including suicides, among adults and children alike. While household firearms can pose a danger to anyone, the inherent curiosity of children makes them particularly susceptible to harm from an unsecured firearm." With awareness of the risk of firearm injuries to children when firearms are in the home, the American Academy of Pediatrics (AAP) firearm safety policy (published in 2012) stated: "the most effective measure to prevent suicide, homicide, and unintentional firearm related injuries is the absence of guns from homes and communities".

If a gun is not removed from the home, safe storage of guns should be recommended. This is defined as having the firearm unloaded, stored, and locked away separately from the ammunition. Safe storage of guns in the home has been shown to reduce both the risk of firearm suicide and unintentional injury to children and youth. A recent modeling study estimated 6–32% of firearm suicide and unintentional injury could be prevented by increasing safe household firearm storage. In an earlier case-control study, firearms in homes with and without safe storage were compared regarding the risk of a shooting involving children. Case firearms were those involved in a shooting incident when a child <20 years old gained access to a firearm and shot himself/herself intentionally or unintentionally or another individual unintentionally. Control firearms were those randomly selected in households matched by age and county as the case firearms. In this study, case firearms were significantly less likely to be stored locked (OR 0.27, 95% CI 0.17, 0.45), less likely to be stored unloaded (OR 0.3, 95% CI 0.16, 0.56), less likely to be stored separately from ammunition (OR 0.45, 95% CI 0.34, 0.93), and less likely to have locked ammunition (OR 0.39, 95% CI 0.23, 0.66) compared to control firearms.

4.5 Physician Counseling and Locking Device Distribution Can Increase Safe Firearm Storage

The GAO (GAO-17-665) evaluated research on programs promoting safe storage of personal firearms in 2017. They found locking device distribution was effective in all five studies they evaluated. One of these was a large cluster randomized trial of office-based counseling versus placebo, in which motivational counseling plus provision of a cable lock increased safe storage of guns by nearly 10%, whereas the no-intervention control group had a decrease of 11%. In an earlier study, distributing free metal gun cabinets to 255 households in Alaska reduced the proportion of unlocked firearms from 95% to 35%, and presence of unlocked ammunition decreased from 89% to 36%. In another community, office-based counseling and gun lock giveaway resulted in either removal of guns from the home or improvement in gun storage. In contrast, only 27% in the control group showed improvement.

The GAO also evaluated seven studies of physician counseling without distribution of locking devices and found mixed results. Three showed positive results, and four showed little or no benefit. The four negative effect studies were all based in primary care settings. In contrast, of the three positive studies, two were in an emergency department setting, and one was in a mental health clinic. However, another pediatric emergency department counseling intervention failed to improve gun safety behavior. Further research is necessary to examine the effectiveness of approaches to firearm counseling alone by healthcare clinicians.

Despite evidence for the effectiveness of firearm safety counseling along with locking device distribution in improving firearm safe storage, there have been legal barriers to physician screening for firearms in the healthcare setting. These include state legislative efforts to prohibit or restrict physician counseling of parents regarding gun ownership and safety. In 2011 Florida enacted the most extensive law of this type, which restricted physicians and other medical staff from asking patients or their families about firearms in the home ("physician gag law"). Physicians who violated the law could be disciplined by the state medical board and fined. After a series of legal challenges and decisions, the US Court of Appeals for the 11th Circuit overturned the Florida law in 2017. This upheld the right of physicians to screen for firearms in the home to provide sound medical advice in this domain. They cited barring physicians from asking patients and families about firearms in the home was a violation of the physician's first amendment rights to free speech. Despite this legal decision, there have been at least 12 other states that have introduced similar legislation; however, none have passed.

4.6   Gun Safety Education for Children

Gun safety education and gun avoidance education, such as the Eddie Eagle GunSafe Program, are designed to teach young children not to handle guns, to leave the scene if they find one, and to report to an adult. The GAO report reviewed four studies of child education programs and concluded that "behavioral skills training did not instill consistent safe firearm habits in young children." One of these studies compared Eddie Eagle and a behavioral skills training program and found both programs effectively taught children to reproduce the gun safety message verbally. The behavioral skills training, but not the Eddie Eagle GunSafe Program, effectively taught children to perform gun safety skills in a role-play setting. However, neither program prevented risky behavior when children were assessed in real-life settings.

4.7   Child Access Prevention Laws

Child access prevention (CAP) laws are intended to prevent children from accessing loaded guns in the home by requiring some form of safe gun storage and by holding gun owners liable for breaches of the state requirements. There are no federal CAP laws in the US. Twenty-five states and the District of Columbia have CAP laws, whereas 25 do not. The laws vary considerably from state to state in a variety of aspects, but they have been categorized into groups based on strength of regulation. Stronger CAP laws include "negligence" laws that hold a gun owner liable simply if a child does or could access a gun. Weaker CAP laws include "recklessness" laws, which hold a gun owner liable only if a gun was given to child and resulted in another person's injury or death by the firearm. Three states, California, Massachusetts, Minnesota, and the District of Columbia have the strongest CAP laws. The gun owner may be charged if the child "may" or "is likely to" access an unsafely stored gun (loaded and unlocked). Eleven states (Connecticut, Florida, Illinois, Iowa, Hawaii, Maryland, New Hampshire, New Jersey, North Carolina, Rhode Island, and Texas) may charge parents if a child accesses an unsafely stored gun. In some states, charges can be brought against the gun-owning adult even in absence of harm or injury (Hawaii, Maryland, New Jersey, and Texas). The weakest CAP laws (recklessness laws) charge gun-owning adults only if the gun owner intentionally, knowingly, or recklessly gives a gun to a child (Colorado, Delaware, Georgia, Indiana, Kentucky, Mississippi, Virginia, and Wisconsin). Compared to recklessness laws, negligence laws have been associated with a 13% relative reduction in unintentional firearm fatalities (95% CI −24%, −1%). The most stringent negligence laws were associated with unintentional firearm fatality reductions of 59% (95% CI −68%, −49%). Sixty-five percent of unintentional firearm deaths are attributable to the absence of the strongest CAP laws – meaning 65% of unintentional firearm deaths could potentially be prevented if all states had the strongest CAP laws.

4.8 Mechanical Safety Mechanisms

Guns currently available for purchase in the United States have a variety of optional mechanical safety mechanisms designed to prevent accidental or unintentional firing. They can be divided into two basic conceptual types: passive (not requiring action by the shooter) and active (requiring action to activate and deactivate the safety mechanism). There are many variations, which are further described in Chap. 12. Passive mechanisms are designed so the gun will only fire when the trigger is pulled. They are engineered so deactivation is not required, and the gun will fire with a trigger pull. These guns are designed not to fire when the gun is dropped, for example. Examples of active safeties are pivot safeties or grip safeties. The user must, respectively, manipulate the pivot safety to fire the gun or depress the grip safety on the handle of the gun to fire. Trigger locks and cable locks are designed to prevent firing while the gun is being stored. It has been noted trigger locks can fail if there is a bullet in the chamber and the trigger is accidentally pulled during installation or removal of the trigger lock. "Smart guns" are engineered to prevent an unauthorized user from pulling the trigger of the gun. These guns are not currently available for sale in the US (see Chap. 8).

In conclusion, while unintentional firearm injuries represent a small proportion of the firearm injuries in children, 5% of fatal and 21% of nonfatal, they are particularly important because they disproportionately affect younger children. Perhaps even more importantly, many of these injuries and deaths are highly preventable. Most of these injuries occur in the home of either the victim or the shooter and involve a child gaining access to an improperly stored gun. Approximately one in three children lives in households with one or more guns; therefore, it is important for healthcare providers to discuss firearm safety with families to decrease unintentional injuries. While the best preventive measure against unintentional firearm injury or death to children is the absence of guns in the home, the ubiquity of guns in the US requires additional preventive strategies. Clinician counseling along with locking device distribution has been shown to increase safe storage practices. Strong "negligence" child access prevention (CAP) laws have also demonstrated an association with decreased unintentional firearm injuries and deaths to children and youth. A multipronged strategy including clinician counseling, locking device distribution, and the adoption of strong state child access prevention laws is necessary to engage families in improving safe firearm storage to decrease unintentional firearm injuries and deaths to children and youth.

Take Home Points
- Annually there are an estimated 110 fatal unintentional childhood firearm fatalities and 20 times that number of nonfatal injuries in the United States. This represents approximately 5% of all fatal firearm injuries and 21% of nonfatal injuries.
- Approximately one-third of American children live in households with one or more guns, and in 21% of these households, at least one gun is stored loaded and unlocked.
- Most unintentional firearm injuries occur in the home with guns stored unlocked and/or loaded.
- Unintentional firearm injuries are highly preventable with removal of firearms from the home or safe storage of firearms in the home.
- Safe storage of guns is effective in preventing these injuries, and physician counseling coupled with locking device distribution increases the frequency of safe storage.
- Child access prevention laws vary by state as there is no federal law; 25 states and the District of Columbia have some form of CAP law.
- Strong child access prevention laws (negligence laws) have been shown to prevent unintentional firearm deaths, whereas weaker CAP laws (recklessness laws) do not.

Suggested Readings

1. Allbright T, Burge S. Improving firearm storage habits: impact of brief office counseling by family physicians. J Am Board Fam Pract. 2003;16:40–6.
2. Azreal D, Cohen J, Salhi C, Miller M. Firearm storage in gun-owning households with children: results of a 2015 national survey. J Urban Health. 2018;95:295–304.
3. Azad HA, Monuteaux MM, Rees CA et al. Child access prevention firearm laws and firearm fatalities among children aged 0 to 14 years 1991–2016, JAMA Pediatr. 2020;174(5):463–69.
4. Barkin S, Finch S, Ip E, et al. Is office-based counseling about media use, timeouts, and firearm storage effective? Results from a cluster-randomized controlled trial. Pediatrics. 2008;122(1):e15–e25.
5. Baxley F, Miller M. Parental misperceptions about children and firearms. Arch Pediatr Adolesc Med. 2006;160(5):542–7.
6. Carbone PS, Clemens CJ, Ball TM. Effectiveness of gun-safety counseling and a gun lock giveaway in a hispanic community. Arch Pediatr Adolesc Med. 2005;159(11):1049–54.
7. Council on Injury, Violence, and Poison Prevention Executive Committee. American Academy of Pediatrics Policy Statement. Firearm-related injuries affecting the pediatric population [Internet]. Pediatrics. 2012;130:e1416–23 Available from: https://pediatrics.aappublications.org/content/pediatrics/130/5/e1416.full.pdf.
8. DiScala C, Sege R. Outcomes in children and young adults who are hospitalized for firearms-related injuries. Pediatrics. 2004;113(5):1306–12.
9. Fleegler EW, Lee LK, Monteaux MC, et al. Firearm legislation and firearm-related fatalities in the United States. JAMA Intern Med. 2013;173(9):732–40.

10. Fowler K, Dahlberg L, Haileyesus T. Firearm injuries in the United States. Prev Med. 2015;79:5–14.
11. Grossman DC, Cummings P, Koepsell TD, et al. Firearm safety counseling in primary care pediatrics: a randomized controlled trial. Pediatrics. 2000;106(1Pt1):22–6.
12. Grossman DC, Mueller BA, Riedy C, et al. Gun storage practices and risk of youth suicide and unintentional firearm injuries. JAMA. 2005;293(6):707–14.
13. Grossman DC, Stafford HA, Koepsell TD, et al. Improving storage in Alaska native villages: a randomized trial of household gun cabinets. Am J Public Health. 2012;102(Suppl 2):S291–7.
14. Hemenway D, Scolnick S. Children and unintentional firearm death. Inj Epidemiol. 2015;2(1):26;1–6.
15. Himle MB, Miltenberger RG, Gatheridge BJ, Flessner CA. An evaluation of two procedures for training skills to prevent gun play in children. Pediatrics. 2004;113(1 Pt 1):70–7.
16. Jenco, M. AAP News February 16, 2017. Federal Court strikes down physician "Gag Law" on guns [Internet]. Available from: https://www.aappublications.org/news/2017/02/16/FloridaGun021617.
17. Jackman G, Farah NM, Kellerman AL, Simon HK. Seeing is believing: what do boys do when they find a real gun? Pediatrics. 2001;107(6):1247–50.
18. Johnston BD, Rivara FP, Droesch RM, et al. Behavior change counseling in the emergency department to reduce injury risk: a randomized controlled trial. Pediatrics. 2002;110:267–74.
19. Kalesan B, Chandana A, Pressley J, et al. The hidden epidemic of firearm injury: increasing firearm injury rates during 2001–2013. Am J Epdemiol. 2017;185(7):546–53.
20. Kalesan B, Dubic S, Vasan S, et al. Racial/ethnic specific trends in pediatric firearm related hospitalizations in the United States, 1998–2011. Matern Child Health. 2016;20:1082–90.
21. Leventhal J, Gaither J, Sege R. Hospitalizations due to firearm injuries in children and adolescents. Pediatrics. 2014;133(2):219–25.
22. Luo M, McIntire M. Children and guns: the hidden toll. The New York Times. September 28, 2013.
23. Medhaven S, Taylor JS, Chandler JM, et al. Firearm legislation stringency and firearm-related fatalities among children in the US. J Am Coll Surg. 2019;229(2):150–7.
24. Miller M, Azreal D, Firearms HD. Violent death in the United States. In: Webster D, Vernick J, editors. Reducing gun violence in America. Baltimore: The Johns Hopkins University Press; 2013.
25. Monuteaux MC, Azreal D, Miller M. Association of increased safe household firearm storage with firearm suicide and unintentional death among US youths. JAMA Pediatr. 2019;173(7):657–62.
26. Nance M, Carr B, Kallan M, et al. Variation in pediatric and adolescent firearm mortality rates in rural and urban US counties. Pediatrics. 2010;125(6):1112–8.
27. Naureckas SM, Galanter C, Naureckas ET, et al. Children's and Women's ability to fire handguns. The Pediatric Practice Research Group. Arch Pediatr Adolesc Med. 1995;149(12):1318–22.
28. Newgard C, Kuppermann N, Holmes J, et al. Gunshot injuries in children served by emergency services. Pediatrics. 2013;132:862–70.
29. Parker K, Horowitz JM, Igielnik R, Oliphant JB, Brown A. The demographics of gun ownership [Internet], Pew Research Center, June 22, 2017. Available from: https://www.pewsocialtrends.org/2017/06/22/americas-complex-relationship-with-guns/.
30. Pickett K, Martin-Storey A, Croswnoe R. State firearm laws, firearm ownership, and safety practices among families of preschool-aged children. Am J Public Health. 2014;104:1080–6.
31. Powell E, Javits E, Tanz R. Incidence and circumstances of nonfatal firearm-related injuries among children and adolescents. Arch Pediatr Adolesc Med. 2001;155:1364–8.
32. Prickett KC, Gutierrez C, Deb S. Family firearm ownership and firearm-related mortality among young children: 1976-2016. Pediatrics. 2019;143(2):E20181171.
33. Reznick S, Smith R, Beard J, et al. Firearm deaths in America: can we learn from 462,000 lives lost? Ann Surg. 2017;266(3):432–40.

34. Safavi A, Rhee P, Viraj P, et al. Children are safer in states with strict firearm laws: a national inpatient sample study. J Trauma Acute Care Surg. 2014;76(1):146–51.
35. Santaella-Tenorio J, Cerda M, Villaveces A, Sandro G. What do we know about the association between firearm legislation and firearm-related injuries? Epidemiol Rev. 2016;38:140–57.
36. Schuster M, Franke T, Bastian A, et al. Firearm storage patterns in US homes with children. Am J Public Health. 2000;90(4):588–94.
37. Scribano P, Nance M, Reilly P, et al. Pediatric nonpowder firearm injuries: outcomes in an urban pediatric setting. Pediatrics. 1997;100(4):E5.
38. Srinivasan S, Mannix R, Lee LK. Epidemiology of paediatric firearm injuries in the USA, 2001–2010. Arch Dis Child. 2014;99(4):331–5.
39. Stevens MM, Olson AL Gaffney CA, et al. A pediatric, practice-based, randomized trial of drinking and smoking prevention and bicycle helmet, gun, and seatbelt safety promotion. Pediatrics. 2002;109(3):490–7.
40. Teret SP, Draisin NA. Personalized guns: using technology to address gun violence [Internet]. The Abell Report. 2014;27(2):1–8. Accessed from: https://abell.org/sites/default/files/publications/Aug2014_Smart_Guns_FINAL.pdf
41. The Small Arms Survey. Guns in the city ed. Small Arms Survey Geneva. Cambridge: Cambridge University Press; 2007.
42. U.S. Government Accountability Office 17-665 September 2017 Personal firearms: programs that promote safe storage and research on their effectiveness [Internet]. Available from: https://www.gao.gov/products/GAO-17-665.

Chapter 5
School Shootings: No Longer Unexpected

Chris A. Rees and Rebekah Mannix

Nation Reels After Gunman Massacres 20 Children at School in Connecticut

By James Baron
December 14, 2012. *The New York Times*

5.1 Defining School Shootings

While there has been some controversy regarding the definition of school shootings, they can be defined broadly as acts of violence carried out with firearms in which schools are deliberately chosen as the site of violence. School shootings may involve students or other school personnel including teachers and other staff; however, students make up 68% of victims in fatal school shootings [1]. Most school shootings are directed, in which assailants (often current or former students) intentionally kill or harm certain individuals [2]. Only 12% of deaths from school shootings are due to random, or so-called "rampage," shootings [3]. Though mass school shootings, in which four or more homicides occur in a single incident [4, 5], receive the majority of media attention, single-victim shootings at schools are more common.

School shootings differ from other mass shootings in the United States (US) in several important ways. First, school shootings often receive immense attention from both media outlets and politicians, often more so than shootings occurring in other venues. It is important to note that this lay press and political attention has often focused on school shootings with multiple victims occurring in majority-White schools; however, as many as 61% of school shootings occur in non-majority-White schools [6]. Second, school shootings occur in an environment that has traditionally been thought to be safe and where the victims are a particularly

C. A. Rees · R. Mannix (✉)
Department of Pediatrics, Division of Emergency Medicine, Boston Children's Hospital, Harvard Medical School, Boston, MA, USA
e-mail: Chris.Rees@childrens.harvard.edu; rebekah.mannix@childrens.harvard.edu

© Springer Nature Switzerland AG 2021
L. K. Lee, E. W. Fleegler (eds.), *Pediatric Firearm Injuries and Fatalities*,
https://doi.org/10.1007/978-3-030-62245-9_5

vulnerable population. Third, school shootings are distinctive in that the assailants are often younger than assailants in other venues. In fact, perpetrators less than 20 years old were responsible for 50% of all school shootings from 1982 to 2018 in the US [7]. Fourth, these events are difficult to study because the resultant injuries and deaths are not specifically labelled with the mechanism of "school shooting" when reported to state and federal agencies [1]. This leads to the inability of identifying school shooting victims in the current state and federal healthcare system and criminal justice data sources.

5.2   Epidemiology of School Shootings

Though mass school shootings such as the events at Columbine High School in Littleton, Colorado, in 1999; Sandy Hook Elementary School in Newtown, Connecticut, in 2012; and Stoneman Douglas High School in Parkland, Florida, in 2018 are truly shocking and capture the world's attention, the majority of firearm deaths in children in the US are not due to mass school shootings [8]. Indeed, school shooting fatalities represent less than 1% of the more than 26,000 children 0–17 years old killed by firearms in the US between 1999 and 2016 [9]. However, firearms are responsible for the vast majority of school-associated fatalities according to the Centers for Disease Control and Prevention (CDC), which has reported that firearm injuries were the cause of death in about 63% of single-victim and 95% of multiple-victim school-associated homicides during 1994–2018 [10].

The US has the highest rates of school shootings in the world, though the high rates of school shootings may simply reflect the overall elevated rates of firearm fatalities in the US compared to other industrialized nations. Between 1966 and 2008, there were 7 school shootings in all of Europe and 44 school shootings in the US [11]. The US has the highest rates of firearm deaths from homicides among the world's 34 most advanced economies [3]. In regard to firearm deaths among children, the US accounts for 90% of all deaths due to firearms [12]. Furthermore, the youth firearm homicide rate in the US is 36 times that of other high-income countries (see Chap. 3) [13].

Even in the US, school shootings represent a relatively new phenomenon in the past 50–60 years, with increasing frequency in the past two decades. From 1966 to 2008, there were only 44 school shootings documented, or 1 event every year on average [11]. An epidemiologic study published in 2013 reported that from 2009 to 2012, there were 42 fatal school shootings in the US, or about 8 events per year on average [3]. Even more recently, data suggest the frequency of school shootings has increased dramatically, with 154 such events happening between 2013 and 2015 alone [14]. This equates to one episode per week on average. Though differences in reporting of school shootings and heightened awareness may account for such increased frequency, alarmingly, the number of school shootings appears to be growing.

Among school shooting events, rampage school shootings are perhaps the most feared and deadly events. Rampage shootings, in contrast to mass shootings in which four or more homicides occur in a single incident, are defined as "an institutional attack [that] takes place on a public stage before an audience, is committed by a member or former member of the institution, and involves multiple victims." Rampage shootings account for only 13% of all school shootings and less than 1% of firearm-related homicides [3, 15].

5.3   Risk Factors for School Shootings

Though there are no centrally uniform reporting or recording of school shootings and there is general underfunding of firearm research, there are documented factors associated with firearm fatalities relevant to school shootings. In general, states with weaker firearm legislation have more firearm-related fatalities [16, 17]. A recent time-series analysis evaluating the relationship between firearm legislation and mass shootings showed state legislation leading to firearm permissiveness was associated with a significant increase in the rates of mass shootings [18]. In a large ecological study using data from the CDC, states with fewer firearm laws had increased rates of firearm-related suicide and firearm-related homicides [17]. States with higher rates of firearm ownership also have higher rates of school shootings and mass shootings in general [4].

Politicians and the media often point to mental illness as a factor potentially related to school shootings [19]. This is based on examples such as the assailant of the Stoneman Douglas High School shooting, who had been evaluated for mental illness prior to carrying out the school shooting. However, this relationship is controversial. A population-based study in the US using data from 1994 to 1999 demonstrated more than half of all school shootings were preceded by some action by the assailants that would have served as warnings for impending violence [1]. In a more recent study evaluating the effect of many factors on school shootings, states with increased budgets for mental healthcare had fewer school shootings [14]. In a study of perpetrators of mass shootings from 1982 to 2018, 54% of assailants had some documented mental health disorder [7]. In contrast, though not estimating firearm-related mortality specifically, a 20-year population-based study in Denmark evaluating mortality of patients with mental health disorders demonstrated persons with mental illness are more likely to be victims, rather than perpetrators, of violence [20].

School shootings may serve as risk factors for future similar events, following contagion patterns or "copycat effect." Using a contagion model applied to school shootings in the US, investigators have found significant evidence of contagion in school shootings, with the period of 13 days following initial school shooting events showing increased rates of school shooting incidents compared to baseline rates [4]. Similarly, a study investigating imitative behaviors after the Columbine High School shooting in 1999 demonstrated a copycat effect with an increase in threats to schools often involving bombs, proportional to days of media coverage for an event [21]. Numerous killers have described taking their inspiration from the Columbine perpetrators.

Lastly, there is some evidence to suggest declines in federal and state funding for education may be associated with increased rates of school shootings. In a review of school shootings from 2013 to 2015, states with lower expenditures for kindergarten through 12th grade had higher rates of school shootings [14]. This is thought to be secondary to overall decreased investment in education resulting in increased violence in schools.

5.4 Protective Factors Against School Shootings

Though interventional studies are lacking, ecological studies have shown several factors to be protective against firearm injuries and deaths, in general, and school shootings, in particular. Most notably, increased legislation targeting the sale, purchase, and storage of firearms in the US has been shown to reduce firearm-related violence. There are more than 300 federal laws in the US regulating the sales, possession, and handling of firearms; however, state-level laws allow for differences in the implementation of federal laws [22].

Regarding the purchase of firearms, states requiring universal background checks prior to the purchase of firearms and ammunition have lower rates of school shootings than states without such laws [14]. Furthermore, requiring permits to purchase firearms may be protective against firearm fatalities in general [16, 17, 23]. Assailants 18–20 years old have been associated with nearly 40% of all school mass casualty fatalities, which has led to the call in many settings to raise the legal age of firearm purchase to 21 years to potentially reduce school shootings [7]. While licensed firearm dealers can only sell handguns to people 21 years and older, they can sell long guns to those 18 years and older. Federal regulation of private sales allows the sale of handguns to those 18 years old and does not regulate by age the sale of long guns [24]. Studies demonstrating the effect of raising the minimum age of legal firearm purchase on school shootings are lacking. Increased firearm legislation has also been shown to reduce the probability of firearms being carried at school and reduce missed days of school due to feeling unsafe at school [25].

Despite evidence suggesting legislation surrounding the purchase of firearms results in reduced school shootings, most firearms used in school shootings are obtained from the assailants' own home, or the home of a friend or relative. This underscores the importance of safe storage and restriction of unsupervised minors to firearms [26]. As a majority of assailants in school shootings are minors, child access protection (CAP) laws, which legislate safe firearm storage practices for firearm owners with children and hold owners criminally liable for children's unsupervised use of firearms, may be an area of targeted research to reduce school shootings. Stringent child access protection laws have been shown to improve firearm storage behaviors [27] and have been associated with decreased firearm-related injuries and deaths [28–31]. The role of child access prevention laws in school shootings has not been described previously. Extreme risk protection order (ERPO) laws, which help prevent a person in crisis from harming themselves or others by temporarily removing guns and prohibiting the purchase of firearms, may be another avenue to prevent access to firearms in an at-risk population.

In the wake of recent school shootings in the US, some have called for arming teachers and other school staff with firearms as a method to reduce such violent acts. Despite such public calls, there is no evidence to suggest this would actually result in reduced firearm violence in schools [32]. Indeed, one study found no association between the presence of school resource officers and the likelihood or frequency of injuries and deaths ("severity of shooting") [6]. Moreover, increased firearm access and possession in general is not associated with reduced violence [33]; thus, the validity of this claim is unclear. Further research is needed to understand the effectiveness of strategies such as school resource officers or arming teachers in preventing the occurrence and mitigating the severity of school shootings, as current evidence does not support these maneuvers. Some authorities have suggested school resources are better directed to other avenues including expert-endorsed school security upgrades (e.g., locks on every classroom door that lock from the inside of the room), evidence-based threat assessments, and trauma-informed emergency planning partnering with local agencies. Others have recommended investment in "school culture" initiatives to ensure safe and equitable schools [34].

5.5 Outcomes After School Shootings

What is often not measured is the psychological trauma among survivors of school shootings. Limited evidence suggests children are often resilient, and few experience long-term dysfunction. However, those who do experience residual psychological trauma often suffer from severe and chronic symptoms of post-traumatic stress disorder, survivor guilt, and acute stress reaction and disorder [35]. Recently there have been suicides among survivors at the Stoneman Douglas High School shooting in Parkland, Florida, suggesting the long-term psychological impact of such tragic acts. Evidence from mass shootings also suggest these events can have at least short-term psychological effects (e.g., increased fears regarding lack of personal safety) on persons living far outside of the affected communities [36]. Those living in the affected communities and those directly affected may also have long-term psychological distress. In 2019 a parent of a victim of the Sandy Hook elementary school shooting committed suicide.

Certain characteristics may confer increased risk of adverse outcomes including demographic factors (e.g., female gender and lower socioeconomic status), higher pre-event trauma exposure and premorbid psychological symptom burden, greater direct and indirect event exposure, and lack of psychosocial resources (e.g., emotional regulation difficulties, experiential avoidance, and low social support). Recently, many US schools have started holding active shooter drills to prepare students for the possible advent of a school shooting. Some US schools are also teaching students how to apply tourniquets for extremity-related trauma (for firearm as well as non-firearm trauma) with the "Stop the Bleed" educational campaign [37]. These drills can possibly lead to psychological distress, including anxiety, among students. The potential benefit and potential harm from these drills have yet to be elucidated.

5.6 Pediatric Clinicians and the School Community

Pediatric clinicians are uniquely positioned to advocate for practical solutions that may improve school safety. Potential areas for advocacy include ensuring school districts partner with local law enforcement, recommending schools have a school safety officer to coordinate school safety planning, and recommending classrooms have doors that lock from the inside. Pediatric and mental health clinicians and school guidance counselors and nurses may also be in a unique position to identify at-risk children and assist with school-associated mental health resources where feasible.

5.7 Future Research on School Shootings

School shooting injuries and deaths have been understudied due to funding bans and difficulty in accurately identifying school shootings. Recently groups like the Firearm Safety Among Children and Teens (FACTS) Consortium, a National Institute for Child Health and Human Development-funded group of scientists and stakeholders, have been created to address gaps in knowledge in firearm-related violence [38]. This Consortium has a research agenda for firearm injury prevention among children. School shootings are a research priority for this group. Only through comprehensive, multifaceted approaches employing rigorous research and meaningful legislation identifying risk factors and preventive strategies can the rise of school shootings in the United States be curbed. Further research on survivors of school shootings is also warranted to identify those at risk for long-term adverse outcomes including depression and suicide.

Take Home Points

- Though school shootings make up a minority of all deaths from firearm violence, they have increased in frequency over the past two decades.
- Weaker state-level firearm legislation, increased state-level firearm ownership, recent school shootings, and declines in federal and state funding for education have been associated with school shootings.
- Increased legislation targeting the sale, purchase, and storage of firearms in the United States has been shown to reduce firearm-related violence and school shootings.
- Comprehensive, multifaceted research and legislation targeting risk factors and preventive strategies are needed to slow the rising rate of school shootings in the United States.
- Pediatricians can work with their school communities to encourage safety practices including:

  - Having all classroom doors have locks that can be secured from inside the classroom
  - Developing school safety plans
  - Collaborating with local police and other safety agencies in the community for school security

- Pediatricians can advocate for stricter state-level firearm legislation as one avenue to decrease youth access to firearms to potentially decrease school shootings.

References

1. Anderson M, Kaufman J, Simon TR, et al. School-associated violent deaths in the United States, 1994–1999. JAMA. 2001;286:2695–702.
2. Newman KS, Fox C, Harding D, Mehta J, Roth W. Rampage: the social roots of school shootings. New York: Perseus; 2004.
3. Shultz JM, Cohen AM, Muschert GW, et al. Fatal school shootings and the epidemiological context of firearm mortality in the United States. Disaster Health. 2013;1:84–101.
4. Towers S, Gomez-Lievano A, Khan M, Mubayi A, Castillo-Chavez C. Contagion in mass killings and school shootings. PLoS One. 2015;10:e0117259.
5. Rocque M, Duwe G. Rampage shootings: an historical, empirical, and theoretical overview. Curr Opin Psychol. 2018;19:28–33.
6. Livingston MD, Rossheim ME, Hall KS. A descriptive analysis of school and school shooter characteristics and the severity of school shootings in the United States, 1999–2018. J Adolesc Health. 2019;64:797–9.
7. Brown JD, Goodin AJ. Mass casualty shooting venues, types of firearms, and age of perpetrators in the United States, 1982–2018. Am J Public Health. 2018;108:1385–7.
8. Gun Violence Archive. Mass shootings [Internet]. 2018. Available from: http://www.gunviolencearchive.org/mass-shooting. Accessed 11 Mar 2019.

9. Fowler KA, Dahlberg LL, Haileyesus T, Gutierrez C, Bacon S. Childhood firearm injuries in the United States. Pediatrics. 2017;140:e20163486.
10. Center for Disease Control and Prevention. School associated violent death study [Internet]. Available from: https://www.cdc.gov/violenceprevention/youthviolence/schoolviolence/SAVD.html. Accessed 11 Mar 2019.
11. Preti A. School shooting as a culturally enforced way of expressing suicidal hostile intentions. J Am Acad Psychiatry Law. 2008;36:544–50.
12. Grinshteyn E, Hemenway D. Violent death rates: the US compared with other high-income OECD countries, 2010. Am J Med. 2016;129:266–73.
13. Richardson EG, Hemenway D. Homicide, suicide, and unintentional firearm fatality: comparing the United States with other high-income countries, 2003. J Trauma. 2011;70:238–43.
14. Kalesan B, Lagast K, Villarreal M, Pino E, Fagan J, Galea S. School shootings during 2013–2015 in the USA. Inj Prev. 2017;23:321–7.
15. Shultz JM, Muschert GW, Dingwall A, Cohen AM. The Sandy Hook Elementary School shooting as tipping point "this time is different". Disaster Health. 2013:165–73.
16. Lee LK, Fleegler EW, Farrell C, Avakame E, Srinivasan S, Hemenway D, Monuteaux MC. Firearm laws and firearm homicides: a systematic review. JAMA Intern Med. 2017;177:106–19.
17. Fleegler EW, Lee LK, Monuteaux MC, Hemenway D, Mannix R. Firearm legislation and firearm-related fatalities in the United States. JAMA Intern Med. 2013;173:732–40.
18. Reeping PM, Cerdá M, Kalesan B, Wiebe DJ, Galea S, Branas CC. State gun laws, gun ownership, and mass shootings in the US: cross sectional time series. BMJ. 2019;364:I542.
19. Rees CA, Lee LK, Fleegler EW, Mannix R. Mass school shootings in the United States: a novel root cause analysis using lay press reports. Clin Pediatr (Phila). 2019;58(13):1423–28.
20. Hiroeh U, Appleby L, Mortensen PB, Dunn G. Death by homicide, suicide, and other unnatural causes in people with mental illness: a population-based study. Lancet. 2001;358:2110–2.
21. Kostinsky S, Bixler EO, Ketti PA. Threats of school violence in Pennsylvania after media coverage of the Columbine High School massacre: examining the role of imitation. Arch Pediatr Adolesc Med. 2001;155:994–1001.
22. Safavi A, Rhee P, Pandit V, et al. Children are safer in states with strict firearm laws: a National Inpatient Sample study. J Trauma Acute Care Surg. 2014;76:146–50.
23. Santaella-Tenorio J, Cerda M, Vellaveces A, Galea S. What do we know about the association between firearm legislation and firearm-related injuries? Epidemiol Rev. 2016;38:140–57.
24. Giffords Law Center to Prevent Gun Violence. Minimum age to purchase and possess [Internet]. Available from: https://lawcenter.giffords.org/gun-laws/policy-areas/who-can-have-a-gun/minimum-age/. Accessed 12 Feb 2020.
25. Ghiani M, Hawkins SS, Baum CF. Gun laws and school safety. J Epidemiol Community Health. 2019;73:509–15.
26. Centers for Disease Control and Prevention. Source of firearms used by students in school-associated violent deaths—United States, 1992–1999. MMWR Morb Mortal Wkly Rep. 2003;52:169–72.
27. Prickett KC, Martin-Storey A, Crosnoe R. State firearm laws, firearm ownership, and safety practices among families of preschool-aged children. Am J Public Health. 2014;104:1080–6.
28. Hahn RA, Bilukha O, Crosby A, et al. Firearms laws and the reduction of violence: a systematic review. Am J Prev Med. 2005;28(2 Suppl):40–71.
29. Hepburn L, Azrael D, Miller M, Hemenway D. The effect of child access prevention laws on unintentional child firearm fatalities, 1979–2000. J Trauma. 2006;61:423–8.
30. Webster DW, Starnes M. Reexamining the association between child access prevention gun laws and unintentional shooting deaths of children. Pediatrics. 2000;106:1466–9.

31. Azad HA, Monuteaux MC, Rees CA, Siegel M, Mannix R, Lee LK, Sheehan KM, Fleegler EW. Child access prevention firearm laws and firearm fatalities among children ages 0–14 years, 1991–2016. JAMA Pediatr. 2020:174(5):463–9.
32. Rajan S, Branas CC. Arming schoolteachers: what do we know? Where do we go from here? Am J Public Health. 2018;108:860–2.
33. Branas CC, Richmond TS, Culhane DP, Ten Have TR, Wiebe D. Investigating the link between gun possession and gun assault. Am J Public Health. 2009;99:2034–40.
34. Everytown for Gun Safety. Keeping our schools safe: a plan for preventing mass school shootings and ending all gun violence in American schools [Internet]. 2020. Available from: https://everytownresearch.org/reports/keeping-our-schools-safe-a-plan-to-stop-mass-shootings-and-end-all-gun-violence-in-american-schools/. Accessed 20 Feb2020.
35. Travers Á, Mcdonagh T, Elklit A. Youth responses to school shootings: a review. Curr Psychiatry Rep. 2018;20:47.
36. Lowe SR, Galea S. The mental health consequences of mass shootings. Trauma Violence Abuse. 2017;18:62–82.
37. Stop the Bleed [Internet]. 2019. Available from: https://www.stopthebleed.org/. Accessed 20 Feb 2020.
38. Cunningham RM, Carter PM, Ranney ML, et al. Prevention of firearm injuries among children and adolescents consensus-driven research agenda from the firearm safety among children and teens (FACTS) consortium. JAMA Pediatr. 2019; [Epub ahead of print]

Chapter 6
Firearm Violence in the Pediatric Population: An International Perspective

Erin Grinshteyn and David Hemenway

Mexico's child vigilantes: The indigenous people of Ayahualtempa are arming their children. Is it for self-defense, or to get attention?

By Kevin Sieff
February 7, 2020. *The Washington Post*

Firearm injuries and deaths are a public health issue not only among the pediatric population in the United States (US) but also in other areas of the world. US rates of firearm homicide, firearm suicide, and unintentional firearm death are much higher than those of other high-income countries. Some countries in the developing world, particularly some in Central and South America, have even higher rates of firearm death than the US. Internationally, relatively little is known about the circumstances of child and adolescent firearm injuries. While there are good data on the number of pediatric firearm deaths in high-income countries, the data are not as good for lower- and middle-income countries. For most countries, the data on the number and circumstances of nonfatal firearm injuries are unavailable or of questionable validity. Mass shootings are also disproportionately high in the US [1, 2]; however, there are no known cross-national studies focusing on school shootings or mass shootings of children and adolescents.

E. Grinshteyn (✉)
Health Professions Department, School of Nursing and Health Professions, University of San Francisco, San Francisco, CA, USA
e-mail: egrinshteyn@usfca.edu

D. Hemenway
Department of Health Policy and Management, Harvard T.H. Chan School of Public Health, Boston, MA, USA
e-mail: hemenway@hsph.harvard.edu

© Springer Nature Switzerland AG 2021
L. K. Lee, E. W. Fleegler (eds.), *Pediatric Firearm Injuries and Fatalities*, https://doi.org/10.1007/978-3-030-62245-9_6

6.1 High-Income Countries

Though few studies have examined firearm violence in the pediatric population cross-nationally, three studies by the same authors provide fatal firearm victimization data comparing children and adolescents in the US to other high-income countries in 2003, 2010, and 2015 [3–5]. The high-income countries for comparison were chosen based on those countries identified by the Organisation for Economic Co-operation and Development (OECD) as high-income countries for the year of each study. Data are from the World Health Organization (WHO). In each year, the US was an outlier, with much higher rates of pediatric firearm death (Table 6.1).

Total Firearm Deaths. The US has about half the population as the other high-income countries combined. In 2015, 7241 American youth 0–24 years old were killed with firearms. By contrast, 685 youth in the other high-income countries combined were killed by firearms. The ratio of US death rates from firearms to death rates from firearms in the other high-income countries was 54 times higher for the 0–4-year-old age group, 21 times higher for the 5–14-year-old age group, and 23 times higher for the 15–24-year-old age group (Table 6.1). It is this last ratio that is most important. In 2015, both in the US and in the combination of other high-income countries, 94% of all firearm deaths in the 0–24-year-old age range occurred to youth 15–24 years old. For young children 0–4 years old, 87 American children were killed by firearms compared to 3 children in all other high-income countries combined. For children 5–14 years old, 356 American children were killed by firearms compared to 31 in the other high-income nations. For youth 5–24 years old, the total firearm deaths were 6798 Americans versus 552 youth in the other high-income countries.

This large difference in firearm fatalities between the US and other high-income countries has been present throughout the twenty-first century. In 2003, there were 7132 American youth (0–24 years old) deaths from firearms, and in 2010, there were 6534. By contrast, in 2003, there were 712 youth in other high-income countries killed by firearms and 515 in 2010.

Table 6.1 Rates of firearm victimization in the United States compared to the other high-income countries [3–5]

Ratio of US death rates to rates of other high-income countries									
	0–4 years old			5–14 years old			15–24 years old		
	2003	2010	2015	2003	2010	2015	2003	2010	2015
Firearm homicide	7.8	22.3	54.5	13.4	18.5	29.1	42.7	49.0	31.1
Non-firearm homicide	4.3	5.2	6.1	1.8	1.4	1.5	3.4	3.1	2.6
Overall homicide	4.4	5.6	6.6	3.6	3.4	3.7	14.2	11.4	13.0
Firearm suicide				8.0	11.2	9.4	8.8	12.5	10.6
Non-firearm suicide				1.2	1.1	1.5	0.6	0.7	0.9
Overall suicide				1.6	1.5	2.2	1.2	1.2	1.6
Unintentional firearm death				10.6	12.2	20.2	11.6	12.6	8.2
Firearm deaths	6.8	33.8	54.5	10.6	14.2	21.1	17.3	22.5	23.3

More American youth aged 0–24 years old are killed in firearm homicides than are killed in firearm suicides. The opposite is true for youth in other high-income countries. In 2015, the relative rates of American youth (15–24 years old) firearm homicide victimization was 31 times higher in the US compared to the high-income nations. Even for firearm suicide, the US rate for those 15–24 years old was more than ten times higher in the US (Table 6.1). In both the US and other high-income countries, the overwhelming majority of youth 0–24 years old killed with firearms were male. In the US, 88% of the victims were male in 2015; for the other high-income countries, the percentage was 91%. We did not find any international studies that compared pediatric gun suicides or gun homicides by their circumstances (e.g., gang-related, intimate partner violence-related, rurality).

6.2   Low- and Middle-Income Countries

There are few cross-national studies examining firearm deaths including low- and middle-income nations. This may be because the mortality data systems are not well developed so the data are not as reliable in these countries [6]. However, some limited information is available. Similar to the high-income countries, among those 0–24 years old, the number of firearm deaths increases rapidly with age and is much higher for males than females [7].

Globally in 2016, there were more firearm homicides than firearm suicides among those 0–24 years old [7]. In 2016, a handful of countries—Honduras, El Salvador, Guatemala, Jamaica, Columbia, Venezuela, Brazil, and occasionally South Africa—were among the leaders in disaggregate pediatric firearm homicide death rates, in all age groups, and among both females and males [7]. The highest rates of firearm homicide victimization occurred in low- and middle-income counties in the Americas. Among the youngest age group of children in 2016, firearm homicide rates per 100,000 male children 0–4 years old were highest in Honduras (1.9), El Salvador (1.6), Guatemala (1.6), Jamaica (1.5), and Columbia (1.4). In contrast, the US firearm homicide rate was 0.5 per 100,000 male children 0–4 years old in 2016.

One study found firearm suicide rates among children were higher in the developing world than among high-income countries—with the exception of the US and Canada [7]. For example, among males aged 10–14 years old, firearm suicide rates per 100,000 were highest in Greenland (9.6), the US (0.78), Albania (0.37), Canada (0.29), and Croatia (0.27). Among males age 15–19 years, firearm suicide rates per 100,000 were highest in Greenland (54.7), Venezuela (10.0), the US (6.4), Argentina (4.88), and Uruguay (3.7). We must note that for countries with a relatively small population like Greenland, where the total population was less than 57,000 in 2019, these rates are unstable and thus must be interpreted with caution though Greenland has historically had one of the highest rates of suicide in the world.

An older study of adolescents and young adults (15–24 years old) in 34 high- and middle-income countries in the early 1990s reported that the US was second to

Finland in firearm suicide and twelfth in overall suicide rates [14]. A more recent study found among 35 high- and middle-income countries, the US had the highest pediatric (10–19 years old) firearm suicide rate and the seventh highest overall suicide rate, following Estonia, New Zealand, Uzbekistan, Kyrgyzstan, Moldova, and Lithuania [8].

6.3   Why Are US Youth at Such High Risk for Firearm Deaths?

The United States has clearly been an outlier in firearm deaths compared to most high-income nations. However, the reasons for this are not well understood, and there have been few international studies comparing risk factors among youth specifically for firearm violence. Here we examine the narrow issue of some risk factors potentially associated with the large differences between the US and the other high-income countries in terms of youth firearm death.

Guns: Not surprisingly, a major risk factor for firearm death is the availability of firearms. It is not possible to have a firearm death if there is no firearm. The US has the most firearms per capita of any high-income country [4]. In 2017, the Small Arms Survey crudely estimated there were over one billion small arms throughout the world globally, of which about 85% were in civilian hands. US civilians accounted for over 45% of the world's civilian-held firearms, which equals approximately 350–400 million firearms. This equates to roughly 120 firearms for every 100 people (man, woman, and child) in the US [9]. Among other high-income countries, there were about 11.5 firearms for every 100 people [9]. The country estimates ranged from a low of 0.16 firearms per 100 people in the Republic of Korea to a second high of 34.7 firearms per 100 people in Canada.

Cross-nationally, many studies have found a strong relationship between levels of household gun ownership (or guns per population) and both firearm homicide and firearm suicide. For example, a recent analysis of 195 countries found estimates of the number of firearms per country were significantly associated with higher rates of firearm homicide and firearm suicide [10]. A study of 26 high-income countries found an association between firearm availability and firearm homicide rates [11], as well as firearm homicide specifically among women [12]. A study including middle-income countries [13] also found a significant relationship between firearms and firearm homicide, even controlling for the possibility of reverse causation—that homicide could lead to increased firearm ownership. Other international studies have found firearm availability is also associated with firearm suicide [14, 15], including one study focusing on adolescents [14].

Many case-control studies of the US population have found having a gun in the home increases the risk of firearm homicide and firearm suicide, with some studies focusing specifically on adolescents [16]. An ecological study in the US focusing on children found firearm availability was associated with homicide, suicide, and unintentional deaths [17]. That study found that firearm availability was associated not only with firearm deaths but also with both overall homicide and overall suicide and was not associated with non-firearm homicide or non-firearm suicide.

Gun Laws: The US has among the weakest gun laws among the high-income countries. Most other high-income countries have national firearm licensing systems and strict laws regulating the acquisition of handguns. Some countries require training courses, character references, verified safe storage practices, lengthy reviews of criminal and health histories, and waiting periods. The US requires none of these practices at the federal level, only requiring that purchasers pass an instant background check when purchasing a firearm through a federally licensed dealer [18].

In recent years, at least four literature reviews have tried to determine the effects of US state gun laws on aspects of firearm-related injuries and deaths [19–22]. The main takeaways are, overall, that stronger gun laws are better than weaker ones for reducing firearm deaths, but it is usually difficult to determine the effect of individual laws on firearm deaths and injuries. The literature does suggest that among the most relevant individual laws for reducing firearm fatalities may be universal background checks, waiting periods, and laws restricting firearm ownership for those with a history of violent misdemeanors and intimate partner violence offenses [23, 24]. While few evaluations focus on the effects on child/youth outcomes, there appears to be solid evidence that child access prevention (CAP) laws in the US reduce self-inflicted shootings of children [25].

Evidence of US Adolescent Violence and Suicidality: Comparing US rates of non-firearm homicide or non-firearm suicide with rates in other countries has sometimes been used to try to determine if Americans are potentially more violent or more suicidal. Contrariwise, it has been argued that if American non-firearm homicide or non-firearm suicide is lower than other countries, it means other countries are just substituting other means of killing for guns. Gun advocates tend to use this as a heads-I-win, tails-you-lose proposition. Either way, it's not the guns. It was only if the non-firearm rates were similar that gun advocates could not readily claim guns were not a risk factor for suicide. For non-firearm suicide, American youth have similar rates compared to youth in other high-income countries (see Table 6.1). In 2015, for example, the 15–24-year-old non-firearm US suicide rate was 90% of the overall rate for the other high-income countries.

In contrast, for non-firearm homicide, US youth have much higher rates than similarly aged youth in other high-income countries. This is even in our youngest children where the non-firearm homicide rates for children 0–4 years old was over six times higher in the US compared to other countries in 2015. If these data are accurate, they indicate a major problem for American children and their caregivers since the perpetrators of infant and toddler homicides are commonly the child's father or the mother's boyfriend [26].

American youth 15–24 years old also have substantially higher rates of non-firearm homicide victimization rates than youth in other high-income countries. While the difference seems large (2.6. times the non-firearm homicide rate of youth in other high-income countries in 2015), they are an order of magnitude less than the difference in firearm homicide (31.1 times the rate). The perpetrators of homicide in this 15–24-year-old age group are typically other youth of similar age. Of course, for those 15–24 years old, there are various reasons why more guns could causally increase not only gun homicides but also non-gun homicides [18]. These reasons include (1) retaliation (guns increase serious violence, leading to retaliation by guns and other methods), (2) lower clearance rates (where there is more gun homicide per criminal justice resources, perpetrators are more likely to get away with murder, and residents grow not to trust the police), (3) reduction in social capital (e.g., more people stay inside and longtime residents move out), (4) a growing tolerance of serious violence, and (5) a more traumatized community with individuals more likely to react violently to signs of disrespect and to perceive innocent actions as signs of disrespect ("hurt people hurt people").

The fact that the US has a larger percentage of its population incarcerated than any other country, high-, middle-, and low-income, might indicate that we are a highly criminal and violent society. It may also suggest that we are a more punitive society than most. Probably a better measure of underlying crime and violence come from cross-national victimization data using comparable questions, such as the International Crime Victim Surveys (ICVS). Such surveys indicate that at least compared to the other high-income countries, the US is an average high-income country in terms of violent (and nonviolent) crimes [27–29]—except for gun crime. Americans do not have especially higher rates of assaults, sexual assaults, robberies, car theft, burglary, or any non-gun crime compared to other high-income countries. It is thus argued that our high incarceration rates may be attributable to other features of our society such as our moralism, punitive attitudes, and structural characteristics of our government. They do not reflect our underlying rates of crime and violence [30].

6.4   Adolescent Risk Factors

The cross-national studies on rates of violent and nonviolent crimes do not provide data by age of the perpetrator or victim, so they do not directly provide comparable data on youth violence. Some studies have compared American youth to youth in other countries about issues, which are often considered risk factors for self-inflicted or non-self-inflicted violence. Data for these studies typically come from the World Health Organization (WHO) collaborative cross-national studies such as the Health Behavior in School-Aged Children (HBSC) and the Global School-based Health Survey (GSHS).

Alcohol Use: Alcohol consumption is a risk factor for violence. The few studies comparing alcohol use among US adolescents to adolescents in other high-income countries have found US adolescents seem consume at the lower end of the spectrum. For example, from HBSC surveys of weekly alcohol use among adolescents aged 11, 13, and 15 years in 28 countries in North America and Europe, American adolescents ranked 24th in 2010 in terms of the percentage consuming alcohol [31]. A study of tenth graders using HBSC data for three countries (the United States,

Canada, the Netherlands) for 2005–2006 found that for most measures of alcoholic drinking, rates were the lowest in the US [32]. Given the findings of these studies, alcohol use is likely not one of the primary risk factors accounting for the increased rates of firearm homicides and firearm suicides in American youth compared to youth in other countries.

Fighting and Bullying: US adolescents also do not appear to be more likely than youth in other countries to engage in either fighting or bullying. One study of those aged 11–16 years in 79 countries from 2003 to 2011 using both HBSC and GSHS data examined rates of four or more episodes of fighting in the past year, as well as bullying victimization. American youth were on the lower end of the distribution among these countries. For example, US youth experienced lower rates of both frequent fighting and bullying victimization compared to youth in Canada and France [33]. A cross-national study of adolescents aged 11,13, and 15 years old examined fighting using HBSC data for 2001–2002 across 35 countries and also found US adolescents at the relatively low end of the spectrum for fighting [34]. A cross-national comparison of bullying across 40 countries using HBSC data found adolescents in the US were in the middle of the range of involvement in bullying among both males and females [35]. An earlier cross-national study of those aged 11,13, and 15 years old in Israel, Ireland, Portugal, Sweden, and the US for 1997–1998 using HBSC data found US adolescents were pretty average in terms of physical fighting, having sustained an injury from fighting, and having bullied others [36]. Based on these findings, it appears that rates of fighting and bullying are not higher in the US compared to other advanced countries. So increased aggressiveness is also likely not a causative factor in the increased rates of firearm deaths in US youth.

Weapon Carrying: This same five-country study found the United States had similar percentages of adolescents who carried a weapon as four other countries (Israel, Ireland, Portugal, and Sweden) [36]. However, another study of seven countries (Belgium-French, Estonia, Israel, Latvia, Macedonia, Portugal, and the United States) using HBSC data for 2001–2002 found the US had the highest percentage of boys and girls who had carried a weapon in the past 30 days (e.g., 22% of boys carried in the US compared to the second high of 19% for Israeli boys). Moreover, among the carriers, the US had the highest percentage of carriers who were carrying firearms (22%) [34].

Violent Media and Violent Video Games: The evidence for a link between violent media use and aggression is remarkably consistent across different countries [37]. Unfortunately, there are no known cross-national studies that include the US on the amount of violent TV and movies watched by adolescents or the time spent playing violent video games. However, HBSC surveys show that US adolescents watch about the same amount of TV (violent and nonviolent combined) as adolescents in 29 other countries and that US adolescents spend relatively less time on the computer (including both gaming and nongaming activities) [38]. In addition, data from a gaming analytics company showed per capita video game revenue for ten countries was higher for Japan and Korea than for the US [39]. It is thus unclear what influence violent media and video games may have on explaining the higher rates of US youth firearm deaths.

Mental Health: We found few cross-national studies on the mental health of American children or youth compared to those in other countries. However, in a study of individuals 18 years and older, from a mix of 17 high- and lower-income countries using the World Health Organization's World Mental Health Surveys, the lifetime prevalence of DSM-IV disorders was highest in the US [40]. An updated version of this study reporting on 28 countries found that more than a third of respondents in the US and four other countries had a lifetime mental health diagnosis [41]. Some of the disorders, especially involving impulse control, often have early age of onset. By contrast, an earlier study of ten countries (Canada, France, Italy, Korea, Lebanon, New Zealand, Puerto Rico, Taiwan, West Germany, the United States) found the US was average in terms of prevalence of major depression and bipolar disorder [42]. A similar study found average US rates for suicide ideation and suicide attempts [43]. Based on these limited data on the mental health of US youth compared to youth in other countries, no conclusions can be made about the contribution of mental health as a risk factor of US youth firearm deaths compared to other countries.

6.5   Research Gaps

Data and research gaps on the issue of firearms and the pediatric populations internationally are enormous. While the quality of the data on the mortality from firearms is considered good in high-income countries, data quality is variable for middle- and low-income nations. Much less is known about morbidity from firearms, with almost nothing known about the circumstances of nonfatal firearm injuries. Cross-national data on household gun ownership is spotty at best, with even less known about adolescent firearm carrying. Comparable cross-national data on many potential adolescent risk factors for firearm injury—e.g., mental health, violent video game play, and firearm use—are largely lacking.

6.6   Conclusions

The Western Hemisphere is home to most of the countries with the worst pediatric firearm injury problems. The United States looks good in comparison to many low-income nations in the Americas but looks terrible when compared to the world's high-income countries. More research on US and international pediatric firearm violence is clearly needed. Compared with many other public health and medical topics, relatively little is known about firearm violence, and firearm studies focused on children and youth in countries other than the US are lacking. The importance of the WHO in organizing the collection of comparable international data is undeniable, as so many of the relevant empirical studies are analyses of WHO-sponsored data collection. But clearly more needs to be done to have accurate and available data for all countries. Only then can robust cross-national studies be conducted to better understand pediatric firearm deaths and injuries in the United States and other countries.

The available evidence suggests that what explains the high US rates of pediatric firearm deaths compared to other high-income countries has little to do with the underlying aggressiveness or mental health of our children. Rather it appears due to the high prevalence of and easy access to highly lethal firearms in the US. The gun question we always get from our international students is why doesn't the US do more to protect its own children from these guns? Acknowledging that we have a serious problem is an important first step, but it is just one step toward a solution. We must work together to find and implement effective ways to protect our children and youth from firearm deaths and injuries.

Take Home Points
- Countries in Central and South America have the highest rates of pediatric firearm deaths.
- Among high-income countries, rates of pediatric firearm deaths are highest in the United States.
- Easy access to firearms appears to be largely responsible for the relatively high rates of firearm violence in the United States.
- More research is needed on pediatric firearm injuries especially from a cross-national perspective.

References

1. Lankford A. Public mass shooters and firearms: a cross-National Study of 171 countries. Violence Vict. 2016;31(2):187–99.
2. Lankford A. Confirmation that the United States has six times its global share of public mass shootings. Econ J Watch. 2019;16(1):69–83.
3. Grinshteyn E, Hemenway D. Violent death rates: the US compared with other high-income OECD countries, 2010. Am J Med. 2016;129(3):266–73.
4. Grinshteyn E, Hemenway D. Violent death rates in the US compared to those of the other high-income countries, 2015. Prev Med. 2019;123:20–6.
5. Richardson EG, Hemenway D. Homicide, suicide, and unintentional firearm fatality: comparing the United States with other high-income countries, 2003. J Trauma Inj Infect Crit Care. 2011;70(1):238–43.
6. Geneva Declaration on Armed Violence and Development. Global Burden of Armed Violence 2015: Every body counts. 2015 May.
7. Global Burden of Disease Pediatrics Collaboration, Kyu HH, Pinho C, Wagner JA, Brown JC, Bertozzi-Villa A, et al. Global and National Burden of diseases and injuries among children and adolescents between 1990 and 2013: findings from the global burden of disease 2013 study. JAMA Pediatr. 2016;170(3):267–87.
8. Glenn CR, Kleiman EM, Kellerman J, Pollak O, Cha CB, Esposito EC, et al. Annual research review: a meta-analytic review of worldwide suicide rates in adolescents. J Child Psychol Psychiatry. 2020;61(3):294–308.

9. Small Arms Survey. Civilian firearms holdings, 2017 [Internet]. Smalls Arms Survey, Weapons and Markets; 2018. Available from: http://www.smallarmssurvey.org/fileadmin/docs/Weapons_and_Markets/Tools/Firearms_holdings/SAS-BP-Civilian-held-firearms-annexe.pdf

10. The Global Burden of Disease 2016 Injury Collaborators, Naghavi M, Marczak LB, Kutz M, Shackelford KA, Arora M, et al. Global mortality from firearms, 1990–2016. JAMA. 2018;320(8):792–814.

11. Hemenway D, Miller M. Firearm availability and homicide rates across 26 high-income countries. J Trauma Inj Infect Crit Care. 2000;49(6):985–8.

12. Hemenway D, Shinoda-Tagawa T, Miller M. Firearm availability and female homicide victimization rates among 25 populous high-income countries. Am Med Womens Assoc. 2002;57(2):100–4.

13. Hoskin AW. Armed Americans: the impact of firearm availability on national homicide rates. Justice Q. 2001;18(3):569–92.

14. Johnson G, Krug E, Potter L. Suicide among adolescents and young adults: a cross-national comparison of 34 countries. Suicide Life Threat Behav. 2000;30(1):74–82.

15. Lester D. The availability of firearms and the use of firearms for suicide: a study of 20 countries. Acta Psychiatr Scand. 1990;81(2):146–7.

16. Anglemyer A, Horvath T, Rutherford G. The accessibility of firearms and risk for suicide and homicide victimization among household members: a systematic review and meta-analysis. Ann Intern Med. 2014;160(2):101–10.

17. Miller M, Azrael D, Hemenway D. Firearm availability and unintentional firearm deaths, suicide, and homicide among 5–14 year olds. J Trauma Inj Infect Crit Care. 2002;52(2):267–75.

18. Hemenway D. Private guns, public health. Paperback ed. Ann Arbor: University of Michigan Press; 2017. p. 360.

19. Fleegler EW, Lee LK, Monuteaux MC, Hemenway D, Mannix R. Firearm legislation and firearm-related fatalities in the United States. JAMA Intern Med. 2013;173(9):732–40.

20. Lee LK, Fleegler EW, Farrell C, Avakame E, Srinivasan S, Hemenway D, et al. Firearm laws and firearm homicides: a systematic review. JAMA Intern Med. 2017;177(1):106–19.

21. Rand Corporation, editor. The science of gun policy: a critical synthesis of research evidence on the effects of gun policies in the United States. Santa Monica: RAND; 2018. 380 p

22. Santaella-Tenorio J, Cerdá M, Villaveces A, Galea S. What do we know about the association between firearm legislation and firearm-related injuries? Epidemiol Rev. 2016;38(1):140–57.

23. Díez C, Kurland RP, Rothman EF, Bair-Merritt M, Fleegler E, Xuan Z, et al. State intimate partner violence–related firearm laws and intimate partner homicide rates in the United States, 1991 to 2015. Ann Intern Med. 2017;167(8):536–43.

24. Siegel M, Pahn M, Xuan Z, Fleegler E, Hemenway D. The impact of state firearm laws on homicide and suicide deaths in the USA, 1991–2016: a panel study. J Gen Intern Med. 2019;34(10):2021–8.

25. Azad HA, Monuteaux MC, Rees CA, Siegel M, Mannix R, Lee LK, Sheehan KM, Fleegler EW. Child Access Prevention Firearm Laws and Firearm Fatalities Among Children Aged 0 to 14 Years, 1991-2016. JAMA Pediatr. 2020;174(5):463–69.

26. Fujiwara T, Barber C, Schaechter J, Hemenway D. Characteristics of infant homicides: findings from a U.S. multisite reporting system. Pediatrics. 2009;124(2):e210–7.

27. Dijk J, van Kesteren J, Smit P. Criminal victimisation in international perspective; key findings from the 2004–2005. Boom Juridische Uitgevers; 2004.

28. Farrington DP, Langan PA, Tonry M. Cross-national studies in crime and justice. US Department of Justice; 2004. Report No.: NCJ 200988.

29. van Kesteren J, Mayhew P, Nieuwbeerta P. Criminal victimisation in seventeen industrialized countries: key findings from the 2000 international crime victims survey. 2000.

30. Tonry M. Why are U.S. incarceration rates so high? Crime Delinquency. 1999;45(4):419–37.

31. de Looze M, Raaijmakers Q, Bogt T t, Bendtsen P, Farhat T, Ferreira M, et al. Decreases in adolescent weekly alcohol use in Europe and North America: evidence from 28 countries from 2002 to 2010. Eur J Pub Health. 2015;25(suppl 2):69–72.

32. Simons-Morton B, Pickett W, Boyce W, ter Bogt TFM, Vollebergh W. Cross-national comparison of adolescent drinking and cannabis use in the United States, Canada, and the Netherlands. Int J Drug Policy. 2010;21(1):64–9.
33. Elgar FJ, McKinnon B, Walsh SD, Freeman J, Donnelly DP, de Matos MG, et al. Structural determinants of youth bullying and fighting in 79 countries. J Adolesc Health. 2015;57(6):643–50.
34. Pickett W. Cross-national study of fighting and weapon carrying as determinants of adolescent injury. Pediatrics. 2005;116(6):e855–63.
35. The HBSC Violence & Injuries Prevention Focus Group, The HBSC Bullying Writing Group, Craig W, Harel-Fisch Y, Fogel-Grinvald H, Dostaler S, et al. A cross-national profile of bullying and victimization among adolescents in 40 countries. Int J Public Health. 2009;54(S2):216–24.
36. Smith-Khuri E, Iachan R, Scheidt PC, Overpeck MD, Gabhainn SN, Pickett W, et al. A cross-national study of violence-related behaviors in adolescents. Arch Pediatr Adolesc Med. 2004;158(6):539–44.
37. Krahé B. Violent media effects on aggression: a commentary from a cross-cultural perspective: violent media effects and culture. Anal Soc Issues Public Policy. 2016;16(1):439–42.
38. Bucksch J, Sigmundova D, Hamrik Z, Troped PJ, Melkevik O, Ahluwalia N, et al. International trends in adolescent screen-time behaviors from 2002 to 2010. J Adolesc Health. 2016;58(4):417–25.
39. Chang A. Why video games aren't causing America's gun problem, in one chart [Internet]. Vox; 2019 Aug. Available from: https://www.vox.com/policy-and-politics/2019/8/5/20755092/gun-shooting-video-game-chart
40. Kessler RC, Angermeyer M, Anthony JC, DE Graaf R, Demyttenaere K, Gasquet I, et al. Lifetime prevalence and age-of-onset distributions of mental disorders in the World Health Organization's world mental health survey initiative. World Psychiatry. 2007;6(3):168–76.
41. Kessler RC, Aguilar-Gaxiola S, Alonso J, Chatterji S, Lee S, Ormel J, et al. The global burden of mental disorders: an update from the WHO world mental health (WMH) surveys. Epidemiol Psichiatr Soc. 2009;18(1):23–33.
42. Weissman MM. Cross-national epidemiology of major depression and bipolar disorder. JAMA. 1996;276(4):293–99.
43. Weissman MM, Bland RC, Canino GJ, Greenwald S, Hwu H-G, Joyce PR, et al. Prevalence of suicide ideation and suicide attempts in nine countries. Psychol Med. 1999;29(1):9–17.

Part II
Interventions

Chapter 7
Talking with Families: Interventions for Health Care Clinicians

Eric W. Fleegler

Community leaders implore parents to ask: Are there guns in the house?

By Rachel Dissell
Updated January 12, 2019; Posted August 23, 2012.
The Plain Dealer

7.1 Introduction

Personal Vignette
I widened my stance, braced the shotgun against my shoulder, aimed down the barrel, and pulled the trigger....

I was 17 years old, at a classmate's house to discuss starting an asphalt driveway resurfacing business. Before we began, he invited me outdoors to do something I had never done before: fire a shotgun. At an old microwave. In the middle of the afternoon with no one else home. The noise and kickback were incredible, and my shot wildly veered into the woods. He laughed and proceeded to shoot the microwave multiple times....

All children in the United States (US), from toddlers through adolescents, have the potential for exposure to firearms. Since the 9/11 attack, which claimed 2977 victims, there have been a staggering 49,568 children, 0–19 years old, killed and another 264,423 injured by firearms in the US [1]. These firearm deaths and injuries occurred just between 2002 and 2018. On the current trajectory of pediatric firearm

E. W. Fleegler (✉)
Department of Pediatrics, Division of Emergency Medicine, Boston Children's Hospital, Harvard Medical School, Boston, MA, USA
e-mail: eric.fleegler@childrens.harvard.edu

© Springer Nature Switzerland AG 2021
L. K. Lee, E. W. Fleegler (eds.), *Pediatric Firearm Injuries and Fatalities*,
https://doi.org/10.1007/978-3-030-62245-9_7

deaths, over 3500 children will be killed by firearms each year—this is equivalent to an entire school bus of children dying every 9 days throughout the year.

In the US, there are an estimated 350–400 million firearms, more than one for every person in the country. And these are only estimates for no one really knows how many guns there are in the US. No national data are collected about firearm sales and few states require registration of firearms. Though the distribution of firearms throughout the US varies, even the states with lowest firearm ownership (e.g., Hawaii and Massachusetts) still have children who needlessly die by guns every year. For this reason, it is imperative that pediatric clinicians make screening and recommendations for safe firearm storage a part of their daily practice.

7.2   Which Families Are Most Likely to Own Guns?

National and state-wide data on firearm ownership are limited by the fact that the majority of states do not require firearm registration. This limits research investigating the demographics of those who own guns. In fact, the most recent large-scale national data on gun ownership, with more than 200,000 surveyed, were collected via the Behavioral Risk Factor Surveillance System (BRFSS) in 2004. Back then, the District of Columbia and state-level firearm ownership ranged from 5.2% in the District of Columbia to 62.8% in Wyoming [2]. Using a well-described methodology for proxy estimation of household firearm ownership rates [3], 1980 and 2016 data estimates suggest that ownership rates have decreased moderately over time. In 2016, the lowest firearm ownership rate of 9% was in Hawaii, New Jersey, and Massachusetts and the highest rate of 65% was in Montana (Fig. 7.1 and Chap. 1, Table 1.1).

Ownership rates significantly vary across the US by region and urbanicity, as well as by the individual characteristics of the owner. From a 2014 national survey of 1711 people, in urban areas, 14.8% of individuals had a gun in the household, while in rural areas, 55.9% had guns. Overall, 35.1% of males owned guns while only 11.7% of females owned guns. By age, only 14.0% of adults less than 35 years old owned guns versus 30.4% over the age of 65 years. White ownership was 39.0%, Black ownership was 18.1%, and Hispanic ownership was 15.2%. Among the low-income households (<$25000/year), 18.0% owned a gun, whereas in high-income households (>$90000/year), 44.0% owned a gun [4]. By political affiliation, 41% of Republicans, 36% of independents, and 16% of Democrats owned a gun [5]. Data from PEW and Gallup in 2019 support these general numbers.

Though the breakdown of firearm ownership has been relatively stable for many years, gun sales dramatically increased during the COVID-19 pandemic. As a result, ownership among different groups may have begun to shift. In March 2020 alone, over 2.5 million guns, including 1.5 million handguns, were sold, an all-time high [6, 7]. By November 2020, an estimated 20 million firearms were sold in the US, beating a former high of 16.6 million guns sold in 2016. Reports from gun store owners suggest that many of these guns were purchased by first-time owners.

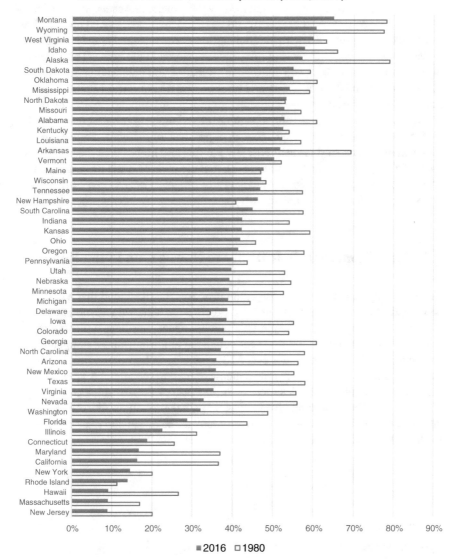

Fig. 7.1 Data from state-level estimates of household firearm ownership, RAND 2020 [6]

Among the 37.4 million households with children in the US, it is estimated that 34% (12.7 million households) have one or more firearms. Among these households, 21% store at least one firearm in the least safe manner, namely loaded and unlocked, and another 50% store a firearm either loaded and locked, or unloaded and unlocked [8]. These unsafe storage practices place 4.5 million and 11.4 million children, respectively, at higher risk of access to and use of a gun, compared to children living in homes either without guns or guns stored in the safest manner. The safest manner of storage, as endorsed by the American Academy of Pediatrics (AAP), is "If you own a firearm, it should be stored unloaded, locked up (lock box, cable lock, or firearm safe), with the ammunition stored separately [and locked]" [9].

Variation also exists in rates of how guns are stored in the home. Thirty percent of firearm owners in the South store firearms loaded and unlocked versus 14–18% in other regions of the US. Urban and rural owners do not differ in rates of unsafe firearm storage. Female owners unsafely store firearms at nearly twice the rate of males (31% vs. 17%). There are no significant variations in unsafe firearm storage by age, race/ethnicity, education, income, or political affiliation. However, the odds of handgun owners storing them unsafely are fourfold higher than those who only own long guns (e.g., rifles) (27% vs. 5%), and the odds of those owning a gun for protection storing them unsafely are sevenfold higher (79% vs. 25%) than other types of gun owners (e.g., hunters) [8].

7.3   How Dangerous Is It Really to Have a Gun in the Home?

Unequivocally, having a gun in the home increases the likelihood that a child will be injured or killed by a gun. Household firearms are a known and modifiable risk factor for death by suicide. People who purchase handguns have a 22-fold higher rate of gun suicide within the first year compared to those who did not purchase a handgun [10]. Among males, for every 10% increase in household firearm ownership rates at the state level, there is an increase of firearm suicides of 3.1 per 100,000. In comparison, among females there is an increase of firearm suicides of 0.4 per 100,000 [11]. While these relative increases may seem small, to illustrate the magnitude of this difference, one needs to only look at the ownership rates and firearm fatality rates in Massachusetts vs. Wyoming [1, 3] (Fig. 7.2).

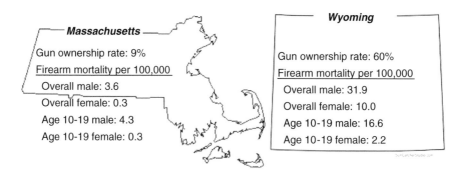

Fig. 7.2 Gun ownership rate, 2016; overall firearm mortality rate, 2018; age 10–19 firearm mortality rate, average 1999–2018 [1, 3]

For over 30 years, studies have shown that access to a gun in the home is associated with increased rates of adolescent suicide [12]. Overall, the risk of suicide for any member of the household where firearms are kept is 2–10 times that of homes without firearms [13, 14]. When a firearm is used in a pediatric suicide, 75% of the time the firearm is owned by the parent or the child themselves [15]. Likewise, in unintentional firearm deaths, the gun used in the shooting originated from the parent 56% of the time with young children and 17% of the time in older teenagers. Among older teenagers, in 43% of the unintentional deaths, the gun was owned by the shooter themselves [15]. These data speak not only to the importance of protecting children from firearms within their own homes, but also of encouraging parents to talk about firearm storage with the owners of the homes their children visit, whether it is a relative, friend, or neighbor.

7.4 Does Storage Matter?

Firearm storage matters – each element of safe storage, namely (1) storing a gun locked, (2) unloaded, (3) storing the ammunition locked, and (4) storing the ammunition separate from the gun, is associated with lower rates of both adolescent suicide and unintentional injuries and fatalities [16]. A simulation model of safe storage suggests that annually up to 135 pediatric lives could be saved and 323 pediatric firearm injuries prevented if even just 20% of parents who currently store their guns unlocked shifted and stored them safely [17].

It is important to realize, and a point to discuss with patients and families, that many gun owners do not store the ammunition locked up; and therefore, a child or young adult with suicidal intent can readily access and load the gun themselves. An analysis of data from the National Violent Death Reporting System (NVDRS) looking at the relationship between gun storage and homicides, suicides, and unintentional deaths shows not only the dangers of storing guns loaded and unlocked, but in the case of suicide, unloaded and unlocked as well. The gun was stored loaded and unlocked in unintentional deaths of children aged 10–14 years and 15–19 years 75% and 66% of the time, respectively. For suicides among children of 10–14 years and 15–19 years, the gun was stored loaded and unlocked (42% and 35%, respectively) or unloaded and unlocked (38% and 39%, respectively) [15]. Added together for pediatric suicides, this data translates to ready access to the gun and ammunition occurred 80% of the time for 10–14 years old and 74% of the time for 15–19 years old.

7.5 What Do Clinicians Believe and Do?

Pediatric primary care clinicians are the number one source of medical contact with children and adolescents and their caregivers. Multiple physician groups, including the AAP [18], the National Academy of Medicine [19], and others recommend that clinicians screen patients for access to firearms and provide concrete recommendations for safe storage if there is a firearm in the home. The AAP's Bright Futures guidelines specifically mention firearm screening and counseling starting at the newborn visit and moving every year through adolescence. What adjusts overtime are the details regarding the content of this counseling. This is because the type and intent of firearm injury change based on the developmental stage of the child or adolescent. For families of younger children, counseling should focus on preventing unintentional injuries, while for teenagers, counseling should focus on suicide prevention. An important universal recommendation that pediatric clinicians can make for all ages includes ideally not having a gun in the home. However, if a gun is present in the home, clinicians should recommend that it is necessary to store all guns unloaded, locked, and separated from the locked ammunition. In addition, parents of preschool and school-aged children should be advised to ask about firearms in the homes their children visit. Pediatric clinicians should speak to adolescents directly about their exposure to and carrying of guns at school/outside of the home, and parents of adolescents should be advised to talk with their teenagers about guns [20].

For the past 30 years, pediatricians have espoused their beliefs that counseling families about firearm safety is important and should be a part of pediatric primary care anticipatory guidance [21]. However, when it comes to firearm counseling, beliefs do not always translate into actions. Though pediatricians recognize the inherent risks associated with guns in the home, they often do not provide routine firearm counseling with any consistency. In a study of Maryland pediatricians in 1992, only 30% said that they had ever spoken to a family about firearm safety, and only 7% counseled at least 50% of their patients [21]. In a survey of pediatricians and family medicine doctors in Washington, only 20% and 8% of practitioners, respectively, counseled more than 5% of their patients about firearms [22]. Fast forward to 2019 and not much has changed – a study of pediatric residents at three different programs showed that 50% essentially never counseled about firearms, and only 15% of them counseled more than 50% of their patients during well-child visits [23]. Rest assured, pediatricians do not differ from their adult counterparts – among internists, 58% report never asking their patients if they have a gun in the home, 77% never discuss ways to reduce the risk for gun-related injury or death, and 62% never discuss the importance of keeping guns in the home away from children [24].

The reasons for the lack of counseling are broad. Some clinicians report fears of confrontation or upsetting their patients and/or caregivers. Others report a lack of comfort with counseling, a lack of training, or uncertainty about what to say. In a study of pediatric residents' beliefs and practices, the majority felt comfortable counseling about gun safety and gun storage, but only 15% were comfortable discussing trigger locks and other safety devices [23]. Others report skepticism that counseling is effective. Uncertainty about physician gag laws and concerns about restrictions on what can be recorded discourage some clinicians (see Chap. 13; spoiler alert – all clinicians in every state can discuss firearms with patients and families). Many report that the significant limitation of time available during the well-child visit impedes these discussions. Some clinicians do not believe that firearms are a major part of their patient's lives; therefore, the counseling does not apply to them. A small percentage of clinicians do not believe that firearm counseling is a part of their work. For some gun owning (and non-gun owning) physicians, their beliefs around the Second Amendment may temper their willingness to have these conversations [24–26].

7.6   What Do Parents Believe About Firearms and Their Children?

One challenge that exists is in parents' perceptions about firearm safety and risks. Though historically most gun owners used firearms for hunting, today over two-thirds of firearm owners overall, and 75% of handgun owners, keep them for personal safety [5]. Major shifts in the belief about the safety of a firearm in the home have occurred in the past two decades. Gallup polls have asked the following question over time "Do you think having a gun in the house makes it a safer place to be or a more dangerous place to be?" In 2000, a third answered "safer" and half "more dangerous." By 2014, the numbers had flipped (Fig. 7.3) [27].

When it comes to guns and children, 75% of gun-owning parents believe that their 4- to 12-year-old children can tell the difference between toy guns and real guns and nearly a quarter believe their child could be trusted with a loaded gun. Even among non-gun owning parents, over half believe their child could differentiate toy versus real guns and 14% could trust their child with a loaded gun. Three quarters of all parents felt their child would not touch a gun if they found one [28].

Reality demonstrates that children have the opposite kind of behavior when they find a gun. Boys in particular appear to have an affinity for guns. A study of 29 small groups of boys 8–12 years old demonstrated that when these boys found a real gun, 74% of them handled the gun and 48% pulled the trigger [29]. This occurred despite the training 90% of these boys had completed called the Eddie Eagle Gunsafe® safety program advocated by the National Rifle Association [30]. This program

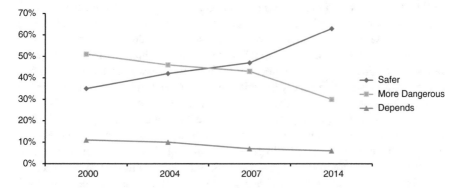

Fig. 7.3 Do you think having a gun in the house makes it a safer place to be or a more dangerous place to be? [27]

instructs children with the following: "If you see a gun, (1) Stop, (2) Don't touch, (3) Run away, (4) Tell a grownup." Good advice, but based on this study, it is unfortunately unlikely to be followed by the majority of boys.

7.7 What Do Parents Believe About Health Clinicians Talking About Firearms?

The vast majority of patients and parents believe that it is ok to for their physician to ask about firearms in the household and to provide firearm safety education. In a study of over 1200 parents, 66% thought a pediatrician should ask about the presence of guns in the household, including 58% of parents who own guns. Seventy five percent of parents felt that pediatricians should advise parents on the safest ways to store firearms in the home, including 71% of gun-owning parents. When asked "If a pediatrician advised me to not have any firearms in the home for child safety, I would…" – the responses were as follows (overall/gun-owning parents): think it over (48%/49%), follow the advice (35%/14%), ignore the advice (11%/22%), and be offended by the advice (8%/14%) [31]. When it comes to talking to other families about guns in their homes, a study of caregivers who had received teaching about ASK (Asking Saves Kids campaign), 96% of caregivers felt that doctors should provide ASK education [32].

Multiple focus groups of gun owners provide insight into some of the beliefs and concerns gun owners have regarding these conversations with their clinicians. Reason for ownership (hunting versus protection) plays a major role in overall perceptions of these conversations. Many owners view the overall risk for firearm injury as low. In truth, this is a matter of opinion with fatality rates around 7.5/100,000 for 10- to 19-year-old children. To place these numbers in context, this rate is actually higher than motor vehicle fatality rates (6.9/100,000), and yet physician advice about seatbelts and safe driving is typically acceptable and expected.

Many gun owners believe that safe firearm storage interferes with personal protection needs, especially for handguns. Devices like trigger locks are considered a nuisance and rarely used. Many parents feel confident in their youth's ability to handle guns safely and do not believe that safe storage would deter suicide. Though gun owners state they are willing to talk to their doctors about firearms, they prefer safe storage education from members of the military or law enforcement [33]. In a nationally representative survey of 1444 gun owners, only 19% rated physicians as excellent or good messengers to teach gun owners about safe gun storage [34].

However, broadly speaking, adult patients are likely more willing to discuss firearms with their doctor than the above data would suggest. In a national survey, nearly 4000 adults were asked, "In general, would you think it is never, sometimes, usually, or always appropriate for physicians and other health professionals to talk to their patients about firearms?" Seventy percent of non-firearm owners and 54% of firearm owners said it is at least sometimes appropriate for clinicians to talk to patients about firearm [35].

7.8 Can You Talk to Your Patients About Guns?

As of 2020, a health care clinician can talk about firearms with their patient in all 50 states. There was a physician gag law in place in Florida from 2011 to 2017, which was ultimately overturned. See Chap. 13 for further details. Twelve other states have attempted to pass laws restricting firearm conversations. Minnesota, Missouri, and Montana have restrictions against laws requiring physicians to ask about guns, but do not prevent the conversation itself. They also have specific limitations on how information can be collected and stored (i.e., standardized questionnaires/data forms).

A health care clinician can document the question asked and the response about firearm ownership and storage in all states. Clinicians can disclose about firearm ownership if there is an imminent concern about safety under the HIPAA exemption stating disclosure "is necessary to prevent or lessen a serious and imminent threat to the health or safety of a person or the public…." In addition, HIPAA regulations state, "No federal law prevents health care providers from warning law enforcement authorities about threats of violence" [36].

7.9 Storage Options

Understanding storage options for firearms is key to moving the conversation from generalizations about safety to actionable change.

As discussed above, storage of firearms outside of the home, and off of the property, is the safest way to keep a gun. Though this is not an option for someone who keeps their gun for home protection, it is an option for hunters and collectors and should be discussed within that context.

Cable/trigger locks: A cable lock blocks either the barrel of the gun and/or the ammunition by preventing a detachable magazine, which holds the bullets, from being attached to the gun. A trigger lock is a two-piece lock that fits over a gun's trigger and trigger guard to prevent a gun from being fired. They are available in versions with keys or combinations and are designed for use on unloaded guns. The cost of these items ranges from $10 to $50. Among some experts, there are concerns that trigger locks can potentially be disabled. Gun owners may find them cumbersome.

Lock box/safe: Lock boxes and gun safes provide the same type of security, namely a place to store a firearm in a locked, ideally unloaded, location. Companies selling these recommend that the lock box should be securely bolted to prevent theft. Lock boxes and safes can be accessed multiple ways including keys, combinations, keypad, biometrics, and radio-frequency indentification (RFID) devices. Makers of biometric access devices state the boxes/safes can be opened in seconds. Safes are typically used for multiple guns or long guns. Costs range from $25 to $350 for lock boxes and $200–$2500 for safes.

Personalized "smart" guns: These firearms are designed to recognize authorized users. The "smart gun" may recognize the authorized user via biometrics embedded into the grip and/or trigger, or they may recognize RFID bracelets or rings that the user wears. These are currently not readily available in the US but have been under development for over a decade and are available in other parts of the world. Please see Chap. 12 for further details.

Transfer possession: An individual may transfer their firearm to another person for safe keeping. This may occur in times of particular concern such as suicidality or may be done at baseline, for instance when there are children in the home. Firearms may be transferred to relatives, non-relatives, police stations, firearm dealers, and shooting ranges. Different states have restrictions on who may receive a firearm; this is especially important in states that require registration of firearms and in states that require background checks beyond the federal laws which only mandate background checks when firearms are sold by legal firearm dealers [37]. There are also some states, which provide regulations and protections related to the transfer back of the firearm, so that an individual who returns a firearm to the owner is not held liable should an injury or fatality occur [38, 39].

Extreme Risk Protection Orders: An Extreme Risk Protection Order (ERPO), also known as a red flag law, is an order from a judge that suspends a person's license to possess or carry a gun. This typically occurs when the family petitions to have a firearm removed from an individual because they believe the individual is at risk of hurting themselves or others. In some states, law enforcement, mental health providers, and others can petition to have a firearm temporarily removed. The immediate removal of the firearm is very brief, 2–3 days, and then an in-person hearing typically determines whether the firearm should be removed for a period typically up to 1 year. As of 2020, 20 states had ERPO laws (Fig. 7.4). Please see Chap. 14 for further details.

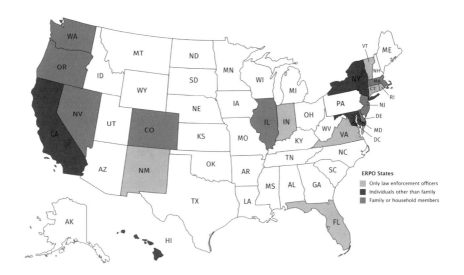

Fig. 7.4 Extreme Risk Protection Orders (ERPO) throughout the US

7.10   What Interventions Work?

There have been 12 studies examining how to intervene with parents and/or adolescents to lower the risk of unsafe firearm exposure or harm [40]. Six of these studies were randomized control trials (RCT). Unfortunately, they are all relatively small and many lack high-quality research methods. The two studies with the highest quality scores were found to improve firearm safety and are described in detail below.

In one RCT involving 124 pediatric practices and a total of 4890 participants, parents/primary caregivers received an intervention that included information about patient-family behavior and concerns related to media use, discipline, and children's exposure to firearms. Practitioners were trained in and provided motivational interviews and instructed families about the use of firearm cable locks and safe storage. Practitioners offered free cable locks to parents who lived in homes with children where guns were stored. Of the families, 470 reported gun ownership. Among these parents, reported use of cable locks at 6-month follow-up increased from 58% to 68% in the intervention group and decreased from 66% to 54% in the control group (odds ratio of increased usage 2.0, $P = 0.001$) [41].

The second RCT involved adolescents who experienced either intentional or unintentional injuries requiring hospitalization at a level 1 trauma center in Seattle, WA. After risk assessment, patients randomized to the intervention arm received care from a social worker and nurse practitioner team. The intervention included care management and motivational interviewing targeting risk behaviors and substance use, as well as pharmacotherapy and cognitive behavioral therapy elements targeting symptoms of post-traumatic stress disorder and depression. Among the 120 randomized adolescents followed for 12 months, 33% reported carrying a weapon at baseline. Carrying dropped from 35% to 7% in the intervention group and 31% to 21% in the usual care group (relative risk 0.31, 95% CI 0.11, 0.90) [42].

Though not as rigorous as the above studies, a quasi-experimental evaluation of a single, in-person message delivered to patients about firearm storage provides an intervention that can readily be incorporated into practices. In two family medicine clinics, 1233 patients were screened for firearm ownership by a nurse after asking basic demographic information. The question was "Does anyone living in your home own a gun?" A total of 156 patients reported guns in their household and were enrolled in the study. Those in the counseling group received verbal counseling from their physician who provided the following advice: "Having a loaded or unlocked gun in your house increases the risk of injury or death to family members, whether by accident or on purpose. I urge you to store your unloaded guns in a locked drawer or cabinet, and out of reach of children." By 2 or 3 months follow-up, among those in the intervention groups, 64% had made a safe firearm storage change, while only 33% in the control group had make a safe change ($P = 0.02$); the odds of making a safe change was 3.0 [43].

7.11   Implementation of Interventions

What does it take to implement these interventions? Analysis of stakeholders' perspectives on implementing firearm safety interventions in pediatrics emphasizes the importance of leveraging existing infrastructures such as electronic medical records as well as brevity of the intervention [44]. Interventions requiring the distribution of firearm locks or lock boxes, though desirable, pose complications of storage space within a practice, cost expenditures and lack of reimbursement, as well as questions of efficacy. But if your clinic is committed to handing out safety devices, families appear to be receptive.

Concerns exist about the appropriateness of talking to parents; the concern of one pediatrician in particular captures this well, "So we're talking about coming into a culture trying to do a very reasonable urban intervention on a mostly rural population that is politically very, very, very charged around gun rights." To lower clinician burden, the notion of screening outside of the examination room (e.g., the waiting room) bundled with other safety questions may be more feasible and acceptable. To make this work within a clinic, staff would require education and training and the availability of hard copies of materials to hand to families could be useful [44].

Teaching kids how to safely use a gun within the context of target shooting or hunting is clearly an important task. However, no known data exist showing that teaching children not to touch a gun and to tell an adult if they see a gun actually works. The Eddie Eagle program mentioned above and the STAR (Straight Talk About Risks) gun-safety programs have not been shown to prevent children from handling guns.

7.12   A Framework for Clinicians to Provide Firearm
Safety Counseling

In 2017, the Massachusetts Attorney General's office assembled a collection of pediatricians, psychiatrists, emergency physicians, public health specialists, law enforcement, lawyers, and other professionals to develop guidelines on how to talk to patients about firearms. The freely available pamphlet "Talking to Patients about Gun Safety" [45], http://www.massmed.org/firearmguidanceforproviders/, emphasizes the following key points (see Fig. 7.5):

1. Most gun owners are knowledgeable and committed to gun safety
2. Focus on health
3. Provide context for the questions
4. Make sure the questions are not accusatory
5. Start with open-ended questions to avoid sounding judgmental (e.g., "Do you have any concerns about the accessibility of your gun?" instead of "Is your gun safely secured?")
6. Meet patients where they are. Where there is a risk, brainstorm together harm reduction measures

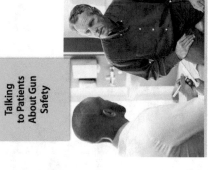

Fig. 7.5 Guide to talking to patients about firearms. From: Talking to Patients About Gun Safety [Internet]. Boston; 2017. Available from: http://www.massmed.org/firearmguidanceforproviders/

b Talking to Patients About Gun Safety

Firearm safety is a public health issue. As such, health care providers are uniquely situated to engage their patients and help prevent injury and death. Of course, most gun owners are responsible and deeply committed to gun safety. Nevertheless, they may have questions about how to keep themselves and their families safe. Some providers may not approach this topic because of concerns about how to talk about guns and what to do when troubling information is gleaned from patients.

This document is designed to provide guidance for talking to patients about guns, and on implications of those discussions for patient privacy and reporting obligations. For specific advice to give patients regarding firearm safety, please see our accompanying handout, "Gun Safety and Your Health."

Are there any legal restrictions on my ability to talk to patients about gun safety?

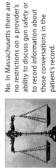

No. In Massachusetts there are no restrictions on a provider's ability to discuss gun safety or to record information about those conversations in the patient's record.

What protected health information *must* I report to law enforcement or to others outside of the provider-patient relationship?

Gunshot wounds

A physician or an administrator at his or her hospital must report all gunshot wounds to the state and local police. Providers should fill out the form provided by the Weapon-Related Injury Surveillance System (WRISS) or contact the State Police's Criminal Information Division and local police.

Abuse and neglect

Most health care providers are required to report any reasonable suspicion of child abuse and neglect, elder abuse, or abuse of a person with disabilities, including if such abuse or neglect involved a gun:

- Report suspected child abuse or neglect to Department of Children and Families.
- Report suspected elder abuse to the Department of Elder Affairs.
- Report suspected abuse of persons with disabilities to the Disabled Persons Protection Commission.

Warning or protecting potential victims

Licensed mental health care providers have a duty to warn or take steps to protect a patient's potential victim(s) if:

- The patient has communicated an explicit threat to kill or inflict serious bodily injury on a reasonably identified potential victim.
- The patient has a history of physical violence and the provider has reason to believe there is a clear and present danger that the patient will kill or inflict serious bodily injury on a reasonably identified potential victim.

In lieu of warning a patient's potential victim(s), a provider fulfills his or her duty by notifying law enforcement or initiating a voluntary or involuntary hospitalization — if these steps would be appropriate under the circumstances.

Court orders and subpoenas

Under state and federal law, providers must respond to court orders, grand jury subpoenas, and some administrative requests by law enforcement. This would most likely come up if a patient is a victim or suspect in a crime.

What protected health information *may* I report to law enforcement or others outside the provider-patient relationship?

Serious and imminent threats

If a health care provider has a good faith belief that information constitutes a serious and imminent threat (to the patient or another person), the Health Insurance Portability and Accountability Act (HIPAA) allows him or her to report that information to any person, including family members and law enforcement officials, who would be reasonably able to prevent or lessen the threat.

Crime on the premises

A provider may report information to law enforcement if he or she believes it constitutes evidence of criminal conduct that occurred on the premises of the health care facility.

Crime in an emergency setting

When responding to a medical emergency, a provider may alert law enforcement to the commission and nature of a crime, as well as its location, victims, and perpetrators.

Minors' records

In most cases, providers can share all protected health information with a minor's parent.

Patient authorized information

A provider may disclose information when a patient has signed a legally permissible written authorization for disclosure.

Fig. 7.5 (continued)

The same group created freely available information sheets that can be given to families entitled "Gun Safety and Your Health," http://www.massmed.org/firearmguidanceforpatients/ (see Fig. 7.6) [46]. Beyond the information about gun safety and health, and the recommendations about safe firearm storage, the pamphlet also discusses how to dispose of an unwanted gun. Options for gun disposal include sale to a dealer, surrender the gun to the police, gun buyback programs, which are sponsored annually, and donation to law enforcement and gun safety training programs.

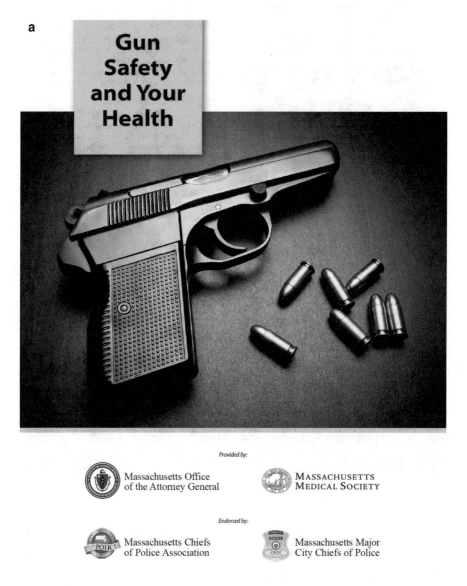

Fig. 7.6 Handout to give to patients about firearm safety. From: Gun Safety and Your Health [Internet]. Boston; 2017. Available from: http://www.massmed.org/firearmguidanceforpatients/

b Gun Safety and Your Health

Gun safety is an important part of your health and the public health. Most gun owners are responsible and deeply committed to gun safety. If you are a gun owner, live in a household where there is a gun, or otherwise might come in contact with guns, the following information may help you keep yourself and those around you safe.

Guns in the home are like any other potentially dangerous household risk, such as chemicals in cleaning supplies, backyard pools, alcohol and cigarettes, prescription medication, or fire hazards. With any of these potential hazards, you can take steps to protect yourself and your family.

Talk to your health care provider about any concerns you might have about gun safety and the potential impact on your health or the health of your loved ones.

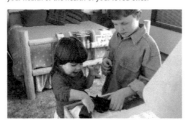

Safe Gun Storage

Safe gun storage is critical to the health and safety of you and your loved ones; it's also the law.

Under Massachusetts law, guns must be stored in a way that makes them impossible to operate by any person other than the owner or lawfully licensed user. This means that stored guns must be securely locked.

An owner may be fined or even imprisoned if his or her firearm is kept in a place where minors could access it. This is particularly important because more than two-thirds of gun-related deaths involving children could have been prevented if guns had been stored locked and unloaded.

The safest way to store a gun in your home is unloaded and securely locked, with the ammunition locked in a separate container.

There are many different options for gun storage, including trigger and cable locks, gun cases, lock boxes, gun cabinets, and gun safes — all of which are widely available online and at various retail locations.

Making a Gun Less Accessible

Guns in the home increase risk under certain circumstances. You may want to take additional steps to keep your family safe if someone in your household:

- Is a young child
- Is a teenager
- Suffers from suicidal thoughts or depression
- Has a history of violence
- Suffers from a condition that results in an altered mental state such as drug addiction or dementia

Because people in these groups are more likely to accidentally or purposely discharge a gun to hurt themselves or others, additional safety steps for your household might include storing a gun at a remote location, making ammunition inaccessible, deactivating the gun, or disposing of an unwanted gun.

Storage at a Remote Location

As long as a gun is properly stored so that it is inaccessible to unlicensed persons, it does not legally need to be kept in the owner's home. For instance, if a gun is primarily used for hunting, it could be stored in another location when not being used for that purpose. Examples of remote locations might include:

- At another licensed person's home
- In a secure storage unit
- In a bonded warehouse for gun storage
- In a second home

An owner could also store the key to access a gun in a remote location.

Making Ammunition Inaccessible

To reduce the chance that someone in the household uses a gun to hurt himself or herself or others, a gun owner can dispose of ammunition or store it in another location, as long as it can't be accessed by someone without a license.

Deactivation

A gunsmith or other certified professional can make changes to a gun so that it can no longer be fired.

Fig. 7.6 (continued)

c

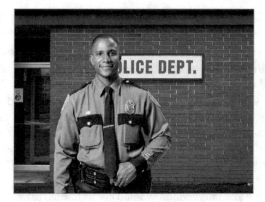

Disposing of an Unwanted Gun

There are several different options for disposing of a gun that is no longer wanted.

Sale to Dealers or Individuals

Guns can be sold to licensed dealers or individuals. This is often the best option for a legally owned firearm, as it allows the owner to be fully compensated for the value of the weapon.

Surrender Programs

In Massachusetts, anyone can surrender a gun to their local police department. To surrender a weapon, a person should contact the local police department to arrange a time to turn it in. The surrender program offers full immunity from prosecution for possessing the firearm.

Gun Buy-Back Programs

Many cities offer gun buy-back programs, during which gun owners receive cash, gift certificates, tax credits, or vouchers in exchange for giving their guns to the local police. Some buy-back programs are anonymous and offer immunity from prosecution for possession.

Contact your local law enforcement officials to find out if there is a buy-back program in your area.

Donation to Training Programs

Some law enforcement agencies and gun safety organizations have limited budgets for purchasing weapons and will accept donations to further their training programs.

What to Do When a Gun Owner Who Is a Friend or Family Member Is at Risk of Violence, Suicide, or Accidental Injury

You may want to talk to your friend or family member about safe storage or gun disposal options, as appropriate.

If your concern relates to mental health or substance use, you may want to recommend counseling or treatment. You can also bring your friend or family member to a primary care physician, mental health counseling center, or local emergency department for evaluation.

If you are concerned that someone you know should not have a gun because he or she might be violent, suicidal, or at risk of accidental injury, you can alert the local police.

The police department may revoke a gun license if the person does not meet the licensing requirements or is otherwise unsuitable for gun ownership.

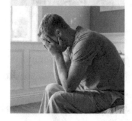

3

Fig. 7.6 (continued)

7.13   Research for Primary Prevention

There is a significant deficit in the knowledge about what interventions work best to reduce both pediatric exposure to unsafely stored firearms and, most importantly, pediatric firearm injuries and deaths. Multiple firearm research groups, including the Firearm Safety Among Children and Teens (FACTS) Consortium and the American Foundation for Firearm Injury Reduction in Medicine (AFFIRM) organization, as well as the American College of Emergency Physicians (ACEP), AAP, and other national groups have put forth research agendas and grants to identify best practices for screening and interventions with patients and families [47–49]. See Chap. 15.

Primary prevention screening and interventions should not be limited to the pediatrician's office. Though clinicians should play an important role in the effort to reduce firearm injuries, as the FACTS consortium describes, it is essential to evaluate the role of school and community-based interventions in primary prevention as well. Engaging caregivers who own firearms is critical for the development of effective prevention strategies [47]. Likewise, research is needed across different regions of the country as attitudes about the role of firearms in the household likely differ. The consideration of scalability and practical implementation is paramount for widespread protection of children.

7.14   My Personal Approach to Firearm Screening and Advice

As a pediatric emergency physician, I do not ask every patient about firearms. I do ask, and I teach my trainees to ask, every patient who comes in with a mental health issue and every patient exposed to violence.

Ideally, I speak to both the patient and their parents separately. With my patients, I use the adolescent conversation approach of starting with safer topics using the HEADDSS acronym: Home, Education, Activities, Drugs, Depression, Sex, Suicide [50]. When I get to the topic of depression and suicide, I ask them directly "Is there a gun in the home?" I explain my reason for asking, "having a gun in the home of a person with depression puts them at higher risk of killing themselves, and I want to help keep you safe." If there is a gun in the home, I ask the patient who owns the gun and how it is stored. I also ask them if they have access to a gun, since data about firearm suicides suggests that of adolescents who commit firearm suicide, 25% use a gun obtained outside of the home [15].

When I speak with the parents as part of the lethal means restrictions conversation, I first ask about how they store medications in their home to provide an overall context for safety planning. I then provide advice about using a locked tackle box to store the medications to provide protection for their child. And then I ask them the same direct questions about firearms that I have asked their children, "Is there a gun in the home?". Regardless of how they answer, I provide the same advice. "The best place to store a gun for the safety of your child is outside of the home, in a safety deposit box or other locked space. If a gun must be stored in the home, for the safety of your child, it is important that the gun is stored locked, unloaded, and separate from the locked ammunition." I provide advice about trigger locks and safety boxes and how to purchase them. I tell them that Massachusetts has laws mandating safe storage of all firearms to prevent access to firearms by children and youth. And I talk about the options of temporarily transfering the firearms to other people including family, friends, gun stores, shooting ranges or law enforcement. Please see Chap. 9 for further details.

One shift, I screened a 12-year-old girl who was acutely suicidal. When I asked about guns in the home, she told me that her brother, a police officer, regularly left his gun on the kitchen table when he came home from work. When I asked the parents if there were any guns in the house, the mom initially said no. I waited silently for 2 seconds. Then her eyes opened wide and her pupils dilated. "Wait! My son is a cop and he doesn't always lock his gun up right when he comes home! I'll talk to him today!"

Take Home Points
- It is difficult to predict which families own guns, and it is difficult to predict which families will store guns safely or unsafely in their homes.
- How firearms are stored in the home makes a difference for risk of injury and death.
- Though clinicians broadly believe in and support screening and providing firearm storage advice, the majority do not regularly provide counseling to their patients.
- The majority of families support health care clinicians discussing firearm safety.
- There are multiple effective approaches to safe firearm storage.
- Health care clinicians can legally talk to their patients about firearms and there are interventions and advice that can be provided effectively to parents and patients.

References

1. Web-based Injury Statistics Query and Reporting System (WISQARS™) [Internet]. Center for Disease Control and Prevention, National Center for Injury Prevention and Control. [cited 2020 Mar 21]. Available from: https://www.cdc.gov/injury/wisqars/fatal.html.
2. Okoro CA, Nelson DE, Mercy JA, Balluz LS, Crosby AE, Mokdad AH. Prevalence of household firearms and firearm-storage practices in the 50 states and the District of Columbia: findings from the behavioral risk factor surveillance system, 2002. Pediatrics. 2005;116(3):e370–6.
3. Terry L. Schell, Samuel Peterson, Brian G. Vegetabile, Adam Scherling, Rosanna Smart, and Andrew R. Morral. State-Level Estimates of Household Firearm Ownership [Internet]. Santa Monica, CA: RAND Corporation, 2020. https://www.rand.org/pubs/tools/TL354.html.
4. Smith TW, Son J. General Social Survey: trends in gun ownership in the United States, 1972–2014 [Internet]. NORD at the University of Chicago. Chicago; 2015. Available from: https://www.norc.org/PDFs/GSS%20Reports/GSS_Trends%20in%20Gun%20Ownership_US_1972-2014.pdf.
5. Parker BYK, Horowitz J, Igielnik R, Oliphant B, Brown A. America's complex relationship with guns [Internet]. Pew Research Center. 2017. Available from: https://www.pewsocial-trends.org/2017/06/22/the-demographics-of-gun-ownership/.
6. Mannix R, Lee LK, Fleegler EW. Coronavirus Disease 2019 (COVID-19) and Firearms in the United States: Will an Epidemic of Suicide Follow? Ann Intern Med. 2020;4:173(3):228–9.
7. Nass, D. How Many Guns Did Amercians Buy Last Month? We're Tracking the Sales Boom. The Trace. [Internet]. 2020. Available from: https://www.thetrace.org/2020/08/gun-sales-estimates/.
8. Azrael D, Cohen J, Salhi C, Miller M. Firearm storage in gun-owning households with children: results of a 2015 National Survey. J Urban Health. 2018;95(3):295–304.
9. Healthychildren.org, American Academy Pediatrics; Gun safety and children [Internet]. Chicago; 2019. Available from: https://www.aap.org/en-us/ImagesGen/Gun Safety 7 x 12 half English_FINAL.jpg.
10. Grassel KM, Wintemute GJ, Wright MA, Romero MP. Association between handgun purchase and mortality from firearm injury. Inj Prev. 2003;9(1):48–52.
11. Siegel M, Rothman EF. Firearm ownership and suicide rates among US men and women, 1981–2013. Am J Public Health. 2016;106(7):1316–22.
12. Brent DA, Perper JA, Allman CJ, Moritz GM, Wartella ME, Zelenak JP. The presence and accessibility of firearms in the homes of adolescent suicides: a case-control study. JAMA. 1991;266(21):2989–95.
13. Dahlberg LL, Ikeda RM, Kresnow M. Guns in the home and risk of a violent death in the home: findings from a national study. Am J Epidemiol. 2004;160(10):929–36.
14. Miller M, Azrael D, Barber C. Suicide mortality in the United States: the importance of attending to method in understanding population-level disparities in the burden of suicide. Annu Rev Public Health. 2012;33(1):393–408.
15. Azad HA, Monuteaux MC, Hoffmann J, Lee LK, Mannix R, Rees CA, et al. Firearm violence in children and teenagers: the source of the firearm. Under Review 2020.
16. Grossman DC, Mueller BA, Riedy C, Dowd MD, Villaveces A, Prodzinski J, et al. Gun storage practices and risk of youth suicide and unintentional firearm injuries. JAMA. 2005;293(6):707–14.
17. Monuteaux MC, Azrael D, Miller M. Association of increased safe household firearm storage with firearm suicide and unintentional death among US youths. JAMA Pediatr. 2019;173(7):657–62.
18. Dowd MD, Sege R. Council on injury, violence and Poison Prevention. Firearm-related injuries affecting the pediatric population. Pediatrics. 2012;130(5):e1416–23.
19. Leshner AI, Altevogt BM, Lee AF, McCoy MA, Kelley PW. Priorities for research to reduce the threat of firearm-related violence. Institute of Medicine and National Research Council. Washington, DC: National Academies Press; 2013. p. 1–109.

20. Hagan JF, Shaw JS, Duncan PM. Bright futures: Guidelines for health supervision of infants, children and adolescents [pocket edition]. 4th ed. Elk Grove Village: American Academy of Pediatrics. 2017.
21. Webster DW, Wilson ME, Duggan AK, Pakula LC. Firearm injury prevention counseling: a study of pediatricians' beliefs and practices. Pediatrics. 1992;89(5 Pt 1):902–7.
22. Grossman DC, Mang K, Rivara FP. Firearm injury prevention counseling by pediatricians and family physicians: practices and beliefs. Arch Pediatr Adolesc Med. 1995;149(9):973–7.
23. Hoopsa K, Crifasi C. Pediatric resident firearm-related anticipatory guidance: why are we still not talking about guns? Prev Med. 2019;124:29–32.
24. Butkus R, Weissman A. Internists' attitudes toward prevention of firearm injury. Ann Intern Med. 2014;160:821–7.
25. Grossman DC, Mang K, Rivara FP. Firearm injury prevention counseling by pediatricians and family physicians. Arch Pediatr Adolesc Med. 1996;149:973–7.
26. Becher EC, Cassel CK, Nelson EA. Physician firearm ownership as a predictor of firearm injury prevention practice. Am J Public Health. 2000;90(10):1626–8.
27. Guns [Internet]. Gallup. 2020 [cited 2020 Mar 30]. Available from: https://news.gallup.com/poll/1645/guns.aspx.
28. Farah MM, Simon HK, Kellermann AL. Firearms in the home: parental perceptions. Pediatrics. 1999;104(5 Part 1):1059–63.
29. Jackman GA, Farah MM, Kellermann AL, Simon HK. Seeing is believing: what do boys do when they find a real gun? J Dev Behav Pediatr. 2001;22(6):1247–50.
30. National Rifle Association. Eddie Eagle gunsafe program [Internet]. 2020 [cited 2020 Mar 27]. Available from: https://eddieeagle.nra.org/.
31. Garbutt JM, Bobenhouse N, Dodd S, Sterke R, Strunk RC. What are parents willing to discuss with their pediatrician about firearm safety? A parental survey. J Pediatr. 2016;179:166–71.
32. Agrawal N, Arevalo S, Castillo C, Lucas AT. Effectiveness of the asking saves kids gun violence prevention campaign in an urban pediatric clinic. Pediatrics. 2018;142:730.
33. Aitken ME, Minster SD, Mullins SH, Hirsch HM, Unni P, Monroe K, et al. Parents' perspectives on safe storage of firearms. J Community Health. 2020;45:469–77.
34. Crifasi CK, Doucette ML, McGinty EE, Webster DW, Barry CL. Storage practices of US gun owners in 2016. Am J Public Health. 2018;108(4):532–7.
35. Betz ME, Azrael D, Barber C, Miller M. Public opinion regarding whether speaking with patients about firearms is appropriate: results of a national survey. Ann Intern Med. 2016;165(8):543–50.
36. Wintemute GJ, Betz ME, Ranney ML. Yes, you can: physicians, patients, and firearms. Ann Intern Med. 2016;165(3):205–13.
37. McCourt AD, Vernick JS, Betz ME, Brandspigel S, Runyan CW. Temporary transfer of firearms from the home to prevent suicide: legal obstacles and recommendations. JAMA Intern Med. 2017;177(1):96–101.
38. Gibbons MJ, Fan MD, Rowhani-Rahbar A, Rivara FP. Legal Liability for Returning Firearms to Suicidal Persons Who Voluntarily Surrender Them in 50 US States. Am J Public Health. 2020;110(5):685–8.
39. Fleegler EW, Madeira JL. First, prevent harm: eliminate firearm transfer liability as a lethal means reduction strategy. Am J Public Health. 2020;110(5):619–20.
40. Roszko PJD, Ameli J, Carter PM, Cunningham RM, Ranney ML. Clinician attitudes, screening practices, and interventions to reduce firearm-related injury. Epidemiol Rev. 2016;38(1):87–110.
41. Barkin SL, Finch SA, Ip EH, Scheindlin B, Craig JA, Steffes J, et al. Is office-based counseling about media use, timeouts, and firearm storage effective? Results from a cluster-randomized, controlled trial. Pediatrics. 2008;122(1):e15–25.
42. Zatzick D, Russo J, Lord SP, Varley C, Wang J, Berliner L, et al. Collaborative care intervention targeting violence risk behaviors, substance use, and posttraumatic stress and depressive symptoms in injured adolescents a randomized clinical trial. JAMA Pediatr. 2014;168(6):532–9.

43. Albright TL, Burge SK. Improving firearm storage habits: impact of brief office counseling by family physicians. J Am Board Fam Pract. 2003;16(1):40–6.
44. Benjamin Wolk C, Van Pelt AE, Jager-Hyman S, Ahmedani BK, Zeber JE, Fein JA, et al. Stakeholder perspectives on implementing a firearm safety intervention in pediatric primary care as a universal suicide prevention strategy: a qualitative study. JAMA Netw Open. 2018;1(7):e185309. 1–12.
45. Talking to Patients About Gun Safety [Internet]. Boston; 2017. Available from: http://www.massmed.org/firearmguidanceforproviders/.
46. Gun safety and Your Health [Internet]. Boston; 2017. Available from: http://www.massmed.org/firearmguidanceforpatients/.
47. Cunningham RM, Carter PM, Ranney ML, Walton M, Zeoli AM, Alpern ER, et al. Prevention of firearm injuries among children and adolescents: consensus-driven research agenda from the firearm safety among children and teens (FACTS) consortium. JAMA Pediatr. 2019;173(8):780–9.
48. AFFIRM [Internet]. American Foundation for Firearm Injury Reduction in Medicine. 2020 [cited 2020 Mar 21]. Available from: https://affirmresearch.org/grants/.
49. Ranney ML, Fletcher J, Alter H, Barsotti C, Bebarta VS, Betz ME, et al. A Consensus-Driven Agenda for Emergency Medicine Firearm Injury Prevention Research. Ann Emerg Med. 2017;69(2):227–40.
50. Goldenring JM, Cohen E. Getting into adolescent heads. Contemp Pediatr [Internet]. 1988;5(7):75–90. Available from: http://contemporarypediatrics.modernmedicine.com/contemporary-pediatrics/news/getting-adolescent-heads.

Chapter 8
Emergency Department and Hospital-Based Interventions

Joel A. Fein

Emergency room doctors speak out on South California gun violence

By Thomas Curwen
August 19, 2013. *Los Angeles Times*

8.1 Introduction

Medical centers, particularly emergency departments (EDs), are frequent touch-points for children and youth exposed to violence in their homes, schools, and communities. Many circumstances place children at risk for firearm injury, and these circumstances vary with age. Young children encountering a firearm in the home can lead to tragic consequences and severe injury or death, whereas older children and adolescents are more at risk for intentional use of a firearm to harm either themselves or others. It is also important to realize that youth age 15–24 years old actually have the highest rate of unintentional firearm deaths, at a rate three times higher than children 5–14 years old. There are antecedents of injury that can be identified during a medical encounter, such as the access to firearms, depression and suicidality, and brewing issues of revenge and retaliation that may offer medical personnel a chance to intervene before severe injury or death. This chapter will describe ED and hospital-based assessment and intervention for youth at risk of firearm injury and will focus on limiting access to firearms, preventing suicide, and reducing the incidence and impact of assaults from peer violence. National medical organizations, including the American Academy of Pediatrics (AAP), the National Academy of Medicine (NAM), the American College of Surgeons (ACS), and the American Medical Association (AMA), have recommended that hospitals utilize a public health approach to incorporate violence prevention into standard practice.

J. A. Fein (✉)
Department of Pediatrics, Children's Hospital of Philadelphia at the University of Pennsylvania School of Medicine, Philadelphia, PA, USA
e-mail: fein@email.chop.edu

© Springer Nature Switzerland AG 2021   111
L. K. Lee, E. W. Fleegler (eds.), *Pediatric Firearm Injuries and Fatalities*,
https://doi.org/10.1007/978-3-030-62245-9_8

In addition to being a frequent touchpoint for youth at risk for firearm violence, medical venues are also relatively "neutral" locations that have the potential to engender trust and build safe linkages to specific interventions. Hospital-based medical clinicians often have access to in-house social service and mental health resources with whom they can connect patients and families. Many hospital systems have established partnerships with community organizations, schools, and other municipal agencies that can promote recovery plans for at-risk youth. It is encouraging that these health-care systems have recognized the vital importance of addressing social determinants of health as part of their mission, with violence prevention and firearm safety as part of that puzzle.

8.2   What Can We Do? A Trauma-Informed Approach

Preventing firearm injury requires a multidisciplinary approach applying a public health model to develop, test, and implement discrete interventions. These efforts are most effective if they are grounded within a trauma-informed care delivery system that mitigates the power dynamic inherent in the clinician-patient relationship and builds the trust needed to create rapid, meaningful connections. Hospital-based clinicians who are versed in the concepts of implicit and explicit bias and understand how prior experiences and traumas shape the way that patients and families experience and react to medical interventions are best poised to initiate and integrate the interventions mentioned in this chapter. Examples of behaviors that put traumatized patients and families more at ease include reducing the perceptions of blame for the injury, safely allowing control at certain medical decision points, and providing clear and nonjudgmental communication about what will transpire during the hospital visit. Despite being a "neutral" venue, the hospital is still quite a foreign, and often threatening, representation of authority. Implementing shared decision-making whenever possible can go a long way toward patient engagement in helpful assessments and referrals.

Medical professionals are accustomed to team-based approaches to care, and these often involve the process of "identify, assess, treat, and refer." Some resources, such as general education about gun safety and suicide hotline information, can be offered universally and do not require more information from the patient and family. Others, such as asking about access to weapons – the strongest risk factor for all types of firearm violence in children – require a sensitivity to patient perceptions of privacy and legal considerations.

8.3 Identification, Assessment, and Interventions for Violence and Firearm Injury

As hospitals have successfully integrated screening for social determinants of health into routine clinical care, clinicians are being trained to assess the risk of child maltreatment, suicide, and intimate partner violence. Instruments used for assessing the risk of firearm access, suicide, and peer violence all contain direct and pointed questions requiring clinicians to introduce concepts of privacy in order to enhance the patients' comfort in responding to these questions. For childhood witnesses to violence and for assault-injured youth in particular, it is also essential not only to heal their external wounds but also to evaluate the potential psychological impact of the event. Posttraumatic stress symptoms (PTSS) are very common after violent injury, and these symptoms can persist over months for a substantial proportion of these youth. It is important to recognize the severity of the injury does not always correlate with the severity of PTS symptoms in children. Rather, the perception of life threat, the pain experienced during and after the event, and other factors may be more pertinent to the trajectory and persistence of these symptoms (please see Chap. 10 for further discussion).

Medical systems utilize a variety of strategies to deliver firearm safety and violence prevention interventions in busy clinical settings, including employing social workers, peer volunteers, and even tablet-based programs that do not require intensive on-site personnel. Technological solutions, such as computerized self-report screening processes, have been designed to ease the burden on clinicians. However, it is also important to introduce the potential to build trust and rapport in order to balance "high-tech" and "high-touch," so clinicians may want to review computerized screening results and discuss the findings with patients and families. It is important to note that each hospital or medical venue must assess its own resources that can be dedicated to prevention programming. Even with limited resources, a hospital or other health-care site can develop community partnerships that enhance and amplify the impact of screening and assessment.

8.3.1 Firearm Safety in the Home

Given our focus on health and safety, medical professionals are well positioned to address known household hazards, with firearms recognized as a clear danger for children and adolescents. If owners keep their firearms locked and unloaded and store the ammunition locked away separately, there is a significantly lower risk of both unintentional pediatric injury and adolescent suicide. In a 2006 study, only one-third of gun-owning parents in pediatric practices reported storing their firearm safely. A subsequent study found almost one-fifth of the respondents in three large cities reported firearms in the home, but only 6% followed the full recommended safety procedures. Even more concerning, a recent study showed a substantial proportion of homes with children who had symptoms of mental illness, such as depression or suicidality, had firearms that were not stored safely.

Most clinicians believe firearm safety counseling is important and appropriate for their clinical role. However, they may feel unprepared or uncomfortable discussing firearm safety with families due to the lack of knowledge or the concern for offending a family or "prying." Fortunately, there are many resources available to help us accomplish this in a natural, comfortable way. The Massachusetts Medical Society has brochures available for families (http://www.massmed.org/firearmguidanceforpatients/) as well as guides for physicians (http://www.massmed.org/firearmguidanceforproviders/) (see Chap. 7).

More importantly, there is no existing law or code preventing clinicians from asking about firearms in the home or their patient's access to firearms, especially if there is a reason they are concerned about the health and welfare of their patient in that regard. Though Florida passed the Firearm Owners' Privacy Act, the firearm "physician gag law," in 2011 placing prohibitions on conversations related to guns, that law was overturned in 2017 (see Chap. 13). The AAP recommends physicians screen for access to firearms in patients at higher risk for injury, including those with mood disorders, a history of substance abuse, or concern for suicidality. In these situations, in particular there is a strong medical indication for the physician to help the family keep their children safe through inquiry about firearm access. In addition, regardless of gun ownership, all families can receive the benefit of gun safety education, including safe storage, tips on how to keep their children safe in the homes of friends or relatives, and safe disposal of firearms. Bright Futures recommends discussing guns in early childhood (age 3 years), middle childhood (age 9 and 10 years), and early adolescence visits (ages 11–14 years). A multicenter study in pediatric primary care found that firearm safety counseling, particularly if coupled with the provision of a free firearm safety device, can significantly increase safe storage behaviors in our patients' homes.

As with any risk behavior counseling, it is important to "meet the family where they are" and learn what steps they can take toward protecting their children from unwanted access to firearms. A home devoid of firearms is clearly the safest situation. If that is not possible, then safe storage practices include using firearm locks, trigger locks, and gun storage cabinets, in addition to removing ammunition from the weapon and storing it in a separate locked location. Because many adults consider the firearm as a means of protection, the conversation may need to address the relative risk of criminal behavior occurring in the home, from which the family requires protection, compared to the risk of unintentional harm or intentional harm, including suicide. However, statistics and numbers do not always counteract unbalanced fears. Having the family member themselves strategize about how they can make their child's environment incrementally safer is a critical first step toward that end.

Some medical sites have begun firearm safety device provision, either on location or in the community, with concomitant improvement of storage practices.

Although more research is needed, a meta-analysis of these types of interventions confirms that families employ safer storage of firearms in the months after receiving a safety device.

8.3.2 Suicide, Self-Harm, and Relationship Violence

It is well known that many patients who die by suicide have had recent contact with the medical system, providing a rationale for routine screening in various medical settings. One study showed nearly one-third of children 11 years and older who completed suicide had visited an ED in the month prior. In preventing firearm-related suicide in children and adolescents, there is a need for validated, brief tools that we can use in busy clinical settings. Medical facilities have incorporated screening tools for depression, such as two-question and nine-question Patient Health Questionnaire (PHQ). For suicide-specific questions, the Ask Suicide-Screening Questions (ASQ) uses four very direct questions about lifetime suicidality and one about current suicidality (Fig. 8.1). The National Institute of Mental Health website provides a clinical pathway designed by the American Academy of Child and Adolescent Psychiatry that helps clinicians incorporate this tool when assessing patients for suicide risk in the ED or hospital. It is freely available at https://www.nimh.nih.gov/research/research-conducted-at-nimh/asq-toolkit-materials/asq-tool/screening-tool_155867.pdf.

The Behavioral Health Screen-Emergency Department (BHS-ED©) assesses suicidality as well as many other risk and protective factors in a computerized, self-administered tool and has had strong acceptance by adolescents in the pediatric setting. Related to suicide risk, four questions are asked in regard to the past year and if the response is "yes," then the questions are asked in regard to the past week, including today: (1) Have you felt that life is not worth living? (2) Have you thought about killing yourself? (3) Did you make a plan to kill yourself? (4) Have you tried to kill yourself? A recent large prospective study through the Pediatric Emergency Care Applied Research Network (PECARN) developed a computerized adaptive screen for suicidal youth (CASSY). This screening tool demonstrated a specificity of 80% and sensitivity of 83% for the prediction of a suicide attempt during a 3-month follow-up period. Many of these brief screening tools are highly sensitive but have low specificity, leading to false positives. Some mental health professionals suggest positive responses to these brief measures be followed-up with longer, more formal assessment by mental health professionals using specific tools such as the Columbia Suicide Severity Rating Scale.

In addition to screening for depression and suicidal ideation, it is also prudent to ask teens about their romantic relationships. As firearms substantially increase the risk of death in situations of intimate partner violence, teens should be asked specifically about their perception of safety within those relationships. It is unfortunate that these relationships may involve emotional and physical violence. One study found approximately 7% of adolescent homicides involved an intimate partner, and

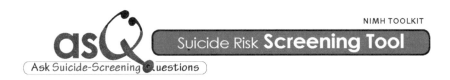

Ask the patient:

1. In the past few weeks, have you wished you were dead? ⚪ Yes ⚪ No

2. In the past few weeks, have you felt that you or your family would be better off if you were dead? ⚪ Yes ⚪ No

3. In the past week, have you been having thoughts about killing yourself? ⚪ Yes ⚪ No

4. Have you ever tried to kill yourself? ⚪ Yes ⚪ No

   If yes, how? _____

   _____

   _____

   When? _____

   _____

If the patient answers **Yes** *to any of the above, ask the following acuity question:*

5. **Are you having thoughts of killing yourself right now?** ⚪ Yes ⚪ No

   If yes, please describe: _____

Next steps:

- If patient answers "No" to all questions 1 through 4, screening is complete (not necessary to ask question #5). No intervention is necessary (*Note: Clinical judgment can always override a negative screen*).
- If patient answers "Yes" to any of questions 1 through 4, or refuses to answer, they are considered a positive screen. Ask question #5 to assess acuity:
  - ☐ "Yes" to question #5 = **acute positive screen** (imminent risk identified)
    - **Patient requires a STAT safety/full mental health evaluation.** Patient cannot leave until evaluated for safety.
    - Keep patient in sight. Remove all dangerous objects from room. Alert physician or clinician responsible for patient's care.
  - ☐ "No" to question #5 = **non-acute positive screen** (potential risk identified)
    - **Patient requires a brief suicide safety assessment to determine if a full mental health evaluation is needed.** Patient cannot leave until evaluated for safety.
    - Alert physician or clinician responsible for patient's care.

Provide resources to all patients

- 24/7 National Suicide Prevention Lifeline 1-800-273-TALK (8255) En Español: 1-888-628-9454
- 24/7 Crisis Text Line: Text "HOME" to 741-741

asQ Suicide Risk Screening Toolkit | NATIONAL INSTITUTE OF MENTAL HEALTH (NIMH) 🩺 **NIH** 6/13/2017

Fig. 8.1 The ASQ suicide screening questions (National Institute of Mental Health)

90% of these victims were female. In addition, young women are sometimes exploited to buy, conceal, store, and hold guns on behalf of men in their lives who are prohibited from purchasing firearms themselves. An organization in Boston known as "Operation LIPSTICK" (Ladies Involved in Putting a Stop to Inner-City Killings) works to educate women about these dangers.

Positive screens for suicidality and intimate partner violence require further a discussion with a clinician to clarify answers and determine the need for further mental health evaluation and treatment and for safety planning (see Chap. 9). Current suicidal thoughts require immediate attention by a mental health professional for safety assessment and potentially inpatient care for stabilization. For children with moderate or severe depression, referral for outpatient treatment, in communication with their primary care physician, should also include lethal means restriction counseling to ensure that there is no access to firearms in their environment. We also know that despite some logistical barriers, pediatric clinicians value the effort to address firearm access in their young patients and are willing to work with their administrators and medical leaders to establish this as a part of their routine practice.

8.3.3 Peer Violence

Assault injury is a common occurrence in school-age children. In 2015, the average rate of ED visits for assault was 267/100,000 patients. For 15–19-year-old teenagers, the rate was more than triple that amount. The average middle school has 600 10–14 year olds, suggesting at least a handful of the children in that school will seek medical care for an assault injury each year. Although rates vary based on age, location, and other risk factors, recent studies suggest that between 11% and 37% of ED patients treated for assault injuries will return to the ED for more serious injuries within 2 years, many within 6 months after the initial ED visit. An unfortunate number of these youth return with injuries involving firearms and other weapons. Each adolescent's visit to a medical facility is an opportunity to learn about and intercede regarding the risk of peer violence. Some programs, such as SafERteens and BHWorks, screen all youth for violence risk, while others utilize a visit due to a violent event as the rationale for assessment and intervention. For those who come to medical attention after a violent event, it is paramount to assess the safety of the patient before he or she leaves the hospital. Many youth will report that either they or other involved parties will continue the fight at the first opportunity. In addition, there are often family or friends of the involved parties who threaten to retaliate as a result of the altercation. Medical personnel, with support of social workers if available, can guide families during the immediate post-injury phase. By establishing the medical system as an ally rather than another traumatic experience, clinicians can potentially enhance connection to services after discharge.

First and foremost, we can allow the patient to tell the story of the event in their own words, as much as they feel comfortable doing. We do not want to force the narrative. Some patients can have increased posttraumatic stress symptoms as they review the event, and others may respond more positively. Another task that can be guided by the hospital team is helping the patient and family report the incident to the police or school authorities as appropriate. This can accomplish a number of goals. Firstly, reporting an incident to police could decrease the likelihood that the child or family will retaliate for the assault, given the fact that they have "transferred" the responsibility to other authorities. That said, youth and family members may consider this reporting more dangerous than helpful by increasing the animosity between involved parties without the expectation of protection by police or the criminal justice system. Secondly, in order for families to receive reimbursement of some of the expenses related to the incident from the Victims' Compensation Assistance Program (VCAP), they need to report the incident to an "appropriate authority," which includes a law enforcement officer, district attorney, campus police, and other agencies. Aside from the medical care we provide, clinicians can also provide connection to community resources, as well as psychosocial support that addresses the emotional toll of the event. In light of this, parents should be encouraged to reach out to school counselors and primary care offices to learn about their options for their child to keep him or her safe, as well as the supportive resources available in communities and schools.

For youth who are seen for assault, various instruments are being developed and validated with the goal of assessing risk of revictimization or reinjury. One recently studied tool is the SaFETy score from the University of Michigan, which asks about *s*erious fighting, *f*riends' weapon carrying, *e*nvironmental exposure to gunshots, and direct *t*hreats with a firearm (Table 8.1). The Children's Hospital of Philadelphia three-item safety tool queries, as part of a comprehensive self-administered computerized questionnaire for adolescents, (1) if the youth feels that the altercation is over, (2) if they or someone they know may retaliate, and (3) if they planned to report the incident to police (as a protective factor against retaliation). The Violence Prevention Emergency Tool (VPET-3) is a seven-item questionnaire that similarly asks questions related to witnessing, crime, or fighting behavior. These questions are as follows: (1) Have you seen a person shoot another person with a real gun? (2) Have you been physically harmed by another person? (3) Have you been injured by someone? (4) Has an angry person chased you? (5) Have you injured someone? (6) Have you stolen anything, sold drugs, or destroyed property? (7) Have you failed a class?

Table 8.1 Items in the SaFETy score for predicting firearm injury risk

S (Serious fighting)	In the past 6 months, including today, how often did you get into a serious physical fight?
F (Friend weapon carrying)	How many of your friends have carried a knife, razor, or gun?
E (Community environment)	In the past 6 months, how often have you heard guns being shot?
T (Firearm threats)	How often, in the past 6 months, including today, has someone pulled a gun on you?

From: Goldstick et al.

Tools that have been validated in the primary care setting include the 5-item FiGHTS screening tool and the 14-item Violence, Injury Protection, and Risk Screen, which has also been validated to assess risk for cyber violence. The five questions of the FiGHTS tool are the following: (1) During the past 12 months, have you been in a physical fight? (2) Is your gender male? (3) During the past 12 months, have you been in a physical fight in which you were injured and had to be treated by a doctor or nurse? (4) During the past 12 months, have you been threatened or injured with a weapon such as a knife or gun on school property? (5) Have you ever smoked cigarettes regularly, that is, at least one cigarette every day for 30 days?

It should be noted that none of these tools provides a certain "score" above or below which the clinician would make a decision about further assessment or referral. However, they do provide important domains that are important to assess to guide that process. Additional efforts have begun to estimate a "risk of violent reinjury assessment" of youth who are seen after assaults; however, more research is needed to fully develop and implement this type of instrument in order to provide a more tailored approach to high-resource interventions.

Similar to those who may be at risk for alcohol or drug use, youth who are deemed at risk for fighting, and therefore, in the current climate, firearm injury, may benefit from brief, contained interventions using motivational interviewing (MI). When done in a nonconfrontational and nonjudgmental manner, MI can help these youth explore their desires to avoid or change risky behaviors. One example of this approach is SafERteens, a screening and 30-minute brief counseling intervention that has been shown to decrease violence and substance use behaviors among teens 14–18 years old who report recent fighting and alcohol use (see Table 8.2).

Table 8.2 Resources for youth violence prevention

Resource	Web site
The Health Alliance for Violence Intervention (HAVI)	www.the HAVI.org
Violence is Preventable: A Best Practices Guide for Launching & Sustaining a Hospital-based Program to Break the Cycle of Violence	www.ncjrs.gov/App/Publications/abstract.aspx?ID=260856
Reinjury Prevention for Youth Presenting with Violence Related Injuries: A Training Curriculum for Trauma Centers	www.stopyouthviolence.ucr.edu
American Academy of Pediatrics "Connected Kids Program: Safe, Strong, Secure"	www.aap.org
University of California at Davis "What Can You Do" Initiative	https://health.ucdavis.edu/what-you-can-do/
SafERteens Youth Violence Prevention Program	www.injurycenter.umich.edu/programs/saferteens
University of Michigan Injury Center "Parents' Guide to Home Firearm Safety"	www.injurycenter.umich.edu
The Center for Violence Prevention at Children's Hospital of Philadelphia	www.chop.edu/violence
Children's Hospital of Philadelphia "After the Injury"	www.aftertheinjury.org
The Society for Advancement of Violence and Injury research "Instrument Library"	https://savirweb.org/aws/SAVIR/pt/sp/instrument-library

Other health-care systems have developed hospital-based violence intervention programs (HVIP) that recruit participants from the hospital (see Chap. 11). These programs extend beyond the patient's initial medical encounter in order to provide or connect the patient directly to services after hospital discharge. Programs are funded through a variety of sources, including hospital operating budgets, philanthropic grants, public sector contracts, and reimbursement for services through Medicaid and Victim of Crime Assistance. HVIPs can either link the youth and family with a community-based organization that carries out the aftercare program or use their own staff members to meet clients and families in community settings. It is optimal for someone from the HVIP to initially meet the patients in the hospital setting to make the connection and mitigate any safety issues that may exist. However, because approximately 90% of youth who have already been injured in a violent event are discharged from the ED rather than admitted to the hospital, many of the clients are recruited after reviews of the medical record system or post-discharge referrals from physicians, nurses, and hospital-based social workers. During the intake process, the patients undergo a comprehensive psychosocial assessment that informs longer-term goals targeting physical and mental health, education, employment, criminal justice, peers, and family relationships. These areas are then addressed through subsequent case management services. In addition to the intensive system navigation guiding the patient and family through the aftermath of the violent event, many programs also provide other services. These include trauma-focused psychoeducation and direct mental health services including cognitive behavioral therapy, group therapy, or linkage to higher-level psychiatric care if needed. Although there is some variability in the way HVIPs deliver the intervention, they are all guided by the tenets of trauma-informed care as described above. Because retaliatory behaviors and reinjury are commonly reported by assault-injured youth and most often occur within the first weeks after the event, some hospital-based programs incorporate or collaborate with "violence interrupter" programs, such as Cure Violence, which employ street-based staff members to prevent retaliation and promote community healing.

HVIPs have been shown to improve mental health outcomes and results in less criminal justice involvement in youth who complete these programs. Studies in high-risk adult patients entering these programs demonstrate lower reinjury rates, decreased violent perpetration, and improved employment. In addition, several economic evaluations indicate these programs could generate substantial cost savings for health-care and criminal justice sectors. Despite these limitations, the Health Alliance for Violence Intervention (HAVI, formerly the National Network of Hospital-Based Violence Intervention Programs) has more than 42 member programs that share best practices and provide training and technical assistance to emerging programs (www.TheHAVI.org – see Table 8.2). The HAVI also promotes collaborative research in order to create more consistent outcome measures, increase sample sizes, and promote fidelity within the interventions. The American College of Surgeons Committee on Trauma has developed guidelines requiring trauma centers to provide prevention programs addressing the most common causes of injury for their catchment population. Careful review of what may work, and more importantly what may potentially do harm, is a critical ingredient in the formulation of such programs.

Many health-care settings do not have the infrastructure to support a hospital-based violence prevention program. For those considering starting such a program, there is a resource monograph available through the National Criminal Justice Reference Service (Table 8.2). However, even when this is not a possibility, there are a growing number of community-based resources to support individual providers who are interested in improving the standard of care for violently injured patients. For example, patients who exhibit or report symptoms of traumatic stress, such as hypervigilance, re-experiencing the event, or intrusive thoughts, can be referred to evidence-based therapies such as trauma-focused cognitive behavioral therapy. These types of therapies can ameliorate these symptoms and bring the child closer to normal daily function. Brief psychoeducation, which allows patients and parents to better recognize developing traumatic stress symptoms and become more in tune with the body's physiologic reactions to these traumatic events, can also be delivered through brief conversations or even through web-delivered content. Other prevention programs and national organizations have developed online resources for physicians with interest in providing violence prevention services. The CDC has developed an online resource titled "Connecting the Dots: An Overview of the Links among Multiple Forms of Violence." (https://www.cdc.gov/violenceprevention/pdf/connecting_the_dots-a.pdf). The CDC has also created a compendium of screening and assessment tools to measure violence-related behaviors, as well as an overview of methods for evaluating youth violence prevention programs.

It is worth noting almost all the research on prevention strategies emphasizing scare tactics, such as trauma bay or morgue tours, suggest these "scared safe" programs are not recommended as a universal intervention for children and teens. One study, published from a hospital-based program, demonstrated some of the youth in the program improved their attitudes toward violence. However, this study suffered from small sample size, selection bias, and a lack of follow-up regarding the persistence of effect or the potential negative emotional or psychological impact of the youth were experiencing. Of note, a Cochrane review of these programs suggest they are ineffective at reducing overall violence risk and in fact are more harmful than helpful for delinquency outcomes.

Finally, a comprehensive dialogue regarding the health system's role in firearm violence prevention can be found in the proceedings of a 2019 National Academy of Science, Engineering and Medicine workshop. This report offers insight into the epidemiology, risk and protective factors, and current health system-based interventions. Many of these have been similarly described in this chapter.

8.3.4 Summary of Important Aspects of Screening and Intervention for Providers in the ED or Hospital Setting

1. ED screening

   (a) Self-harm or suicidality
   (b) Relationship violence and intimate partner violence (IPV) exposure
   (c) Firearm access or exposure

2. ED-based interventions

   (a) Transparency regarding limits of confidentiality
   (b) Discussion of means restriction and harm reduction practices for firearm access
   (c) Motivational interviewing (MI) and counseling by hospital staff or on-site community-based personnel
   (d) Involvement of social workers if needed

3. Hospital-based interventions

   (a) Initiation of community-based services through hospital-based violence intervention program (HVIP)
   (b) Training in trauma-informed approaches to patients and families exposed to violence
   (c) Partnerships increasing communication with primary care providers, schools, and other support networks
   (d) Support from hospital administration for educational initiatives that promote violence prevention policy efforts

8.4 Conclusions

Firearm injury, whether unintentional or intentional, is tragic and life-changing and as witnessed by health-care providers has motivated them to intervene. The issue is clearly "in our lane," and we are all obligated to address it using all our capacity and resources. Clinicians can often identify situations heralding impending firearm injury, such as unsafely stored weapons, depression and suicidality, and lower-level peer violence. This provides us the opportunity, at various touchpoints, to screen for risk and protective factors and apply assorted interventions in the health-care setting that can reduce or even remove these tragic events from our patients' lived experiences.

Take Home Points
- Medical centers are frequent, neutral touchpoints for children and youth at risk for experiencing or being exposed to violence, which affords an opportunity to intervene.
- Trauma-informed approaches, which include reducing blame and increasing control for patients and families, optimize the potential for successful interventions.
- "Locked and loaded" is only half of the story for child safety – locked, unloaded, and locked ammunition stored separately is the best option short of keeping the firearm out of the home entirely.
- Routine inquiry about suicidality, intimate partner violence (IPV), and firearm carrying/access is best if done universally, to avoid perceptions of "profiling" or stigma.
- Violence prevention programs which rely on scare tactics or require considerable exposure to others' traumatic experiences are not recommended as violence prevention strategies.
- Hospital-Based Violence Intervention Programs (HVIPs) are gaining in popularity but require significant investments and strong partnerships with community services to be effective.

Suggested Readings

1. Adhia A, Kernic M, Hemenway D, Vavilala M, Rivara F. Intimate partner homicide of adolescents. JAMA Pediatr. 2019;173(6):571–7.
2. Ahmedani B, Simon G, Stewart C, Beck A, Waitzfelder B, Rossom R, et al. Health care contacts in the year before suicide death. J Gen Intern Med. 2014;29(6):870–7.
3. Barkin S, Finch S, Ip E, Scheindlin B, Craig J, Steffes J, et al. Is office-based counseling about media use, timeouts, and firearm storage effective? Results from a cluster-randomized, controlled trial. Pediatrics. 2008;122(1):e15–25.
4. Becher EC, Christakis NA. Firearm injury prevention counseling: are we missing the mark? Pediatrics. 1999;104(3):530–5.
5. Butts J, Gouvis Roman C, Bostwick L, Porter J. Cure violence: a public health model to reduce gun violence. Annu Rev Public Health. 2015;36:39–53.
6. Carter PM, Walton MA, Roehler DR, Goldstick J, Zimmerman MA, Blow FC, et al. Firearm violence among high-risk emergency department youth after an assault injury. Pediatrics. 2015;135(5):805–15.
7. Chong VE, Smith R, Garcia A, Lee WS, Ashley L, Marks A, et al. Hospital-centered violence intervention programs: a cost-effectiveness analysis. Am J Surg. 2015;209(4):597–603.
8. Conway PM, Erlangsen A, Teasdale TW, Jakobsen IS, Larsen KJ. Predictive validity of the Columbia-suicide severity rating scale for short-term suicidal behavior: a Danish study of adolescents at a high risk of suicide. Arch Suicide Res. 2016;21(3):455–69.

 9. Cunningham R, Knox L, Fein J, Harrison S, Frisch K, Walton M, et al. Before and after the Trauma Bay: the prevention of violent injury among youth. Ann Emerg Med. 2008;53(4):490–500.
10. Cunningham RM, Walton MA, Goldstein A, Chermack ST, Shope JT, Raymond Bingham C, et al. Three-month follow-up of brief computerized and therapist interventions for alcohol and violence among teens. Acad Emerg Med. 2009;16(11):1193–207.
11. Dahlberg LL, Toal SB, Swahn M, Behrens CB. Measuring violence-related attitudes, behaviors, and influences among youths: a compendium of assessment tools. 2nd ed. Atlanta: Centers for Disease Control and Prevention, National Center for injury Prev Control; 2005.
12. David-Ferdon C, Haileyesus T, Liu Y, Simon T, Kresnow M. Nonfatal assaults among persons aged 10–24 years — United States, 2001–2015. Centers for Disease Control and Prevention MMWR. 2018;67(5):141–5.
13. Daviss W, Mooney D, Racusin R, Ford J, Fleischer A, McHugo G. Predicting posttraumatic stress after hospitalization for pediatric injury. J Am Acad Child Adolesc Psychiatry. 2000;39(5):576–83.
14. De Vries APJ, Kassam-Adams N, Cnaan A, Sherman-Slate E, Gallagher PR, Winston FK. Looking beyond the physical injury: posttraumatic stress disorder in children and parents after pediatric traffic injury. Pediatrics. 1999;104(6):1293–9.
15. Dowd MD, Sege R. Firearm-related injuries affecting the pediatric population. Pediatrics. 2012;130(5):e1416–e23.
16. DuRant R, Barkin S, Craig J, Weiley V, Ip E, Wasserman R. Firearm ownership and storage patterns among families with children who receive well-child care in pediatric offices. Pediatrics. 2007;119(6):e1271–9.
17. Fein JA, Kassam-Adams N, Gavin M, Huang R, Blanchard D, Datner EM. Persistence of posttraumatic stress in violently injured youth seen in the emergency department. Arch Pediatr Adolesc Med. 2002;156(8):836–40.
18. Fein JA, Kassam-Adams N, Vu T, Datner EM. Emergency department evaluation of acute stress disorder symptoms in violently injured youths. Ann Emerg Med. 2001;38(4):391–6.
19. Fein JA, Pailler M, Barg FK, Wintersteen M, Hayes K, Tien A, et al. Feasibility and effects of a web-based adolescent psychiatric assessment administered by clinical staff in the pediatric emergency department. Arch Pediatr Adolesc Med. 2010;164(12):1112–7.
20. Fischer K, Bakes K, Corbin T, Fein J, Harris E, James T, et al. Trauma-informed care for violently injured patients in the emergency department. Ann Emerg Med. 2019;73(2):193–202.
21. Fischer K, Schwimmer H, Purtle J, Roman D, Cosgrove S, Current J, et al. A content analysis of hospitals' community health needs assessments in the most violent U.S. cities. J Community Health. 2018;43:259–62.
22. Fowler K, Dahlberg L, Haileyesus T, Gutierrez C, Bacon S. Childhood firearm injuries in the United States. Pediatrics. 2017;140(1):1–11.
23. Gairin I, House A, Owens D. Attendance at the accident and emergency department in the year before suicide: retrospective study. Br J Psychiatry. 2003;183:28–33.
24. Gipson P, Agarwala P, Opperman K, Horwitz A, King C. Columbia-suicide severity rating scale: predictive validity with adolescent psychiatric emergency patients. Pediatr Emerg Care. 2015;31(2):88–94.
25. Goldberg AJ, Toto JM, Kulp HR, Lloyd ME, Gaughan JP, Seamon MJ, et al. An analysis of inner-city students' attitudes towards violence before and after participation in the "Cradle to grave" programme. Injury. 2010;41(1):110–5.
26. Goldstick JE, Carter PM, Walton MA, et al. Development of the SaFETy score: a clinical screening tool for predicting future firearm violence risk. Ann Intern Med. 2017;166(10):707–14.
27. Grossman DC, Mueller BA, Riedy C, et al. Gun storage practices and risk of youth suicide and unintentional firearm injuries. JAMA. 2005;293(6):707–14.
28. Hayes DN, Sege R. FiGHTS: a preliminary screening tool for adolescent firearms-carrying. Ann Emerg Med. 2003;42(6):798–807.

29. Health Research & Educational Trust. Hospital approaches to interrupt the cycle of violence. Chicago: Health Research & Educational Trust; 2015.
30. Hettema J, Steele J, Miller W. Motivational interviewing. Annu Rev Clin Psychol. 2005;1:91–111.
31. Hildenbrand AK, Kassam-Adams N, Barakat LP, Kohser KL, Ciesla JA, Delahanty DL, Fein JA, Ragsdale LB, Marsac ML. Posttraumatic Stress in Children After Injury: The Role of Acute Pain and Opioid Medication Use. Pediatr Emerg Care. 2020;36(10): e549–e557.
32. Juillard C, Smith R, Anaya N, Garcia A, Kahn JG, Dicker RA. Saving lives and saving money: hospital-based violence intervention is cost-effective. J Trauma Acute Care Surg. 2015;78(2):252–8.
33. Karraker N, Cunningham RK, Becker MG, Fein JA, Knox LM, editors. Violence is preventable: a best practices guide for launching and sustaining a hospital-based program to break the cycle of violence. Office of Victims of Crime, Office of Justice Programs, U.S. Department of Justice; 2011.
34. King CA, Grupp-Phelan J, Brent D, Dean JM, Webb M, Bridge JA, Spirito A, Chernick LS, Mahabee-Gittens EM, Mistry RD, Rea M, Keller A, Rogers A, Shenoi R, Cwik M, Busby DR, Casper TC; Pediatric Emergency Care Applied Research Network. Predicting 3-month risk for adolescent suicide attempts among pediatric emergency department patients. J Child Psychol Psychiatry. 2019;60(10):1055–64.
35. Ko SJ, Ford JD, Kassam-Adams N, Berkowitz SJ, Wilson C, Wong M, et al. Creating trauma-informed systems: child welfare, education, first responders, health care, juvenile justice. Prof Psychol Res Pract. 2008;39(4):396–404.
36. Kramer E, Dodington J, Hunt A, Henderson T, Nwabuo A, Dicker R, et al. Violent reinjury risk assessment instrument (VRRAI) for hospital-based violence intervention programs. J Surg Res. 2017;217:177-86.e2.
37. Lowe SR, Galea S, Uddin M, Koenen KC. Trajectories of posttraumatic stress among urban residents. Am J Community Psychol. 2014;53(1-2):159–72.
38. Manual for Compensation Assistance Pennsylvania Victims Compensation Assistance Program [Internet]. In: Pennsylvania Commission on Crime and Delinquency. 2018. Available from: https://www.pccd.pa.gov/Victim-Services/Documents/2018%20VCAP%20Manual.pdf.
39. Marsac ML, Kassam-Adams N, Hildenbrand AK, Nicholls E, Winston FK, Leff SS, et al. Implementing a trauma-informed approach in pediatric health care networks. JAMA Pediatr. 2016;170(1):70–7.
40. National Academies of Sciences Engineering and Medicine. Health systems interventions to prevent firearm injuries and death: proceedings of a workshop. Washington, DC: The National Academies Press; 2019.
41. Nonfatal Injury Data [Internet]. National Center for Injury Prevention and Control, Department of Health and Human Services. 2017. Available from: https://www.cdc.gov/injury/wisqars/nonfatal.html.
42. Pailler M, Fein JA. Computerized behavioral health screening in the emergency department. Pediatr Ann. 2009;38(3):156–60.
43. Pallin R, Spitzer S, Ranney M, Betz M, Wintemute G. Preventing firearm-related death and injury. Ann Intern Med. 2019;170(11):ITC81-ITC96.
44. Petrosino A, Turpin-Petrosino C, Hollis-Peel ME, Lavenberg JG. 'Scared Straight' and other juvenile awareness programs for preventing juvenile delinquency. Cochrane Database Syst Rev. 2013;20(4):CD002796.
45. Price J, Thompson A, Khubchandani J, Wiblishauser M, Dowling J, Teeple K. Perceived roles of emergency department physicians regarding anticipatory guidance on firearm safety. J Emerg Med. 2013;44(5):1007–16.
46. Purtle J, Cheney R, Wiebe DJ, Dicker R. Scared safe? Abandoning the use of fear in urban violence prevention programmes. Inj Prev. 2015;21(2):140–1.

47. Purtle J, Rich LJ, Bloom SL, Rich JA, Corbin TJ. Cost-benefit analysis simulation of a hospital-based violence intervention program. Am J Prev Med. 2015;48(2):162–9.
48. Rich J. Wrong place, wrong time: trauma and violence in the lives of young black men. Baltimore: Johns Hopkins University Press; 2009. p. 232.
49. Rowhani-Rahbar A, Simonetti J, Rivara F. Effectiveness of interventions to promote safe firearm storage. Epidemiol Rev. 2016;38:111–24.
50. Schwebel D, Lewis T, Simon T, Elliott M, Toomey S, Tortolero S, et al. Prevalence and correlates of firearm ownership in the homes of fifth graders: Birmingham, AL, Houston, TX, and Los Angeles, CA. Health Educ Behav. 2014;41(3):299–306.
51. Scott J, Azrael D, Miller M. Firearm Storage in Homes With Children With Self-Harm Risk Factors. Pediatrics. 2018;141(3):e20172600.
52. Sigel E. Violence risk screening: predicting cyber violence perpetration and victimization. J Adolesc Health. 2013;52:S53.
53. Simonetti J, Rowhani-Rahbar A, King C, Bennett E, Rivara F. Evaluation of a community-based safe firearm and ammunition storage intervention. Inj Prev. 2018;34:218–23.
54. UC Davis Health. What you can do initiative [Internet]. Available from: https://health.ucdavis.edu/what-you-can-do/.
55. Vasiliadis H, Ngamini-Ngui A, Lesage A. Factors associated with suicide in the month following contact with different types of health services in Quebec. Psychiatr Serv. 2015;66(2):121–6.
56. Walton MA, Chermack ST, Shope JT, Bingham CR, Zimmerman MA, Blow FC, et al. Effects of a brief intervention for reducing violence and alcohol misuse among adolescents: a randomized controlled trial. JAMA. 2010;304(5):527–35.
57. Weiss D, Kassam-Adams N, Murray C, Kohser KL, Fein JA, Winston FK, et al. Application of a framework to implement trauma-informed care throughout a pediatric health care network. J Contin Educ Heal Prof. 2017;37(1):55–60.
58. Wiebe DJ, Blackstone MM, Mollen CJ, Culyba AJ, Fein JA. Self-reported violence-related outcomes for adolescents within eight weeks of emergency department treatment for assault injury. J Adolesc Health. 2011;49(4):440–2.
59. Winston F, Kassam-Adams N. AfterTheInjury.org: Center for Injury and Prevention- Children's Hospital of Philadelphia; 2014. Available from: https://www.aftertheinjury.org/.
60. Wolk C, Van Pelt A, Jager-Hyman S, Ahmedani B, Zeber J, Fein J, et al. Stakeholder perspectives on implementing a firearm safety intervention in pediatric primary care as a universal suicide prevention strategy: a qualitative study. JAMA Network Open. 2018;1(7):e185309.

Chapter 9
Depression and Means Restriction

Zheala Qayyum and Cynthia Wilson

Second Parkland survivor to die by suicide is identified.
Mental health town hall Wednesday

By Monique O. Madan and David J. Neal
March 26, 2019. *Miami Herald*

9.1 Background

Depression is arguably one of the earliest described and most widely known psychiatric illnesses. It is often discussed in colloquial terms as having a down mood or a bad day. However, true clinical depressive disorders are distinct and diagnosable health conditions. The *Diagnostic and Statistical Manual of Mental Disorders, Fifth Edition: DSM-5* criteria for major depressive disorder are well defined and include many describable physical symptoms. The *DSM-5* defines major depressive disorder as depressed mood or loss of interest in daily activities for at least a period of 2 weeks representing a change from baseline and causing social, occupational, or educational dysfunction. A minimum of five of nine symptoms are required for diagnosis (see Table 9.1). The *DSM-5* further describes varying severities of illness as well as specifiers including anxious distress, melancholic features, psychotic features, peripartum onset, or seasonal pattern (for a full list, see the *DSM-5*) [1].

Other related diagnoses include persistent depressive disorder, bipolar disorder, depressive disorder due to another medical condition, and other depressive conditions. Persistent depressive disorder is a milder but more chronic form of

Z. Qayyum (✉)
Department of Psychiatry & Behavioral Sciences, Boston Children's Hospital,
Harvard Medical School, Boston, MA, USA

Department of Psychiatry, Yale University School of Medicine, New Haven, CT, USA
e-mail: zheala.qayyum@childrens.harvard.edu

C. Wilson
Department of Psychiatry, Yale University, New Haven, CT, USA

Table 9.1 Depression symptoms (five of nine required for depression diagnosis) [1]

1	Depressed mood or irritability most of the day nearly every day by either subjective report or observation by others
2	Decreased interest or pleasure in activities most days
3	Significant changes in weight or changes in appetite
4	Changes in sleep
5	Change in activity
6	Fatigue or loss of energy
7	Feelings of guilt and worthlessness
8	Diminished ability to concentrate
9	Suicidality

depression. Manic episodes consist of periods of time with symptoms including, but not limited to, decreased need for sleep, elevated or irritable mood, increased energy, and risk-taking behaviors. An individual with both manic and depressive episodes potentially has bipolar affective disorder. Children and adolescents can present with some or all the symptoms described. However, they can also manifest as greater levels of anger and irritability, increased emotional responses to small stressors, chronic low self-esteem and hopelessness, and unexplained aches, pain, and physical ailments without clear medical cause. Children and adolescents will not always describe their feelings as sadness, and clinicians must rely more on their professional inclinations and experience and less on subjective reports.

9.2 Depression Prevalence

The World Health Organization (WHO) indicates 10–20% of children worldwide experience a mental health condition. Neuropsychiatric conditions are the number one cause of disability for children and adolescents worldwide [2]. They estimate the global prevalence of depression in youth 15–19 years old is approximately 4.4% in females and 3.2% in males [3]. A 2015 meta-analysis reported a worldwide prevalence of 13.4% of any mental health condition in children and adolescents and 2.6% specifically for depression [4].

In the US, the Centers for Disease Control and Prevention (CDC) estimates 3.2% of children and youth 3–17 years old have been diagnosed with depression. This disorder often co-occurs with other mental health conditions common in childhood such as anxiety and attention deficit hyperactivity disorder (ADHD) [5]. Rates of depression in children increase with increasing age. The incidence in children 6–11 years old ranges from 0.5% to 0.75%. This increases eightfold for youth 12–18 years old, with the incidence of depression ranging from 2% to 4%. In the US, 80% of children with depression obtain mental health treatment, although there is a great deal of regional variability in the availability and types of mental health providers [5].

There are ethnic and racial disparities in rates of completed suicide in the US for youth. Understanding these ethnic and racial differences is crucial to understanding and implementing suicide prevention efforts. While American Indian and Alaskan Natives make up 1.3% of the US general population, their youth have the greatest rates of completed suicide. This is followed by rates for White youth, then Hispanic, Asian, Native Hawaiian, and Pacific Islanders and with the lowest rates in Black youth [6]. Since death records do not include one's sexual orientation or gender identity, the rates of completed suicide in LGBTQ youth is unknown. However, LGBTQ youth are known to be four to six times at greater risk of attempting suicide needing medical attention from a doctor or a nurse compared to heterosexual youth [7]. Ethic and racial and LGBTQ disparities warrant further research and attention and should factor into suicide risk assessments.

Although psychological and pharmacological treatments exist for depression, this condition can be treatment-resistant. Overall, up to 5–8% of patients with mental health disorders will attempt suicide [8]. The estimated prevalence of suicidal ideation, plans, and attempts among 13–18 year olds are 12.1%, 4.0%, and 4.1%, respectively [9]. Depression plays a role in more than one-half of all suicide attempts, and the lifetime risk of suicide among patients with untreated depression is nearly 20% [10]. In youth 15–29 years old, it was the second leading cause of death internationally and is the second leading cause of death in the US as well [11]. From 1999 to 2017, US suicide rates for 10–14 year old youth doubled and for 15–24 year old youth rates have increased approximately 50% [12].

9.3 Depression and Firearm Suicide

While depression and suicide have been described throughout antiquity, a consideration of how depression and risk of suicide relates to firearm ownership is a newer phenomenon. Worldwide, there are at least 875 million firearms, and 75% of them are owned by civilians [13]. The proportion of suicides involving firearms varies both by country and by gender. In the US, the proportion of suicides involving firearms was 56% for men and 31% in females in 2017 [14]. Given this large proportion of suicide by firearms, the association of firearm ownership and risk of suicide is a very important consideration.

Examining 2017 fatality data, in children 10–14 years old, suffocation was by far the most common means of suicide at 54%. However, firearms accounted for 36% of suicides in this age group. In 15–24 year olds, firearms account for approximately half of all suicides. In females, firearms are the mechanism of suicide in 17% of children 10–14 years old and increases to 26% in 15–24 year olds. Males are more likely than females across the life span to commit suicide by use of firearms. Boys 10–14 years old were almost equally as likely to commit suicide by suffocation and by firearms (51% vs. 44%). For males 15–24 years old, more than half (52%) of suicides are caused by firearms [15].

9.4   Comorbid Risk Factors

While depression and other mental health disorders are known to be risk factors for suicide, there are also many other notable risk factors. Suicide at times is an impulsive act in times of distress, without any known or diagnosable mental health condition. Other factors known to increase the risk of suicide include comorbid psychiatric diagnoses, family history of suicide, history of adverse child experiences and trauma, previous suicide attempts, use of alcohol and substance use, hopelessness, social isolation, financial and relationship losses, local epidemics, physical illness, recent discharge from an inpatient unit, exposure to the suicide of others, and easy access to lethal means. All these factors should be taken into account, and each risk factor should be also considered as part of the cumulative risk assessment.

As discussed in Chap. 2, firearms are quick, highly lethal, and irreversible; and therefore, are a major risk factor for those with any mental health disorder or other risk factors for suicide. The majority of suicidality is transitory, involves little planning, and are related to a short-term crisis. If youth can survive this crisis without access to lethal means, it is likely that they will opt not to make a suicide attempt. Even in situations in which another method of suicide is attempted, other means have a much lower lethality and can provide time for the individual to change their mind. Suicide attempts by non-firearm means, like an overdose, also allow time for the individual to tell someone and for medical care to be sought. Firearms often do not allow an individual to change his/her mind or obtain subsequent medical care. For comparison, almost 90% of suicide attempts with a firearm are fatal, compared to less than 5% with cutting or drug overdose [16]. While it is a common misperception that suicide is inevitable, it is known that the majority of people who survive a suicide attempt do not go on to die by suicide [17]. It is therefore crucial to take of the high lethality of firearms and firearm access into account when performing a risk assessment.

9.5   Inquiry by Medical Clinicians into Firearms in the Home and Clinical Considerations

Clinicians have an obligation to ensure the safety of their patients. Inquiring about the presence and storage of firearms in the household should constitute an integral part of any risk assessment for all patients (see Chaps. 7 & 8). However, greater exploration is warranted in cases of minors and young adults who have depression, anxiety, increased impulsivity, and disruptive and self-injurious behaviors. Particular attention should be paid to those with any previous suicide attempts. These assessments should incorporate identifying factors increasing the risk of suicide or self-injury; enhancing factors that promote safety; direct inquiry about suicidal thoughts, intent, plans, and aborted attempts; appropriate assessment of risk level; and thorough documentation (SAFE-T) (Table 9.2) [18, 19].

Table 9.2 Suicide Assessment Five-Step Evaluation and Triage (SAFE-T)

Identify risk factors: note those that can be modified to reduce risk
Identify protective factors: note those that can be enhanced
Conduct suicide inquiry: suicidal thoughts, plans, behavior, and intent
Determine risk level/intervention: determine risk – choose appropriate intervention to address and reduce risk
Document: assessment of risk, rationale, intervention, and follow-up

Used with permission of the Substance Abuse and Mental Health Services Administration (SAMHSA)

Many families and patients are cooperative with providing this critical information when the screening is presented as a standard part of providing optimal clinical care and in the context of anticipatory guidance for preventive health. Still, other families can be sensitive to the stigma around mental health and especially suicide. It is helpful for the clinician to explore the family's psychiatric history and their prior contact with mental health care to be able to provide more knowledge-informed care. At times, challenging experiences in the past may predispose the family in being guarded about seeking mental health treatment for their children. It can be helpful to frame psychiatric treatment as part of comprehensive medical care. Also, a family's cultural and religious ideology and perspective is important to respect and explore as it pertains to their hopes and fears about their child's mental health and their expectations about treatment and care.

It is also imperative to understand and respect the family's views and motivation for gun ownership. Some families may feel strongly about keeping firearms at home, or it may be the cultural and family norm. At other times, the guardian's professional or occupational responsibilities may necessitate firearm ownership, such as military families and those in law enforcement. It is important to understand the family's views and perspective in order to best delineate a safety plan that can realistically be followed by the patient and the family.

Clinicians should inquire the parent/caregiver of the pediatric patient directly about the type and number or firearms at home. This includes asking about firearms physically inside the home as well as those that may be easily accessible in other places (e.g., car, outdoor shed on the same property, relative's home). The use of handguns for suicide in adolescents doubled in urban and rural settings between 2005 to 2015, whereas long guns have been implicated in adolescent suicide in more rural settings [20].

Inquiries should include:

1. Where the firearms are stored

   - If stored in a safe, the type of safe and how it is secured (e.g., keylock, biometric lock)
   - If stored locked, what type of lock used (e.g., trigger lock)

2. Whether the firearms are loaded
3. Where the ammunition is stored (i.e., loaded in the gun, separately from the gun) and if locked away

Gun ownership has been shown to impact the mental health of children and adolescents in a gun owner's home. There is increased risk of aggression and aggressive thoughts [21]. A not widely discussed topic is the psychological effects of gun ownership in the home. One 2018 study reported gun ownership had adverse mental health effects on adolescents. This was found especially in females, with increased rates of depression in homes with gun ownership as well as feeling less safe in school [22]. Clinicians should discuss with families the increased safety risk access to firearms adds to depressed youth with suicidal ideation.

In adults with depression, a firearm in the home is also an increased risk factor for suicide. The lasting psychological effects on a child of the death of a parent, especially due to suicide, cannot be underestimated. We must also consider other secondary effects on children and adolescents when they lose a parent to suicide and do everything possible to minimize this risk. An additional consideration is that depression can affect attention, concentration, and motivation. It is likely given these symptoms, even if adults with depression did not consider the use of firearms to kill themselves, they potentially would not be as vigilant to these safety practices. This then increases the risk of unintentional injury to those around them. This also applies to the vigilance required when handling or cleaning a gun. Guns in the home also increase the risk of gun-related violence. While there are twice as many suicides in the US as homicides in the general population, it is still an important consideration.

9.6   Legal Considerations

It is important for clinicians to be aware of their own state laws and legislation regarding firearms. Federal laws impose minimum age restrictions on the sales of firearms, but do not regulate the storage of firearms, which relies on state legislation. Licensed dealers may not sell handguns and ammunition to individuals less than 21 years old, and long guns and ammunition may not be sold to individuals less than 18 years old. Remarkably, unlicensed sellers have lower restrictions: they may not sell handguns to individuals less than 18 years old, and there are no restrictions on the sale of long guns by age. Multiple state laws regulate the purchase and possession of handguns and long guns at different ages (for an up-to-date complete list by state, see Giffords Law Center to Prevent Gun Violence and statefirearmlaws.org) [23].

Child access prevention (CAP) laws vary by state, as there are no federal CAP laws. As of 2020, 25 states have some form of CAP law including 9 states with recklessness laws and 16 with varying forms of negligence laws (Fig. 9.1). Recklessness laws hold a firearm owner liable if a child injures another person, only if someone provided the firearm to the child. Of the three negligence law types, the narrowest are the "Child Uses" laws, which hold a firearm owner liable if a child accesses and uses an improperly stored firearm. The next type of negligence laws are the "Child Accesses" laws, which apply if a child accesses an improperly stored firearm, even if the child does not actually use the firearm. The final, most stringent type of negligence laws are the "Child Could Access" laws, which apply if a child

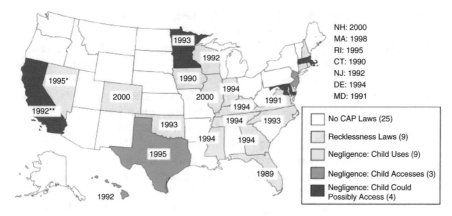

Fig. 9.1 Child access prevention laws by state, from Azad et al. [24]; used with permission

could potentially access an improperly stored firearm, regardless of whether they actually do. Recklessness laws do not appear to reduce the risk of child firearm fatalities, but negligence laws are associated with a 13% reduction in all-intent firearm fatalities, a 15% reduction in firearm homicides, a 12% reduction in firearm suicides, and a 13% reduction in unintentional firearm fatalities among children 0–14 years old [24]. Many states also require gunlocks, trigger locks, and other locking devices for the firearm to be provided at the time of firearm sale as another form of legislation focused on child safety.

Another category of law focuses on reducing high-risk individuals from owning or purchasing firearms. These extreme risk protection order (ERPO) laws prohibit the possession of firearms for persons who are imminent risk of harming themselves or others. In 2017, five states had these laws, and as of February 2020, 18 states had passed ERPO laws (see Fig. 7.4). These laws primarily allow family members to petition the courts to remove a firearm from a person they feel is at high risk of harm to themselves or others. If a judge agrees, the firearm may be removed up to 1 year, and the restriction may be reconsidered at that time. In some states, law enforcement and mental health providers may petition for removal. Knowledge of this law among clinicians and laypersons is important to potentially remove firearms from an individual at risk for suicide.

The voluntary transfer of firearms when a person is suicidal is another option. Though on the surface this is a straightforward manner of lethal means reduction, this option has challenges as well. First, the firearm owner must be willing to transfer (temporarily) the firearm during a crisis period. They may typically transfer the firearms to a family member, friend, gun retailer, or law enforcement organization. These transfers are only allowed for a limited period (1–30 days) depending on the state. Second, among the 20 states and the District of Columbia mandating universal background checks, only 14 states allow exemptions for transfers during suicide crisis periods. Third, there are potential concerns about liability associated with the transfer back of firearms, i.e., what if the person hurts themselves when the gun is given back? In reality, the liability is quite low because (1) the law places the legal responsibility of suicide on the person who attempted or killed themselves and (2) it is very difficult to sue people and organizations trying to do the right thing in these circumstances [25, 26]. Laws regarding seizures of weapons are limited to four states (CT, NY, IN, CA) as of 2020, allowing the police to obtain a warrant for removal of weapons from those who pose a risk to themselves or others. Firearm safety warrants can be obtained from the court when there is imminent risk of personal injury in these cases. Clinicians should utilize these resources if they feel the young patient is at risk for harming themselves or others [27].

An important consideration regarding state laws is if concerns for the safety of minors will warrant removal of weapons, since minors are not legally the owners of these firearms. In such circumstances, the clinician should explore options such as the recommendation for temporary removal of firearms from the home. In instances where the risk of suicide or harm to the minor is significant and state laws do not allow for removal of firearms from the home, child protective services in the state can be a source of support for the clinician in ensuring the safety of the minor. Additionally, when there is grave concern for suicidal ideation or depressive symptoms causing significant impairment of function or judgment, the youth may be legally committed for psychiatric evaluation or treatment in order to keep them safe. These laws for psychiatric commitment also vary across states in terms of who can request a psychiatric evaluation or commit the youth, as well as the length of psychiatric commitment.

9.7 Proposed Recommendations and Interventions for Primary Care Clinicians and Mental Health Clinicians

Primary care clinicians are often the first point of contact for families who have concerns about depressive symptoms or behavioral changes in their children. In times of crisis, initial calls for support and guidance are commonly made to primary care offices. Other times the family may not be aware of a patient's depression. In these instances, as well as when the parents have mental health concerns, the primary care clinician may be one of the first to make this diagnosis. However, for a sizeable portion of teen suicides, there has been no previous history of depression or prior indications of psychopathology. Among a cohort of 813 adolescents with initial suicide attempts, 29 (3.6%) died by suicide. Of these 29 youth, 20 died in the initial attempt (69%), and in these cases, 85% had used a gun [28]. It is therefore important for clinicians to make depression screening, risk assessment, and counseling regarding firearms, especially around safe storage, a standard part of clinical practice, regardless of a previous or known diagnosis of depression in the adolescent or young adult.

Incorporating depression screening regularly can facilitate early identification of youth who need referrals for mental health services. Beck's Depression Inventory and Asking Suicide-Screening Questions (ASQ) (see Fig. 8.1) screening tools are validated tools that can be utilized in the primary care setting [29, 30]. Mental health clinicians should focus on thorough risk assessments and safety planning to ensure the safety of the minor. In severe cases, when depressive symptoms are worsening or in the presence of expressed or implied suicidal ideation, the minor should be referred to a psychiatric facility or an emergency department for further evaluation for a higher level of psychiatric care.

Emergency department visits, and outpatient and inpatient psychiatric treatments are all venues for developing and revising safety plans for patients. This can be done by emergency department and mental health clinicians. However, it is best when these safety plans are initiated at the time of assessment and not at the time of a crisis. Safety plans should be written in a way that is easy for the patient and family to understand and follow. These should include coping strategies the minor can use when experiencing a suicidal crisis, as well as a commitment to the treatment process and staying alive.

The initial step is to work with the minor to identify the stressors and warning signs leading to worsening depressive symptoms that can progress to suicidal ideation. The patient should then identify coping strategies that can be used for self-regulation as well as strategies requiring the presence of supportive family members and friends. Specifically knowing how to contact supportive family members and friends as well utilizing crisis hotlines is important to document for each patient.

Means restriction should be discussed with families of children and youth with depression and risk of suicidal ideation by primary care, emergency department, and mental health clinicians. Low lethality means (e.g., pills) as well as high lethality means (e.g. firearms) should both be addressed. Unnecessary medications should be removed from the home, and other medications should be locked up in the home. Psycho-education should focus on safety planning not only for youth who have expressed suicidal ideation and have mood disorders, but also for those who are impulsive, have comorbid substance use disorders which may worsen impulsive behaviors, have anxiety or psychotic disorders, or exhibit disruptive and aggressive behaviors.

It is important to highlight that securing and locking up weapons does not differ much in households with kids having self-harm risk factors and those without. Approximately 7% of US children (4.6 million) live in homes in which at least one firearm is stored loaded and unlocked [31]. In a study by Scott et al., only 1 in 3 gun-owning parents keep their weapons secured whether their child had depression or other mental health concerns. In these cases, only 34.9% household stored the firearms locked and unloaded when their child had self-harm risk factors compared to 31.8% households with children who did not have a mental health history [32].

There may be legitimate concerns raised by families who own firearms regarding the need for protection in the home. While it is reasonable to have these concerns, studies have shown that for every one burglar/stranger shot in self-defense within the home, there are 37 suicides [33]. The risks and benefits should be thoughtfully explored and discussed with the family, since parents may underestimate the suicide risk of the child [34]. The immediate time period after discharge from a psychiatric hospitalization is a time that is high risk for suicide [35]. Recommendations should be made for removal of firearms in this immediate time frame to minimize the risk. This can be arranged by having the firearms stored temporarily at different locations, including with other family members. Parents in law enforcement also can lock and leave their firearms at their duty station and not bring them home. However, if parents are not able to remove the firearm from the physical home, then all necessary efforts should be made to ensure safe firearm storage.

It is important to note that not all families may be forthcoming about disclosing ownership of firearms, particularly in instances where they may feel judged by the clinical team, whom they perceive as having a personal or political agenda differing from their own point of view. Other families may receive the information and recommendation for firearm removal from the home but may not comply. In a study by Brent et al. in 2000, only one-quarter of families complied with the recommendation to remove firearms. This was particularly true for families who acquired firearms for protection and tended to store them loaded. However, the study also showed parents were three times as likely to remove firearms if their child had made a recent suicide attempt. This may be explained by the parental realization of the possibility of subsequent suicide attempts in their child or the possibility of suicide becoming a tangible reality.

It is often not common practice to counsel parents about the risks of firearms to those who do not own firearms at the time of contact or initial assessment. Given the understanding that parents may not be forthright about gun ownership, this should be reconsidered. It is imperative to directly communicate the risks of gun acquisition to parents of minors with depression at the outset, highlighting the compounding effect impulsivity paired with access can have in elevating suicide risk. It is also important to continue discussions of means restrictions, for guns and other means of suicide, at subsequent health visits. This allows for a continued open discussion, affording the parents the opportunity to weigh the risks against the benefits of gun ownership in the context of having an at-risk minor at home.

9.8 Approaches to Harm Prevention for Firearm Ownership

Firearms in the home are known to be a risk factor for intentional and unintentional injury in children and adolescents, including suicide. There is some evidence that depressive symptoms in parents increase the rates of gun ownership and decrease the rates of having the guns in the home stored securely, unloaded and locked, especially when the depressed parent is the mother [36]. Children and adolescents do not have fully developed frontal lobes and tend to be more impulsive than adults. In addition, they cannot always accurately assess risk and are drawn to risk taking behaviors. Thus, depression in children and adolescents is a risk factor for suicidal ideation, and while thoughts may be fleeting, increased impulsivity and access to highly lethal means such as firearms greatly increase this risk and are avoidable.

The only way to minimize this risk of death or injury from firearms is to eliminate firearms in the home and remove external access to firearms for the patient. Where there are firearms, there will always be potential danger to children and adolescents for self-harm. If complete removal of the firearm is not achievable by the family, then recommendations should be made for safely storing the firearm(s) in the home. Safe storage techniques include keeping firearms locked in a safe and storing the ammunition locked away separately. These techniques are the next best method to reduce this risk of self-harm by firearm. This applies not only to children and adolescents who live in the home but also to children and adolescents visiting the homes of friends or family members.

In order to engage the patient and family effectively, the clinician must meet them where they are – both mentally and emotionally, about their attitudes toward mental health, as well as about gun safety. This includes understanding the parent or family's reason for owning a gun and for why it is stored the way they report. Respect and understanding when openly expressed can help the clinician and family work toward a safety plan that can be agreed upon and most importantly followed to keep the child or adolescent safe. Reducing access to lethal means is a key component of any safety plan. Parents may show greater willingness to lock up firearms based on the clinician's advice rather than removing them [34].

Helping parents with concrete measures for safe forearm storage and ongoing counseling about firearm safety can be very helpful. This can also facilitate their engagement and adherence to mental health treatment and related recommendations. The safety plan for secure firearm storage in the home of a youth with depression and suicidal ideation should focus on minimizing access, particularly when the minor feels overwhelmed, in a crisis, or acts impulsively in the direction of self-harm or suicide.

There are also technological advances in gun safety and storage. These include biometric safes and smart gun technology, which prevent access to weapons by non-firearm owners. Biometric and keypad access gun boxes and safes can provide access to a firearm in seconds. Biometric locks and safes range in price. As a result, firearm owners might not have universal access to these due to local availability and cost. The so-called smart guns can recognize the owner and cannot be used by non-owners (e.g., adolescents). Unfortunately, these are not currently available for sale in the US but are available in Europe (see Chap. 12).

Provisions of safety devices for gun storage, such a gunlock boxes and gun safes, have been shown to improve safer firearm storage practices [37]. Inexpensive interventions such as providing families with trigger locks and working toward a plan to keep the firearms hidden and inaccessible to the minor can also be beneficial. It is important to educate families that parental perceptions of their children and adolescents' lack of awareness of the home location of firearms or where keys or combinations are kept may be inaccurate. In other words, parents may think their children does not know where the guns and keys to the safes and locks are – when in fact the children do. This necessitates greater vigilance on the part of parents if they chose to keep guns in the home [38]. These are all important aspects of preventing the child or teen from unauthorized use of the gun to commit suicide.

Another important aspect when considering access to firearms in depressed youth is related to relatives with firearms. Most firearms used in adolescent suicide belonged to family members, most commonly their parents, but in some instances, firearms were accessed from friends, roommates, or close relatives [39, 40]. Hence, it is important to know about close relatives with firearms in their home and to inquire about other places from where the minor can access firearms.

9.9   Practical Tips for Primary Care Clinicians

For the pediatric primary care clinician, we recommend including the following screening and anticipatory guidance tools for suicide harm prevention:

1. *Depression screening*: Standardized screening instruments like ASQ, Beck's Depression Inventory
2. *Other risk screening*: ADHD, impulsivity, substance use, psychosis, parental mental illness, prior suicide attempt
3. *Safety planning*: Limit access to firearms including recommendations for removal, lock box for medications, SAFE-T, national suicide hotline number (1-800-273-8255/text HOME to 741741), Crisis hotline 211
4. *Discussion points for lethal means restriction*:

   - Are there firearms at home? *Discussion about risk to the minor and recommendation for removal and storage elsewhere.*
   - If family maintains that firearms remain stored at home: Where and how are they stored? *Recommend storing firearm unloaded, with firearm and ammunition locked away separately.*
   - What kind of safe or lock box is used? Where are the keys and combination code and who has access? *Recommend safe storage and biometric locks.*
   - Where is the ammunition stored? *Should be stored and locked separately.*
   - Are there friends or relatives with firearms that minor has access to? *Recommendations for closer supervision and monitoring of visits and access to these households.*
   - Is there great risk to the minor that is not mitigated with these safety measures? *Emergency psychiatric evaluation, contact local law enforcement for support in removal of firearms.*

9.10   Conclusions

Children and adolescents are a vulnerable population who are at risk for suicide as one possible outcome if they have depression. Still it must be remembered that 50% of patients who commit suicide did not have a known history of mental illness. Suicide attempts with firearms have significantly greater lethality than other means of suicide. It is incumbent upon primary care and mental health clinicians to ensure the safety of these youth and to work with the patient and their family to limit their access to firearms. Understanding the family's motivation and perspectives for owning firearms is also important in providing appropriate psycho-education about recognizing worsening depressive symptoms suicidal ideation and around safe firearm storage. In instances where the clinician has significant concerns about the presence of firearms in the home of a youth at risk for suicide, knowledge of state laws can assist them in taking appropriate actions in ensuring their safety.

Take Home Points
- Depression and other mental health disorders are risk factors for suicide; however, 50% of individuals who commit suicide had no prior history of a mental health disorder.
- Firearms are a common means for suicide in children and youth, and there is increased use in teenagers and young adults and in males.
- Firearms are the most lethal mechanism of suicide attempts, resulting in fatality >90% of the time. Unlike other means, firearm suicide attempts usually do not allow the individual time to tell someone or seek medical care.
- Lethal means restriction for firearms ideally with removal of firearms from the home, as well as removal of other means (e.g., medications), is one important primary prevention strategy for youth suicide.
- Primary care, emergency medicine, and mental health clinicians should screen for suicide risk factors and firearm access and provide guidance on lethal means restriction as part of suicide harm prevention.
- Knowledge of state laws (e.g., extreme risk protection order laws) can assist providers in taking appropriate action, including the possible removal of firearms from the home, to decrease the risk of firearm suicide for potentially at-risk youth.

References

1. American Psychiatric Association. Diagnostic and statistical manual of mental disorders. 5th ed. Arlington: American Psychiatric Publishing; 2013.
2. World Health Organization. Improving the mental and brain health of children and adolescents [Internet]. https://www.who.int/mental_health/maternal-child/child_adolescent/en/. Accessed 19 Sept 2019.
3. Depression and Other Common Mental Disorders: Global Health Estimates. Geneva: World Health Organization; 2017. Licence: CC BY-NC-SA 3.0 IGO.
4. Polanczyk GV, Salum GA, Sugaya LS, Caye A, Rohde LA. Annual research review: a meta-analysis of the worldwide prevalence of mental disorders in children and adolescents. J Child Psychol Psychiatry Allied Discip. 2015;56:345–65.
5. Center for Disease Control and Prevention. Data and Statistics on Children's Mental Health [Internet]. https://www.cdc.gov/childrensmentalhealth/data.html. Accessed 19 Sept 2019.

6. Suicide Prevention Resource Center. Racial and Ethnic Disparities [Internet]. http://www.sprc.org/racial-ethnic-disparities. Accessed 10 Mar 2020.
7. Aranmolate R, Bogan DR, Hoard T, Mawson AR. Suicide risk factors among LGBTQ youth: review. JSM Schizophr. 2017;2(2):1011.
8. Bråtvik L. Suicide risk and mental disorders. Int J Environ Res Public Health. 2018;15(9):2028.
9. Nock MK, Green JG, Hwang I, McLaughlin KA, Sampson NA, Zaslavsky AM, et al. Prevalence, correlates, and treatment of lifetime suicidal behavior among adolescents: results from the national comorbidity survey replication adolescent supplement. JAMA Psychiat. 2013;70(3):300–10.
10. Petersen TJ. Handbook of depression. Gotlib IH, Hammen CL, editor. Guilford Press: London; 2002. p. 624. Psychol Med. 2003.
11. World Health Organization. Depression [Internet]. January 2020. https://www.who.int/en/news-room/fact-sheets/detail/depression. Accessed 19 Sept 2019.
12. Hedegaard H, Curtin SC, Warner M. Suicide rates in the United States continue to increase [Internet]. NCHS Data Brief, no 309. Hyattsville, MD: National Center for Health Statistics. 2018 https://www.cdc.gov/nchs/products/databriefs/db309.htm. Accessed 19 Sept 2019.
13. World Health Organization. Guns, knives and pesticides: reducing access to lethal means [Internet]. 2009. https://apps.who.int/iris/bitstream/handle/10665/44060/9789241597739_eng.pdf.
14. National Institute of Mental Health. Suicide [Internet]. https://www.nimh.nih.gov/health/statistics/suicide.shtml#part_154971. Accessed 8 Mar 2020.
15. Center for Disease Control and Prevention. WISQARS [Internet]. https://webappa.cdc.gov/sasweb/ncipc/mortrate.html.
16. Conner A, Azrael D, Miller M. Suicide case-fatality rates in the United States, 2007 to 2014 a nationwide population-based study. Ann Intern Med. 2019;171(12):885–95.
17. Owens D, Horrocks J, House A. Fatal and non-fatal repetition of self-harm. Systematic review. Br J Psychiatry. 2002;181:193–9.
18. Shaffer D, Pfeffer CR, Bernet W, Arnold V, Beitchman J, Benson RS, et al. Practice parameter for the assessment and treatment of children and adolescents with suicidal behavior. J Am Acad Child Adolesc Psychiatry. 2001;40(7 Suppl):24S–51S.
19. SAFE-T [Internet]. https://www.integration.samhsa.gov/images/res/SAFE_T.pdf.
20. Hanlon TJ, Barber C, Azrael D, Miller M. Type of firearm used in suicides: findings from 13 states in the national violent death reporting system, 2005–2015. J Adolesc Health. 2019;65(3):366–70.
21. Benjamin AJ, Kepes S, Bushman BJ. Effects of weapons on aggressive thoughts, angry feelings, hostile appraisals, and aggressive behavior: a meta-analytic review of the weapons effect literature. Personal Soc Psychol Rev. 2018;22(4):347–77.
22. Kim J. Beyond the trigger: the mental health consequences of in-home firearm access among children of gun owners. Soc Sci Med. 2018;203:51–9.
23. Giffords Law Center to Prevent Gun Violence. Minimum Age to Purchase & Possess [Internet]. https://lawcenter.giffords.org/gun-laws/policy-areas/who-can-have-a-gun/minimum-age/
24. Azad HA, Monteaux MC, Rees CA, Siegel M, Mannix R, Lee LK, Sheehan KM, Fleegler EW. Child Access Prevention Firearm Laws and Firearm Fatalities Among Children Aged 0 to 14 Years, 1991-2016. JAMA Pediatr. 2020;174(5):463–469.
25. Gibbons MJ, Fan MD, Rowhani-Rahbar A, Rivara FP. Legal Liability for Returning Firearms to Suicidal Persons Who Voluntarily Surrender Them in 50 US States. Am J Public Health. 2020;110(5):685–688.
26. Fleegler EW, Madeira JL. First, prevent harm: eliminate firearm transfer liability as a lethal means reduction strategy. American journal of public health. 2020 May 1;110(5):619–20.
27. Rose V. OLR Research Report. Summary of Conneticut gun laws [Internet]. 2013 https://www.cga.ct.gov/2013/rpt/2013-R-0001.html.
28. McKean AJS, Pabbati CP, Geske JR, Bostwick JM. Rethinking lethality in youth suicide attempts: first suicide attempt outcomes in youth ages 10 to 24. J Am Acad Child Adolesc Psychiatry. 2018;57(10):786–91.

29. National Institute of Mental Health. Ask Suicide-Screening Questions (ASQ) Toolkit [Internet]. https://www.nimh.nih.gov/research/research-conducted-at-nimh/asq-toolkit-materials/index.shtml.
30. Beck AT, Ward CH, Mendelson M, Mock J, Erbaugh J. An inventory for measuring depression. Arch Gen Psychiatry. 1961;4:561–71.
31. Azrael D, Cohen J, Salhi C, Miller M. Firearm storage in gun-owning households with children: results of a 2015 national survey. J Urban Heal. 2018;95(3):295–304.
32. Scott J, Azrael D, Miller M. Firearm storage in homes with children with self-harm risk factors. Pediatrics. 2018;141(3):e20172600.
33. Kellermann AL, Reay DT. Protection or peril? An analysis of firearm-related deaths in the home. N Engl J Med. 1986;314(24):1557–60.
34. Brent DA, Baugher M, Birmaher B, Kolko DJ, Bridge J. Compliance with recommendations to remove firearms in families participating in a clinical trial for adolescent depression. J Am Acad Child Adolesc Psychiatry. 2000;39(10):1220–6.
35. Chung DT, Ryan CJ, Hadzi-Pavlovic D, Singh SP, Stanton C, Large MM. Suicide rates after discharge from psychiatric facilities: a systematic review and meta-analysis. JAMA Psychiat. 2017;74(7):694–702.
36. Morrissey TW. Parents' depressive symptoms and gun, fire, and motor vehicle safety practices. Matern Child Health J. 2016;20(4):799–807.
37. Carbone PS, Clemens CJ, Ball TM. Effectiveness of gun-safety counseling and a gun lock giveaway in a Hispanic community. Arch Pediatr Adolesc Med. 2005;159(11):1049–54.
38. Baxley F, Miller M. Parental misperceptions about children and firearms. Arch Pediatr Adolesc Med. 2006;160(5):542–7.
39. Johnson RM, Barber C, Azrael D, Clark DE, Hemenway D. Who are the owners of firearms used in adolescent suicides? Suicide Life-Threatening Behav. 2010;40(6):609–11.
40. Wright MA, Wintemute GJ, Claire BE. Gun suicide by young people in California: descriptive epidemiology and gun ownership. J Adolesc Health. 2008;43(6):619–22.

Chapter 10
Caring for Pediatric Patients After Gun Violence

Judy Schaechter and Michael P. Hirsh

> Hidden toll of Chicago's gun violence: $447 million in hospital bills over seven years
>
> By Jennifer Smith Richards, Annie Sweeney, and Jason Meisner July 21, 2017. *Chicago Tribune*

Firearm injury, prevention and treatment are under-researched and incompletely understood. This is particularly true for pediatric firearm injuries. The evidence to guide clinicians in the posthospitalization care for children and adolescents after exposure to firearm injury is very limited. Thus, care for youth after shootings is guided by other available evidence, mostly from similar traumas, clinical expertise, and the individual needs of presenting patients and families.

Care for a child or adolescent after gun violence considers the physical, developmental, behavioral, and psychosocial needs of the patient, the family, and the community. Physical needs will vary based on injury characteristics including injury location, severity, and physical sequelae, as well as the patient's premorbid condition and developmental stage. Psychosocial considerations are also diverse and particularly influenced by the intent and circumstances of the gun violence, as well as by individual, systemic and environmental characteristics, including supports, stressors, and resilience.

The treating clinician can optimize short- and long-term outcomes with careful assessment of the patient's comprehensive needs, facilitation of collaboration among the patient's multidisciplinary support team, and ongoing communication with the family. The primary care clinician is positioned to coordinate and prioritize needed services, including rehabilitative medicine, pain management, home health,

J. Schaechter (✉)
Department of Pediatrics, University of Miami, Miller School of Medicine, Miami, FL, USA
e-mail: jschaechter@miami.edu

M. P. Hirsh
Department of Surgery, University of Massachusetts Medical School, Worcester, MA, USA
e-mail: Michael.Hirsh@umassmemorial.org

© Springer Nature Switzerland AG 2021
L. K. Lee, E. W. Fleegler (eds.), *Pediatric Firearm Injuries and Fatalities*,
https://doi.org/10.1007/978-3-030-62245-9_10

physical therapy, occupational therapy, psychology, psychiatry, surgical follow-up, and organ-specific consultants. Integration with social supports, inclusive of school, friends, and faith-based networks can help families with healing. Medical care and social system navigation after a violent injury can be challenging, even more so for those with lower socioeconomic status and complex medical needs, such as patients requiring new ambulation or respiratory supports, ramps and other physical alterations to their home. Primary care clinicians can assist families to find needed social work services, transportation, and parental respite care.

Gun violence is an extremely disruptive trauma – both physically and emotionally. It causes tearing of tissue, permanently destroys organ function, changes relationships, and upends psychological well-being. All these things can impact a child's developmental trajectory and long-term physical and emotional health. Aiding families by identifying strengths, increasing resilience, and assisting children in reaching their full potential is of utmost importance. Health-care clinicians can help families chart a new, adjusted course and support them through unexpected challenges.

10.1 Physical Healing

10.1.1 The Wound

Firearm injury is frequently fatal. Over 90% of suicide attempts with a firearm end in death. The case fatality rate for firearm assault injury is 22%, far higher than other serious traumas or assaults by other means. For those who survive a shooting, post-hospitalization management of these injuries can be complex and may not result in complete physical healing and return to prior levels of independent functioning. The injury location and initial tissue damage can help to predict physical consequences. While some superficial wounds may affect physical function minimally, nearly half of children hospitalized with non-fatal injuries were discharged with a disability. Gunshot injuries of the extremities are the most frequent cause of short-term disability, although nerve palsies, joint limitations, and chronic pain may also not resolve quickly. Long-term physical disability is most frequently associated with central nervous system injury. Penetrating brain trauma can result in seizure disorders, paralysis, headache, and cognitive changes, and up to 27% of patients have associated eye injuries.

10.1.2 Infection Risk, Prevention, and Management

Traumatically injured patients are at increased risk of infection due to impaired host defenses and tissue violation from the penetrating gunshot wound. The readmission rate after firearm injury for children under 18 years old is 6.2%, higher than the national average of 5.7% for all postoperative patients. Infection is among the most common reasons for hospital readmission.

Children injured by firearms will often be discharged with incompletely healed wounds. Injured sites may require lengthy secondary intention closure. Families should be well-apprised in the care of such wounds. Some caregivers may require home health assistance for dressing changes and drainage checks. The primary care clinician coordinates close communication with the surgical team, home health, and family members to be certain the correct techniques are used to prevent infection and the site is assessed frequently, whether in person or via telehealth. Such attention may hasten healing and reduce the frequency of hospital readmission due to infection.

Infection risk exists for secondary sites as well. People injured by firearms experience more pressure ulcer episodes per year than those similarly injured in motor vehicle crashes. Follow-up medical assessments of firearm-injured children should include full-body inspection with attention to thinning, reddening, or warmth of the skin, particularly in dependent areas. Partnership with families is essential, to help caregivers assist with the necessary frequent position changes and use of appropriate cushioning. Patients who can move independently or with assistance should be encouraged to do so as early and often as possible.

10.1.3   Pain Management

Optimal treatment of pain not only affects how a child feels but also is critical to the recovery process. Pain and infection risk are linked, as poorly controlled pain may lead to splinting, inadequate aeration, and poor clearance of pulmonary secretions, placing patients at risk of secondary pneumonia. Pain has also been associated with increased incidence of PTSD and depression. Despite these concerns, there is evidence that a significant proportion of trauma patients, and children in particular, receive inadequate pain control, both at the time of injury and later in their recovery course.

Postoperative pain management is usually initiated by the surgical team. Discharge planning should consider the need for adequate pain control in balance with attention to inherent potential risks of the medications prescribed. Follow-up is necessary to assure appropriate adherence and adjustment of tapers, if necessary. Pain inhibits healing physically and psychologically. Even a year after injury, half of adult trauma patients still experience pain, and a quarter use pain control medications. While children's experience of pain after firearm injury is understudied compared to adults, there is consensus that pain assessment and treatment is a disparity health issue. The pain management needs of very young children and underrepresented minorities are even more underestimated, and they more frequently receive insufficient pain medication.

Attention to how implicit bias in the assessment and prescription of pain medications for children is essential. Pain assessments by care providers correlates poorly with patient self-assessment. Injury severity scores are also not predictive of pain. However, parental estimates of pain do strongly correlate with both the child's assessment and pain scoring tools. Several pain-level screening tools have been validated in verbal and preverbal children (e.g., Faces/FPS-R, color analog, FLACC). Clinicians seeking to reduce bias, more accurately determine pain, and follow change over time are encouraged to utilize these validated tools.

Finding the right treatment is also key. A year after presenting trauma, 12.5% of adolescent patients (12–18 years old) continued to use prescription opioids. The leading predictors of prolonged opioid use were pre-trauma marijuana use and higher pain score at the time of injury. Increased awareness and state regulations aim to reduce overall opioid prescriptions, number of pills dispensed, and prescription refills. In addition, alternative medications are available and often preferable, particularly in the outpatient setting. A randomized controlled clinical trial for the treatment of pain after acute musculoskeletal injury in children (6–17 years old) which compared acetaminophen/codeine and ibuprofen concluded pain relief was best achieved with ibuprofen, whereas codeine approximated acetaminophen in its effect.

Narcotics, both strong and effective, may sometimes be needed to treat pain. If opioids are used, the course should be brief, with an identified transition to alternative pain management either before discharge or soon after in the outpatient setting. In the setting of depression or past suicide attempts, all medications should be kept locked away from children and administered by an adult to the injured child as needed. Consultation with a pain treatment specialist and consideration of methodologies such as nerve blocks and vibratory stimulation can be considered. Pain management is not solely pharmacological, but may also incorporate non-pharmacologic treatments, including acupressure/acupuncture, hypnosis, mindfulness, massage, distraction, hot/cold applications, and other complementary therapies. Alternative and multimodal treatments are particularly important for patients with chronic pain and phantom pain.

Mental health issues are associated with pain. Depression, anxiety, and pain can be interrelated and disruptive of function, and interfere with sleep and social and academic activities. In such cases, management of the affective disorder is essential to pain relief. The primary care clinician will assess patients for pain and comorbidities thoroughly as part of the physical and mental recovery after a firearm injury.

10.1.4   Functional Disabilities

Chronic sequelae are common and vary by location and severity of the injury. Gunshot wounds may lead to amputations or limb impairment, including paralysis and limp, brain damage, personality change, and dependence on assist devices, including, but not limited to, tracheostomies, ventilators, feeding tubes, gastrostomy bags, and urinary catheters. Patients with pulmonary and neurologic injury often experience recurrent pneumonias, particularly due to aspiration. Nonambulatory and paraplegic patients are at high risk for decubitus ulcers. Rapid growth during childhood and adolescence merits frequent reassessment of wheelchair fit or accommodation of other assist devices. Patients with damage to the genitourinary system face complications of more frequent urinary tract infections and vesicoureteral reflux. High functioning patients with brain damage and/or personality changes may present with increased risk taking, such as drug use, aggression and interpersonal conflicts, unsafe sex, and injury recidivism. Thus, connection to a medical home, where the patient is known and receives close follow-up, with rapid and careful attention to concerns is essential. Medical visits may be advised more frequently than those recommended for healthy children to attend to physical, emotional, and social needs. Anticipatory care is essential.

10.1.5 The Bullet

A retained bullet fragment (RBF) is associated with mood disorder and dysfunction in patients. Parents may experience anxiety that displacement could result in increased tissue injury. As bullets are comprised primarily of lead, a concern receiving increasing attention is whether the risk of lead due to retained bullet(s) should be monitored. Cases of lead toxicity requiring debridement and chelation have been reported. More recently, lead-level surveillance among adults found 5% of the highest lead levels (>80 ug/dl) were in persons with RBFs. Persons with elevated lead levels associated with RBF were significantly younger (16–24 years old) than those with lead elevations related to occupational exposures. Given these findings and that symptoms of lead toxicity may be nonspecific, baseline and periodic lead level screening and a heightened index of clinical suspicion regarding symptoms are warranted.

10.2 Mental Health, Development, and Behavior After Gunshot Wounds

Trauma, and most significantly, the experience of violence, are associated with elevated rates of mood disorders, including depression, anxiety, and post-traumatic stress disorder (PTSD), as well as substance abuse. In such cases, substance abuse may be a form of self-medication for the internalizing conditions or untreated physical pain. The importance of periodic screening for depression, anxiety, PTSD, and substance use is heightened in these patients. Patients with affective disorders and brain damage or living in stressed environments may present with flat affect and based on cultural norms and individual factors may verbally deny their symptoms. Validated screening tools such as the PHQ-9, Columbia Depression Inventory, SCARED, GAD, and CPSS can help providers establish a baseline and track progress or challenge over time, including in response to therapeutic adjustments.

10.2.1 Depression and Anxiety

Trauma is associated with both intrinsic and extrinsic behavioral changes. Risk and expression may vary by gender, socioeconomic supports, developmental stage, and the severity, context, and chronicity of the traumatic insult. Mental health conditions prior to the injury as well as family history of mental health concerns may affect outcomes. Depression and anxiety are frequent comorbidities of violent trauma. There is a significant risk of suicidality, which should be screened for directly. Both require careful assessment and treatment, sometime multimodal, inclusive of medication, counseling, supportive sleep, and activity routines. Social and spiritual connections may help many patients. Depression and anxiety may exist in the same patient. Panic attacks often complicate anxiety. The astute clinician will screen for these and be alert to physical manifestations such as vital sign changes and symptoms such as chest tightness, palpitations, and dizziness.

Treatment plans for patients who screen positively on mental health disorder screening should be individually tailored and attuned to symptom severity. They should also consider the patient's ability to access effective counseling (such as cognitive behavioral therapy, family functional therapy) and the patient and caregivers' acceptance of both medical management and counseling. Clinicians caring for patients with gunshot wounds will need to be cognizant of community resources, including locations for sliding fee psychology, social work, support groups, bereavement centers, and engaged clergy.

10.2.2 Developmental Considerations

Child development begins before birth and continues into young adulthood. Trauma, be it psychological or physical, can disrupt or even regress the normal developmental trajectory. Successive developmental milestones come in rapid succession when children are very young. Delays in development may be more difficult to detect as children progress through the school-age years and adolescence. Physical injury will cause delays in fine and gross motor function. Cognitive injury will require careful assessment through psychoeducational testing, often without an established baseline for patients who were never tested before. Emotional disruption may present with developmental delay and functional changes, such as irritability, sensitivity, concentration and attention disorders, enuresis, and sleep issues. Young patients may demonstrate attachment problems. The effects of trauma extend throughout childhood and into adulthood, though the expression in older children and adolescents may differ.

10.2.3 Behavior Changes After Gunshot Wounds

School avoidance may also occur among victims of gun violence. The reasons for this are self-evident if a recent shooting took place at a child's school or at another school in the vicinity or even if reported through the media. Such avoidance may also occur for firearm injury victims who were shot elsewhere. Such survivors may have multiple concerns, such as reluctance to answer questions about the shooting, the circumstances, the nature of their injuries, or to face people they believe may have been involved in the shooting. They may feel social pressures related to their altered condition, be that due to physical, emotional, or cognitive change. Siblings and peers who lost a friend may also present with school avoidance and social anxiety. These children should be assessed and supported. Health-care clinicians can work with schools to assist in the return of a patient and help other student with adjustment after a shooting in their community. Changing of schools may sometimes be necessary, though such decisions ought to incorporate the desires of the patient and consider the additional burdens this kind of change might place on families.

10.2.4 Post-traumatic Stress Disorder

The prevalence of post-traumatic stress disorder (PTSD) following pediatric gunshot wounds is not well established but may be the most common psychological consequence of such events. In a study of children 7–17 years old who experienced unintentional trauma, nearly 30% reported symptoms consistent with full or partial PTSD. Another study found for children experiencing even mild or moderate physical trauma, 38% will still have symptoms of PTSD at 18 months post-event. Half of children exposed to violence, even in the absence of physical injury, report symptoms of PTSD.

When asked, children will often describe intrusive thoughts, including nightmares, flashbacks, and triggers, which seem like the event is real or repeating. They may have difficulty concentrating and sleeping and be emotionally labile. For many victims, the firearm injury was neither an isolated event nor the first trauma they experienced. The injury may have occurred in a context of family or community violence. Such exposures are associated with more pre-injury psychopathology as well as higher levels of parental distress, at times inhibiting a caretaker's ability to support the child.

Shootings and intimidation with violence may be common in a patient's environment, though they are neither normative nor part of an emotionally healthy life. Some patients live with a clustering of toxic stress risk factors, including shelter instability, food scarcity, family drug use, violence, mental health challenges and racism. Patients should be screened for other adverse childhood experiences (ACEs), which can impede recovery. PTSD screening tools, such as the Clinician-Administered PTSD Scale for Children and Adolescents (CAPS-CA) or Child PTSD Symptom Scale (CPSS), are useful. Some have found that screening tools at injury presentation or before discharge may predict likelihood for PTSD.

Children live within families and generally thrive when those families are supportive and have emotional stability. The family environment can moderate the likelihood of PTSD and other child developmental outcomes. Assessment of parental PTSD, depression, and functioning and connection to care if warranted helps the child. Family-focused interventions can increase youth resilience in the context of trauma.

10.2.5 Grief and Adjustment

Firearm injury can change everything – relationships, family integrity, sense of security, and life plans. Even children and youth with relatively minor firearm injuries can experience major life changes. Patients who had planned on a college sports scholarship may no longer be able to run or throw long. Dancers may be immobilized. Budding engineers or premed students may have debilitating headaches or difficulties with concentration. The challenge of adjusting goals and expectations will require time, resilience, and encouragement. The pediatric clinician can assist an adjusting patient with community resources and supports.

Children injured by firearms are often not the only victims in the shooting event. A child shot by a friend or family may lose that person to the same shooting event, to the court system, or to revenge violence. Mass shootings cause the deaths of multiple people, many of whom were acquaintances or have shared similarities and common experiences. Patients may develop "survivor's guilt" and may ask themselves why they lived when someone else didn't. They may fear they will be targeted again. They may harbor anger that they were not protected. Research has not yet elucidated all the varied reactions, adaptations to the stages of grief, or how one's childhood development colors those emotional experiences. It is critical that witnesses to shootings and those on either side of a gun are supported with counseling, friends, trusted adults, time and space to heal, and wherever possible, action steps to prevent continued violence.

10.3 When the Child Is Also the Shooter

When young children less than 10 years old are shot, the most common offender is the child himself or someone close to him, including siblings, other relatives, and friends. Self-inflicted gunshot wounds may be intentional or unintentional. There is little to no research on the effect of nonfatally shooting oneself. The effect of shooting a family member, be that a sibling, a parent, or a cousin, can be devastating. Adults who experienced shooting someone as children have described the long-term effects on the family and themselves, including drug use, school drop-out, and unrelenting guilt in the media. These anecdotes stand alone, as there is no research on the long-term outcomes for child offenders in family or friend shootings.

10.3.1 After a Suicide Attempt

Two-thirds of all firearm deaths are suicides (see Chap. 2). Though the proportion is less in children, suicide remains the second leading cause of death for children 1–18 years old, and over 40% of all suicides involve a firearm. Most youth who attempt suicide by firearm do so with a weapon kept in the home or by a family member. Suicide attempts by firearm are fatal over 90% of the time. When it is not fatal, attention must be paid to the surviving child's depression and risk for subsequent attempts. Adolescents who attempted suicide with a firearm and survived are more likely to commit suicide and die, compared to teens who attempted with other means. Such patients can benefit from a combination of medication, counseling, exercise, social supports, school connectivity, and close follow-up. Family should be counseled about means restriction to eliminate any future access to firearms, be it the weapon that was used, others in the home, or guns kept by family and friends in homes where the child or adolescent visits. In addition, family should be counseled about means restriction for other mechanisms of committing suicide (e.g., medications, knives) (see Chap. 9).

A nonfatal suicide attempt may be highly disfiguring, particularly to the head and neck if that is where the youth shot himself/herself. Beyond the physical care needed, patients may struggle with self-blame and adjustment to their losses. Return to their prior school and other social environments may be complicated by questions and judgment from others or their perception of that judgment. Clinicians may help families by alerting them to risks and augmenting resilience factors.

After a firearm suicide, classmates and acquaintances will experience a range of emotions. There is evidence that youth exposed to firearm suicide by a peer have a higher risk of mood disorders and suicidality. Counseling and bereavement services are warranted. The community should be alert to subsequent suicides or the so-called copycat effects. Clinician recommendations should include alertness to warning signs, availability of counseling, and recommendations to remove or lock firearms once accessible to youth.

10.4 Secondary Victims

10.4.1 Siblings

Pediatric gunshot wounds often have many secondary victims. As with other diseases, the lives of siblings change dramatically when parental attention is focused on the death or severe injury of a child and the subsequent long-term care. The emotional and physical toll on parents may be consuming and thus further distance them from the uninjured child or children in the family. The family of a child shot in community violence may move, disrupting school, peer relationships, and support for siblings as well. Clinicians can support siblings of shooting violence by assessing their experiences and mental health and encouraging parents to respond to their needs and spend one-on-one time together.

10.4.2 Witnesses

Witnessing firearm violence may be up close and direct, such as seeing a friend or family member shot. Yet, that is not the only means of witnessing trauma. Children can be "close" through any sensory or cognitive exposure. They may have heard the gunshot and the argument, encountered a warning sign left unreported, or been with the victim shortly before the shooting. Witnesses can be affected even when the victim is removed by one or several degrees, including someone in the same school or on the team who attended the same house of worship or lived in the same community or of a similar age. The prevalence of youth witnesses to shootings has been reported as high as 5%. Gun violence has been called "epidemic;" the contagion affects both primary and secondary pediatric patients. While there is scant research on secondary victims and witnesses, primary care clinicians can incorporate assessment and therapeutics into their care. In an era of immediate and round-the-clock media coverage amplifying messages to children and teens, the very definition of witnessing violence has changed starkly. Mass murders, law enforcement brutality and racially-targeted attacks, even if geographically distant, become our own witnessed experiences. We know the names and repeatedly relive the violence. Pediatricians can facillitate dialogue to help patients struggling with recent events, racism, feelings of rage, helplessness or despair. Healing, while never easy, will come only after assessing the injury and finding a path forward together.

10.4.3 Family Violence

Family and community violence do not routinely make the headlines, but these events far too often wound and scar youth in the long term. Parental violence may lead to firearm death within a family and/or separation due to arrest and incarceration of a family perpetrator. Some children have multiple family members who have already been shot, either as the direct target or the result of being in the wrong place at the wrong time. The chronicity of such violence is somewhat understudied, but is likely akin to other forms of community and family violence, which result in higher levels of fatalism, internalizing and externalizing symptoms. Children shot due to family violence may lose loved caretakers and be separated from siblings and peers, which compounds their experience of psychosocial trauma. The pediatric clinician's understanding of family and long-term involvement can be crucial to ultimate outcome.

10.4.4 Disparities

Firearm injury is a disparity health issue. Children and young adolescents are more likely to be injured by unintentional gun fire than adults and teens. In contrast, young adults are at higher risk of intentional gun assault. The leading cause of death for Black male youth is gun injury – Black males are killed at a rate 15 times higher than for White males. There is clear and concerning evidence that Black youth are at higher risk for disparate treatment by law enforcement, far too often with fatal result. Black and Hispanic males are more likely than White peers to be injured by firearms and to require hospitalization for their injuries. Black adolescent males have more extensive injuries and a higher case fatality rate than White counterparts.

As previously mentioned, pain management differs for Black patients, who typically receive less treatment than White or Hispanic patients. Posthospitalization, White patients are transferred to a rehabilitation facility more often, while Black and Hispanic patients are discharged to home. As outpatients, Black adults demonstrate less utilization of rehabilitation services and ambulatory visits after a trauma.

People who live in high poverty concentration areas have higher risks of firearm violence. Poverty also affects access to and utilization of care. While one study showed equivalent prescribing for home health services across racial groups for those with insurance, Hispanic patients without insurance were offered significantly fewer services. Caring for a child with significant needs and medical appointments is stressful for any parent, but impoverished families face additional challenges caring for a child after a firearm injury. Families living in or near poverty often work, or work more than one job. Time off and transportation required for medical care add additional strain. Trust with care providers is essential. This may begin with understanding the family's concerns and stressors. Primary care clinicians can give emotional support as well as tangible assistance: writing letters when eviction looms, continuation of the electricity if it is threatened, and connecting families with community support organizations. Clinicians can also connect families with social support groups for those affected by gun violence. Keeping children on health insurance is a critical need. Families will need help applying for Supplemental Security Income (SSI), which can be an arduous task even for the most savvy families. All families are affected by gun violence, but not all families are treated the same nor experience the same threats. Working with families through challenges is essential to aid the pediatric gunshot wound patient.

10.5 Conclusions

Firearm injury is among the leading causes of pediatric death and acquired disability. Treatment begins with emergency care for tissue damage, but it doesn't end there. Injured patients are at risk for acute and chronic psychological sequelae, complicated by differences in developmental stage, pre-injury conditions, access to supports and resources, and individual characteristics. Posthospitalization, patients benefit from a wraparound, whole-child approach which incorporates their physical, mental health, behavioral, and social needs. The primary care clinician tends to patients' immediate and ongoing health-care needs, provides coordination of multidisciplinary services, comprehensively assesses patient supports and social context, utilizes validated screening tools, is aware of potential for bias, and adjusts management as children grow. While family, friends, and the community are partners in recovery, they may also be secondary (or even primary) victims of gun violence and thus potentially limited in their abilities to support the injured patient. As leaders in child health, pediatric clinicians can assist in family and community recovery, as well as the prevention of subsequent and future events.

Take Home Points
- Injuries and deaths related to gun violence have long-term physical, developmental, behavioral, and psychosocial consequences for the child and family.
- The primary care clinician is an integral part of the child's larger family and community network to ensure long-term care for physical, developmental, and mental health consequences after firearm injury.
- Physical injuries can result in chronic pain and long-term disability requiring rehabilitation and assistive devices for the child.
- Psychosocial effects, including changes in behavior and PTSD, are influenced by the intent and circumstances of the shooting event as well as the child's personal, family, and environmental history.
- Racial and socioeconomic disparities in children and youth experiencing gun violence and injuries and in the care after these injuries should be recognized and addressed.
- Optimizing short- and long-term outcomes with careful assessment of the patient's comprehensive needs, facilitation of collaboration among the patient's multidisciplinary support team, and ongoing communication with the family is an important role of the primary care clinician.
- Pediatric clinicians can be involved in family and community recovery as well as efforts toward prevention of future firearm injuries and deaths to their patients and community.

Suggested Readings

1. Crossen EJ, Lewis B, Hoffman BD. Preventing gun injuries in children. Pediatr Rev. 2015;36(2):43–51.
2. Gardner HG, Quinlan KP, Ewald MB, Ebel BE, Lichenstein R, Melzer-Lange MD, et al. Firearm-related injuries affecting the pediatric population. Pediatrics. 2012;130(5):e1416–23.
3. Hoffmann JA, Farrell CA, Monuteaux MC, Fleegler EW, Lee LK. Association of Pediatric Suicide with county-level poverty in the United States, 2007–2016. JAMA Pediatr. 2020;174(3):287–94.

4. Karb RA, Subramanian SV, Fleegler EW. County poverty concentration and disparities in unintentional injury deaths: a fourteen-year analysis of 1.6 million U.S. fatalities. PLoS One. 2016;11(5):e0153516.
5. Leventhal JM, Gaither JR, Sege R. Hospitalizations due to firearm injuries in children and adolescents. Pediatrics. 2014;133(2):219–25.
6. Olson LM, Christoffel KK, O'Connor KG. Pediatricians' involvement in gun injury prevention. Inj Prev. 2007;13(2):99–104.
7. Petty JK, Henry MCW, Nance ML, Ford HR. Firearm injuries and children: position statement of the American Pediatric Surgical Association. J Pediatr Surg. 2019;54(7):1269–76.
8. Vella MA, Warshauer A, Tortorello G, Fernandez-Moure J, Giacolone J, Chen B, et al. Long-term functional, psychological, emotional, and social outcomes in survivors of firearm injuries. JAMA Surg. 2019;155(1):1–9
9. Wintemute GJ. The epidemiology of firearm violence in the twenty-first century United States. Annu Rev Public Health. 2015;36(1):5–19.

Chapter 11
Violence Intervention Advocacy Program and Community Interventions

Elizabeth C. Pino, Francesca Fontin, and Elizabeth Dugan

Is violence a contagious disease?

By Felice J. Freyer
February 27, 2017. *The Boston Globe*

11.1 Introduction

Hospital-based interventions currently in practice for youth victims of firearm violence are included in Chap. 8. In this chapter, we present the program goals, accomplishments, and practical details of a single hospital-based violence intervention program (HVIP), the Violence Intervention Advocacy Program (VIAP) at Boston Medical Center (BMC). Created in 2006, the VIAP was one of the eight founding members of the National Network of Hospital-Based Violence Intervention Programs (NNHVIP), now known as the Health Alliance for Violence Intervention (HAVI). In its over 13 years of existence, the VIAP has continually sought out improved ways to assist victims of violence in Boston by engaging stakeholders at the hospital, community, and local government levels. These VIAP partners and associated community outreach initiatives will be discussed further in this chapter.

Each HVIP in the HAVI dictates its own criteria for inclusion into their program, with some programs including victims of assault in addition to victims of penetrating (gunshot or stab wound) injury and others imposing an upper age limit to restrict program focus to youth victims of violence [1, 2]. At BMC, all victims of penetrating injury treated in the emergency department (ED) are eligible to receive or decline VIAP services to aid in their physical and emotional recovery [3]. Among VIAP's pediatric victims of violence, we observe specific trends in demographics and injury type, allowing our partners in local government and community outreach

Elizabeth C. Pino and Francesca Fontin contributed equally.

E. C. Pino · F. Fontin · E. Dugan (✉)
Department of Emergency Medicine, Boston Medical Center, Boston, MA, USA
e-mail: Elizabeth.pino@bmc.org; francesca.fontin2@bmc.org; Elizabeth.Dugan@bmc.org

© Springer Nature Switzerland AG 2021   157
L. K. Lee, E. W. Fleegler (eds.), *Pediatric Firearm Injuries and Fatalities*,
https://doi.org/10.1007/978-3-030-62245-9_11

to target youth at high risk for violence. Further, we recognize the unique and often challenging cases pediatric clients present to their case managers and partners in injury recovery. In this chapter, we will present a complicated pediatric case study of an 18-year-old gunshot victim, whose injury recovery required integration of several facets of VIAP services and hospital partners.

11.2   The Boston Violence Intervention Advocacy Program (VIAP)

In 2006, the City of Boston experienced a resurgence of youth violence, with a more than doubling of the number of nonfatal shootings and firearm homicides over a 3-year period [4]. According to the Centers for Disease Control and Prevention (CDC), from 2001 through 2006, homicide was the second leading cause of death among youth aged 10–24 years in Massachusetts, with firearm deaths accounting for 71.9% of all deaths [5]. Among Black youth aged 10–24 years over the same time period in Massachusetts, homicide was the leading cause of death with firearm deaths accounting for 84.8% of all deaths [5]. Gun violence occurring in just 5.1% of Boston's geography generated 53% of fatal and near-fatal shootings [4]. BMC treats approximately 70% of the gunshot and stab wound victims in Boston [6].

In June 2006, the BMC Violence Intervention Advocacy Program (VIAP) was established with funding from the mayor of Boston and with support from Thea James, MD, and other Boston stakeholders. Previous observational and analytical studies have demonstrated the positive, mitigating effects of HVIPs [1, 2, 7–11]. Like other HVIPs, BMC's VIAP is an ED-centered program taking advantage of the short time window after a traumatic injury when the victim of violence is at a crossroads and may be more amenable to an intervention or "teachable moment" [1, 12, 13]. While in the ED, those who have been violently injured report that their thoughts are either to change their way of life or to retaliate. Without HVIPs, most emergency departments treat the physical wounds of victims of violence but neglect the factors that could potentially lead to revictimization or future perpetration of violence [1]. Particularly for young victims, those who survive their injuries are often underserved by traditional health-care systems and are ill-prepared to address their emotional and social needs, both in the hospital and after discharge [1, 14].

BMC's VIAP recruits employees from the Boston communities commonly served by the VIAP and trains them as violence intervention advocates. VIAP Advocates attempt to contact all victims (or legal guardians of victims) of penetrating trauma treated in the BMC ED. Based on a peer advocate model, VIAP uses a trauma-informed care approach to assist in the physical and emotional recovery from violent trauma. Trauma-informed care is an approach integrating knowledge about the effects of, and recovery from, the neurobiological and psychosocial effects of trauma. In trauma-informed care, symptoms are not seen as pathology, but as attempts to cope and survive [1, 15]. This approach acknowledges each violent injury traumatizes many people beyond the direct victim, including siblings, partners, parents, children, friends, and others in the community.

The first point of contact with VIAP for victims of violent injury is in the ED with the VIAP Trauma Response Team, formerly part of the Boston Street Worker Program (discussed in depth in Sect. 3.1). VIAP employs two trauma response street workers who respond to victims of violence and their families on an on-call, 24-hour basis to deliver immediate psychological first aid in the ED. The Trauma Response Team provides immediate response to violent trauma incidents and provides crisis intervention, safety planning, and resources for victims and their families after ED discharge. This team has proven to be a valuable asset for VIAP and BMC for stabilization of these tense situations.

Following the immediate crisis management in the ED, victims are then assigned both a VIAP Advocate and a mental health clinician from the BMC Community Violence Response Team (CVRT) (discussed in 3.2). Most gunshot and stab wound victims are admitted to the hospital, enabling advocates and mental health professionals to make initial contact and develop a relationship during daily visits while they are inpatients. During this time, VIAP Advocates develop relationships with victims of violence and their families, conduct needs assessments, and begin to create plans to address identified needs. CVRT clinicians provide crisis intervention, psycho-education, counseling, and therapeutic support. If a victim is discharged from the ED, outreach is done through follow-up phone calls. However, due to numerous reasons, such as transience, homelessness, or incarceration, advocates are not able to connect with everyone. Once patients are discharged from the hospital, advocates maintain case management relationships with their clients who choose to participate in the program. They provide support to address individual needs, and promote trauma recovery, and behavioral change while incorporating violence prevention messages [3]. CVRT clinicians work in conjunction with VIAP Advocates to provide ongoing counseling, trauma-focused cognitive behavioral therapy, and referrals to community partners. Through client services, VIAP Advocates aim to address the social determinants of health that could hinder recovery and lead to reinjury, in addition to addressing the physical and mental health of the client.

Clients afflicted by serious injuries, temporary or permanent disability as a result of their injuries, or limited access to caregivers face additional barriers to recovery after discharge to their homes. To address this gap in care, VIAP employs a registered nurse to make home visits (discussed in 3.3) to interested clients in need, alongside client advocates. VIAP also offers support services to family members of clients and family survivors of homicide victims. Family Support Advocates and CVRT clinicians provide intensive support to family members of VIAP clients, particularly caregivers, by offering information, referrals, and ongoing coordination of any needed services. VIAP does not limit the amount of time a client and their family can receive services; the work continues as long as a client or family is willing to engage. On average, participation in the program continues for 1 year (see Fig. 11.1 for a flowchart of VIAP procedures and services).

Pediatric clients, which the VIAP defines as 24 years old or younger, comprise 44% of the 5558 total victims of violence from the inception of the VIAP in 2006 through the year 2018 (Fig. 11.2a). Compared to adult clients, a greater percentage of pediatric clients were either Black or Hispanic (Fig. 11.2b), and more than half of VIAP pediatric clients were victims of gunshot wounds versus stab wounds,

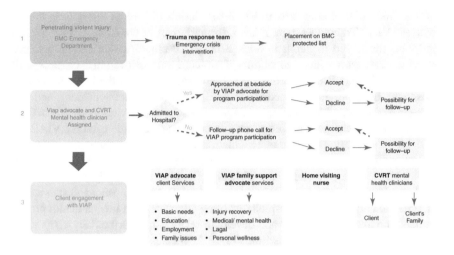

Fig. 11.1 Flowchart of the Boston Violence Intervention Advocacy Program (VIAP) procedures and services

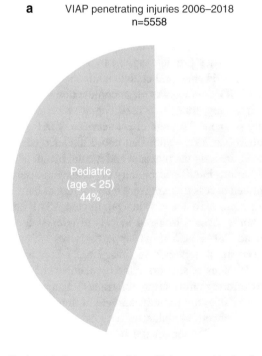

Fig. 11.2 Distribution (**a**), demographics (**b**), and injury type (**c**) of pediatric and adult penetrating injuries with the Boston Violence Intervention Advocacy Program (VIAP), 2006–2018. Graphs represent all penetrating injuries seen by the VIAP from 2006 to 2018. Victims of multiple injuries are represented more than once in the data. Pediatric clients are defined as those aged < 25 years old at the time of injury

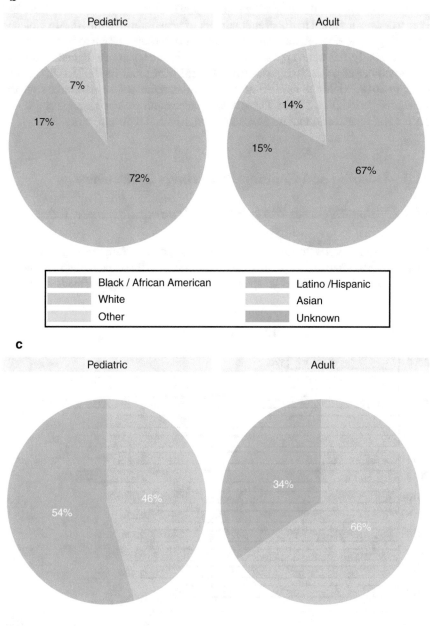

Fig. 11.2 (continued)

compared to only a third of adult clients (54% versus 34%) (Fig. 11.2c). Through the efforts of the VIAP and coordinated initiatives in the City of Boston, there has been a downward trend in the overall number of penetrating injuries due to violence presenting to the BMC ED over the 12 full years of VIAP program data (Fig. 11.3a). Most strikingly, this trend appears to exclusively be the result of a dramatic decrease in the number of pediatric injuries from 295 (53% of total) in 2007 to 91 (26% of total) in 2018, while the number of adult injuries remained largely static over the same time period (Fig. 11.3b). These data suggest youth violence is preventable and HVIPs and related community programs save lives and reduce reinjury.

11.3   Hospital and Community Partners in Recovery

11.3.1   Boston Street Workers/VIAP Trauma Response Team

In December 2008, the Boston Foundation established StreetSafe Boston as a violence prevention and intervention program aimed at dramatically reducing gun violence in the city. StreetSafe deployed 25 street workers into the 5 neighborhoods of Boston

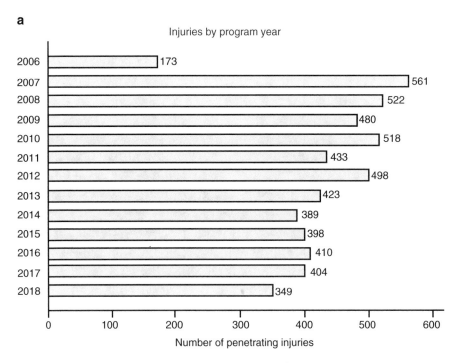

a

Injuries by program year

Year	Number of penetrating injuries
2006	173
2007	561
2008	522
2009	480
2010	518
2011	433
2012	498
2013	423
2014	389
2015	398
2016	410
2017	404
2018	349

Number of penetrating injuries

Fig. 11.3 Total penetrating injuries by program year of the Boston Violence Intervention Advocacy Program (VIAP), overall (**a**) and by age group (**b**), 2006–2018. Graphs represent all penetrating injuries seen by the VIAP from 2006 to 2018. Victims of multiple injuries are represented more than once in the data. Pediatric clients are defined as those aged < 25 years old at the time of injury

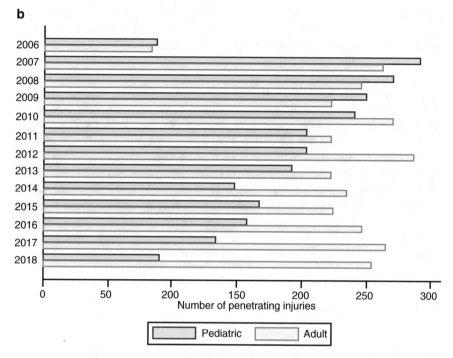

Fig. 11.3 (continued)

most afflicted by violence. This program engaged with young people deemed most at risk for committing violent offenses, which became a model intervention strategy used around the country [16, 17]. StreetSafe Boston was designed to build on the legacy of the Boston Miracle, which is credited with sparking an unprecedented drop in urban crime during the 1990s. During this time, a similar strategy placing street workers into sections of the city where violence was particularly high was implemented [18].

By 2015, StreetSafe was absorbed by the City of Boston's own Boston Street Worker Program to create a unified network of trained street workers. The street workers' role is to engage hard-to-reach, high-risk youth and to help them with issues such as substance abuse, court involvement, teen violence, sexuality, etc., through a service delivery system including intervention and advocacy. These high-risk youths typically avoid social support and do not make use of traditional youth service agencies. Thus, the Boston Street Worker Program is designed to reach these youths who are not being reached by traditional sources [19].

11.3.2   Community Violence Response Team (CVRT)

In 2010, when the community voiced concerns that mental health resources were lacking for victims of violence and their families, BMC responded by establishing the CVRT. Masters-level mental health counselors provide crisis intervention and trauma-focused mental health counseling to adults, adolescents, and children. The

CVRT clinician provides ongoing therapeutic support at the bedside in the hospital and upon discharge to the patient as well as any family members or friends impacted by violence. CVRT also provides these services to families affected by homicide.

All CVRT services are free to clients and are paid for from reparations offered through the victims' fund of the federal Victims of Crime Act (VOCA). This also provides funding for state- and community-based organizations to offer free mental health counseling and other specialized services. This fund is essential to provide clients with the services and support they need to recover from trauma without having to navigate insurance coverage and without the requirement to establish a mental health diagnosis in the client's medical record. Stigma against those with mental illness, or of mental health treatment in general, is particularly pronounced among members of racial and ethnic minorities, who are similarly less likely to seek mental health treatment [20, 21]. The standard of care for clients of CVRT has been especially designed to most effectively reach and help those impacted by violence, who most often are uninsured and racial and ethnic minorities [13].

11.3.3 Home Visiting Nurse

Many clients who are discharged home after violent injury have inadequate access to caregivers, follow-up medical care and supplies, and a limited understanding of how to care for complicated wounds (see Chap. 10). Further, many victims of violence fear leaving their homes after injury to attend medical appointments over concerns of facing the perpetrator of their injuries within their own community or of subsequent threats to their lives. To address this gap in care for our clients, in 2017, the VIAP implemented a home visiting nurse program to ensure clients continue a successful road to physical recovery once they return home.

While most studies evaluating the effectiveness of home-based care programs focus on homebound geriatric populations [22, 23] or newborn infants and their mothers [24–26], the results are incontrovertible among these and other high-risk patient populations [27, 28]. Implementation of a home visiting nurse program reduces hospital admission rates, repeat emergency department visits, and 30-day readmission rates [22, 23, 28]. Importantly, the experiences of patients receiving home nurse care are overwhelmingly positive, with particular emphasis placed on feeling respected and supported, and not patronized or judged, highlighting the critical importance of the nurse-client relationship [26, 29].

VIAP employs one home visiting nurse to visit 1 day per week, while the remainder of the week she serves as an overnight intensive medical care unit nurse at BMC. This allows her to form a continuing relationship with clients from their hospital admission to their discharge and beyond, with check-in phone calls and home visits when needed. She provides consultation, education, medical care, and supplies. In her professional medical opinion and through client self-report, her interventions prevent a repeat visit to the hospital in 90% of cases.

11.3.4 Neighborhood Trauma Teams (NTT)

Incidents of interpersonal violence extend well beyond the violently injured individual and permeate many aspects of community life that influence health. Overseen by the Boston Public Health Commission (BPHC), Neighborhood Trauma Teams (NTTs) were created in 2017 to offer immediate support from a continuum of providers to Boston residents impacted by community violence. In the aftermath of neighborhood violence, community health centers, hospitals, and community groups coordinate an immediate response and sustained recovery for all those affected. When a victim of penetrating injury arrives at BMC, the VIAP is the first point of contact for communication and collaboration with community partners who then deploy teams to specific neighborhoods. Support for individuals and families include ongoing behavioral health services, vigils, and memorial and funeral services. At the community level, NTTs offer coping/healing groups and trauma education and support. Access to a support hotline is available 24 hours a day, 365 days a year.

This model was designed with input from over 350 community residents and providers through several neighborhood listening sessions hosted by the BPHC, incorporating the services and assistance that residents and communities need most following a violent or traumatic event. The NTTs are supported through a combination of city funding and grants from Boston Children's Hospital and Partners HealthCare System. To ensure a focus on children and youth exposed to violence, BPHC programs have trained approximately 2500 youth workers, over 100 clinicians, 50 public school employees, and 200 maternal and child health workers to recognize and respond appropriately to trauma [30].

11.4 Local and National Outreach

11.4.1 Boston Public Schools: Succeed Boston

Succeed Boston (formerly called the Counseling and Intervention Center and the Barron Center) is a short-term counseling and intervention program serving students who have violated the most serious offenses of the Boston Public Schools Code of Conduct, such as carrying weapons into school and other expellable offenses. This program provides individual and group counseling services, substance abuse education and treatment, restorative circles, and academic support. It also provides students with the social-emotional skill building they need to assess risk, consider potential consequences, and improve decision-making.

VIAP Advocates have partnered with Succeed Boston to deliver workshops to address a variety of issues surrounding the capability of proven-risk youths to grow and elevate their lives. During these group sessions, advocates create an open and safe space for students in grades 6–12 to have a dialogue with professionals regarding intergenerational trauma, grieving after a traumatic event, negative and positive influences, resiliency, and medical emergencies. The sessions conclude with a hospital tour. Each session is facilitated by a guest speaker from a community organization and a VIAP Advocate. With this local outreach initiative, the VIAP hopes to strengthen communities beset by violence and intervene before these high-risk youths become victims of violent injury.

11.4.2   Trainings: Trauma-Informed Care Simulation and Violence Prevention Professional (VPP)

The VIAP team has emerged as a resource for training and education for medical professionals at BMC and for victim advocates nationwide. At BMC, advocates present the psycho-educational components of trauma-informed care to nurses, doctors, and medical residents, followed by small group trainings through stations in a simulation center where VIAP staff act out scenarios that commonly arise with gunshot and stabbing victims admitted to the hospital. The objective is to educate staff and give them tools to employ a trauma-informed care approach. The use of the simulation lab and role-playing these scenarios give the medical staff the opportunity to receive critical feedback while practicing the skills learned.

At the national level, VIAP Advocates also participate in facilitating HAVI-sponsored Violence Prevention Professionals (VPPs) training programs for frontline violence intervention workers. The goal is to standardize training for staff doing violence prevention work around the country and to make those who successfully complete the training eligible for reimbursement for their peer counseling services.

11.5   Pediatric Case Study of a Gunshot Victim

11.5.1   Presenting Trauma

Carlos, an 18-year-old Hispanic male with a past medical history of learning disabilities due to lead exposure, and a gang affiliation at the time of the injury, presented to the BMC ED at 11:20 PM with a gunshot wound to his left temple. This resulted in bilateral globe rupture, with poor prognosis for his vision. Upon admission to the pediatric intensive care unit, medical personnel learned that Carlos was riding as a passenger in a car with his older brother Juan, a known associate of the same gang. Juan, the driver of the vehicle, was shot and pronounced dead on the scene. A bystander had called 911 and applied first aid to Carlos until emergency medical services arrived and transported him to the BMC ED. At this time, Carlos was unaware that his brother had died at the scene.

Later that night, Carlos' mother, Rosa, an undocumented immigrant with a history of the Department of Children and Families (DCF) involvement, alcoholism, and a former victim of domestic violence, arrived to the ED heavily intoxicated. Rosa was in recovery and one year sober from alcohol when she received a call from BMC that her son was in the ED. This news led her to relapse, and she arrived at the hospital inebriated. In addition to Carlos and Juan, Rosa also had a 24-year-old son and two younger daughters, aged 17 and 11 years. When Rosa arrived to the ED, she was under the impression that it was Juan who was shot and receiving care at BMC, as the caller from BMC did not specify which of her children was injured. After learning it was in fact Carlos in the hospital, Rosa also became increasingly concerned about the welfare of Juan.

11.5.2   Trauma Response Team

The VIAP Trauma Response Team supervisor was notified of the incident and arrived at BMC. He approached Rosa in the ED where he introduced himself and helped her regain some composure. The trauma response supervisor expedited the waiting time to meet with Carlos' doctors regarding his medical condition, but observed that it was difficult for Rosa to process the information while she was still uncertain about Juan's whereabouts. VIAP's home visiting nurse was present on the floor as a charge nurse. She observed Rosa upset and tearful on the floor of the waiting room. She alerted the VIAP trauma response supervisor, who made sure he was present when Boston Police Department detectives informed Rosa her son Juan died at the scene. The VIAP trauma response supervisor also secured a more private location in the hospital for Rosa to grieve the loss of Juan until she was ready to see Carlos. In addition, VIAP staff connected the family with the Louis D. Brown Peace Institute, VIAP's partner organization in the community that assists families impacted by murder and trauma with burial and funeral services. He also notified Rosa that representatives from the VIAP and CVRT would contact her within the day and provide services for Carlos and his family.

11.5.3   Recovery Weeks 1–2: Inpatient Stay

On the following morning, Carlos was assigned a VIAP Advocate and a VIAP Family Support Advocate, as well as a mental health clinician from CVRT. Eventually, a second CVRT clinician was added to the case to work exclusively with Carlos, so that the other clinician could work exclusively with Rosa and other family members. During the first few days, Carlos was irritable and withdrawn from social interaction. Medical personnel had explained to him that given the extent of his injuries, he would likely experience a complete loss of vision. They discussed medical options with him, including surgical procedures on both eyes and the various possible outcomes. After speaking with him, alongside Rosa and a Spanish language interpreter, consent was given for the surgery.

The VIAP home visiting nurse and other nurses helped Carlos regain some independence during his stay at BMC. They gradually introduced and explained aspects of Carlos' routine that he could achieve independently, such as adding tangible markers that would lead him to the restroom independently.

11.5.3.1 Partners in Recovery: VIAP Advocates and CVRT Clinicians

Carlos' VIAP Advocate recognized that Carlos was withdrawn and untrusting of medical staff. He checked in with Carlos often and spent the beginning of their working relationship sitting with him and having casual conversations with Carlos and his CVRT clinician in order to build rapport. Once the advocate established a relationship, he provided stabilization services: he helped Carlos file for victim's compensation and social security benefits. He expressed that first establishing a relationship with Carlos helped in providing services later in his recovery.

For days, Carlos had been asking medical staff about his brother's status. He had suspected his brother was killed in the shooting, but it was never confirmed to him by family or medical staff. Rosa feared revealing Juan's death to Carlos would have an adverse effect on his recovery. Rosa's CVRT clinician and the pediatric social worker, however, expressed concerns to Rosa that the longer it took to reveal the news to Carlos, the angrier and more withdrawn he could become once he discovered the fate of his brother. Rosa agreed and was able to communicate with Carlos about Juan's death, with the support of both CVRT clinicians and the social worker.

Carlos' VIAP Advocate and CVRT clinician continued their working relationships with him during his stay. His advocate and CVRT clinician attempted to lighten Carlos' mood through casual conversations and by listening to music. Appointments were arranged also with the Art Lab, BMC's collaboration with Boston University's College of Fine Arts. Carlos was able to use the Art Lab as a therapeutic, creative outlet to make and play music. The CVRT clinician helped Carlos adjust to walking without vision by coaxing him out of his room and walking laps around the pediatric floor. During these walks, they would have conversations about his concerns regarding his discharge and life changes to help him process his emotions.

Often, the CVRT clinician and VIAP Advocate felt compelled to speak with medical staff about their behavior toward Carlos, as he had developed a mistrust of several medical staff due to their judgmental tone when addressing him. Nurses complained he smelled of marijuana and had an irritable demeanor. The Family Support Advocate observed there was a negative perception of Carlos as a violent adult instead of a traumatized adolescent. The CVRT clinician recalled one nurse declaring "there is a reason he was shot." Advocates were concerned that the circumstances surrounding Carlos' injury affected the quality of his care and diminished the compassion of those caring for him. They explained to medical staff that Carlos' marijuana use was a coping mechanism to deal with his trauma, and his irritable demeanor was a symptom of grief over his deceased brother and his own newly altered life circumstances. The CVRT mental health clinician and VIAP Advocate reminded staff to be trauma-informed and to understand that Carlos' speculated history with violence should not be a factor in the quality of care he receives.

During one incident, Carlos had not bathed for several days following his surgery, and medical staff complained of his smell. When Carlos' mental health clinician approached him regarding his hygiene, Carlos explained he was reluctant to shower because he was afraid that water would enter through his eye sockets. She addressed these concerns and encouraged Carlos to bathe again. Before she approached him, no other member of the medical staff had asked him his reasons for not bathing.

11.5.3.2 Partners in Recovery: VIAP Family Support

Rosa often drank heavily and was very tearful while at Carlos' bedside. VIAP Advocates and medical staff observed the interactions between Rosa and her son at this time. They determined Rosa's mourning process and her anxiety negatively affected Carlos' personal grieving process. At this point, the initial CVRT mental health clinician had been exclusively working with Rosa and the rest of Carlos' family. However, the clinician found she had little time to devote to Carlos. CVRT determined a second mental health clinician would be necessary to work with Carlos in this case to ensure that he and his family would receive the appropriate amount of support they needed.

According to the VIAP Family Support Advocate, Rosa felt as if sometimes medical staff shut her out in relation to Carlos' care management because he was 18 years old and legally an adult. Often in the first few days of Carlos' care, medical professionals would bypass Rosa and speak to Carlos privately about his conditions. Rosa expressed to the Family Support Advocate that in their family's culture, she, the mother, takes care of everything in the family. Furthermore, although Carlos had just turned 18 a few months earlier, Rosa was still taking care of all her son's matters. Due to Carlos' learning disabilities, he had dropped out of school in the eighth grade and couldn't fully comprehend his diagnosis or prognosis without help. The Family Support Advocate helped Rosa advocate to be present during all future conversations regarding Carlos' medical care and also provided a referral to BMC's food bank to help combat the family's food insecurity.

VIAP and CVRT each helped Rosa with her relapse with alcohol. During Carlos' hospitalization, Rosa had come in the hospital intoxicated many times. During one incident, public safety was called when she attempted to see Carlos. Medical personnel had refused for her to see Carlos while inebriated. She pulled a knife out to her neck and threatened suicide if she didn't see her son. Rosa was coaxed back to the trauma room where she was sedated and would obtain a mental health consult once she was sober, in order to be discharged. Rosa understood, and the next day, she was cleared to leave the hospital. The Family Support Advocate and Carlos' VIAP Advocate spoke to medical personnel on behalf of Rosa. They explained the events that had transpired, including numerous previous incidents in which she was intoxicated, but didn't pose a risk for violence. During this conversation, the advocates explained that Rosa had gone through a traumatic event, which had changed the trajectory of her life and had triggered her relapse. Despite these events, Rosa had always attempted to be by her son's side. Advocates reminded medical personnel to be mindful of her trauma and to use a trauma-informed care approach.

Rosa continued to visit Carlos while under the influence and sought help for her alcohol dependence issue. Before her incident with public safety, she worked with VIAP's Family Support Advocate to contact her recovery program, which had previously helped her maintain her sobriety. Rosa told the program in confidence that she had broken her sobriety. In response, the program filed a 51A report on her to DCF for relapsing while in the care of two minors and removed her from the program. The Family Support Advocate helped Rosa navigate the legal system, while her CVRT mental health clinician directed her recovery and assisted with crisis management. While Rosa was fluent in English, she felt much more comfortable communicating in Spanish. Her mental health clinician believed that being able to communicate with Rosa in her native language considerably strengthened their relationship and helped Rosa to trust her with sensitive information.

11.5.4 Recovery Week 2–Month 7: Discharge Home

Carlos was discharged home from BMC after a 14-day inpatient stay. Prior to discharge, his VIAP Advocate made efforts to manage a variety of issues to ensure as smooth a transition as possible back home. He visited Carlos' residence and helped rearrange furniture so he could better navigate through his home. The advocate helped Carlos apply for a state-sponsored chauffer program that assists people with disabilities who are unable to use traditional public transportation. He also located a rehabilitation program for the blind and visually impaired that would aid in his adjustment to vision loss and transition toward independent living.

Carlos' mental health clinician and VIAP Advocate discussed next steps with him and brought him to a meeting with the admissions director of the rehabilitation program for the vision impaired. The program mainly served an older population with a higher socioeconomic background who had gradually lost their vision. Carlos' advocates observed the director used a lot of judgmental language when addressing him. The admissions director made comments about Carlos' marijuana usage and the circumstances surrounding his injury. These comments made Carlos feel uncomfortable, and the impact of her choice of language and her bias toward Carlos was evident. Carlos expressed his concerns to his advocates. His VIAP Advocate later phoned the admissions provider and explained to her that she was not acting in a trauma-informed manner. She apologized for her behavior. However, this first impression was enough for Carlos to decide not to attend the program.

During the next several months, the CVRT mental health clinician and VIAP Advocate continued to engage with Carlos on his journey to recovery. They frequently conducted home visits to catch up with him using light conversations. Carlos' advocate would pick him up and bring him to his appointments. Carlos' advocates recognized he spent most of his time at home listening to music and smoking marijuana. He didn't make many efforts to make decisions regarding his health and his life, despite words of encouragement and attempts to support him in creating plans to move forward in his life. The two later discussed pulling back from services, believing that their work in helping Carlos was inadvertently enabling him to become inactive and promoting his reliance on them to do things for him. They explained to him they would continue to check in on him periodically and would be available to assist him when he was ready to participate in his own plan to recover and move forward.

11.5.5   Continuing Recovery: 8 Months–1 Year Post-injury

Carlos returned to the ED 8 months after initial discharge for seizure activity. He was diagnosed with further brain and skull injuries as a result of this initial gunshot wound. He returned to BMC several days later for surgery to repair the base of his skull and his sinus defect. Carlos' mental health clinician and VIAP Advocate visited him during his inpatient stay. Carlos expressed frustrations with returning to BMC as well as his fear of his current diagnosis and upcoming surgery. They validated his feelings and kept him in good spirits before the procedure.

During this time, VIAP assigned a new Family Support Advocate who is a native Spanish speaker, which helped the team break down some of the cultural barriers that existed with Carlos and his family. Rosa's mental health clinician still met with her intermittently, especially during follow-up appointments. She was able to help often during breakdowns, crisis situations, and addressing substance use. The new VIAP Family Support Advocate accompanied Rosa to medical appointments and assisted her with other case management tasks.

Carlos was discharged home after a 3-week inpatient hospital stay following surgery. His VIAP Advocate discussed follow-up care with Carlos and encouraged him not to use marijuana while taking his new prescriptions. When he checked in with Carlos via phone 1-month postop, the visiting nurse had removed his IV, and he was making a positive recovery. However, a month after the call, Carlos was back in the ED for alcohol intoxication. He had been binge drinking and his friend observed him vomiting blood. Carlos' VIAP Advocate and mental health clinician used this moment as an opportunity to address his lifestyle behaviors. Carlos explained he was binge drinking because he couldn't celebrate his birthday while recovering at home with an IV. His advocates each individually expressed to him the dangers of binge drinking with a traumatic brain injury. The VIAP Advocate had also noticed Carlos had been recently spending the majority of his disability checks on marijuana. He discussed with Carlos his spending habits and instead suggested he put his funds toward a savings account to track how he spends his money. Carlos was having difficulty planning to move forward and was not ready to or interested in participating in concrete services to support any changes. His VIAP team decided to step back to allow some time for him to reflect and decide how and if he wanted support or services.

Months later, Carlos called his VIAP Advocate to inform him that he had enrolled in the program for the blind that they had together visited the previous year. Carlos enrolled on his own and was expecting to begin the program in the following weeks. Carlos is currently attending the program for the blind. The VIAP and CVRT are actively engaged in supporting him as he learns to navigate the world around him and continues to recover.

11.5.6 Discussion

More than 1300 pediatric firearm injuries have presented to the BMC ED over the 14-year history of the VIAP, 20% of which involve gunshot injuries to the head or neck. For pediatric patients younger than 20 years old in the United States, on average, about 20 youth are hospitalized due to firearm injuries every day [31]. Higher levels of violence are more likely to occur in neighborhoods with high unemployment or poverty, gang activity, drug sales, and instability [32]. Further, minority youth hold greater risks for intentional firearm injuries resulting in hospitalizations or deaths compared to their White counterparts, irrespective of neighborhood income level [31]. Carlos' case highlights the complexities of working with a pediatric gunshot survivor and his family. At the root of firearm injuries like Carlos' lies unaddressed social determinants of health that have led to his penetrating injury. The VIAP aims to address these social determinants of health as part of the emotional and physical recovery from injury, using a trauma-informed approach centered on patient advocacy.

Compared to other high-income nations that have better overall health, the United States invests far more money in providing clinical services than in addressing social, economic, and behavioral factors that powerfully affect health and mortality [33]. The clinical manifestations seen by health-care providers are consequences of upstream systemic and structural barriers to health. Social determinants of health include factors like socioeconomic status, education, neighborhood and physical environment, employment, and social support networks, as well as access to health care [34]. As was the case with Carlos, addressing the social determinants of health is often at the forefront of VIAP client advocacy services. It would have been difficult or impossible for Carlos to recover from his life-altering injury without addressing the stress experienced by his family, substance use of his primary caregiver, food insecurity, access to quality mental health care free of cost, or educational opportunities as a person with blindness. As part of its mission as a safety net hospital, BMC seeks to address social determinants of health for its patients and has taken an important first step by collecting information on these factors as part of a patient's general medical history [35].

While the health-care clinician's first contact with a pediatric patient may be in the ED following a firearm injury, the trauma experienced by that patient usually spans years before this incident. The majority of pediatric youth who have survived some form of intentional injury have witnessed a form of violence in their youth prior to their injury and are more likely to witness additional violent events after being discharged from their initial injury [1]. Witnessing community violence is a proven risk factor for anxiety, depression, aggression, and substance abuse [1]. In a study of over 8000 children from sixth to eighth grade, those who have experienced large amounts of community violence were much more likely to carry a gun, become involved in a gang, use marijuana, and binge drink, as well as be more likely to have an injury as a result of fighting [1, 36]. These significant traumatic events cause not only physical wounds but also neurobiological and psychosocial stress reactions altering their behavior [37]. Pediatric patients may withdraw socially and emotionally, display hypervigilance and hyperarousal, and develop symptoms of PTSD, anxiety, and depression [1, 37, 38]. In addition, pediatric patients who are gang affiliated or perceive themselves to have few life possibilities may combine their symptoms of trauma with "street code" rules to regain a sense of safety. These actions include carrying weapons, seeking vengeance/retaliation, and coping through the pain of injury with substance use [1, 37, 39].

To engage with pediatric firearm patients, VIAP staff use a trauma-informed care approach centered on patient advocacy. This set of principles acknowledges the previous traumatic experiences of a client, or patient, may affect the way they act in response to the medical care that they receive and helps survivors rebuild a sense of control and empowerment [38, 40]. Often, a patient outwardly showing signs of aggression or noncompliance is actually demonstrating the effects of trauma [38, 40]. Further, it is known that the racial and ethnic biases (both implicit and explicit) of health-care clinicians can negatively affect the quality of care for minorities [41–43]. Victims of firearm injury may be stigmatized even further as a criminal or "bad person," which influences the treatment they receive from medical and nonmedical staff [37, 38, 44]. Throughout Carlos' pathway to recovery, VIAP Advocates and CVRT clinicians utilized a trauma-informed approach to his care and the care of his family. Importantly, VIAP staff continually advocated for Carlos and Rosa, by reminding and educating hospital and community partners in Carlos' care to be trauma-informed and to attempt to remove their biases against Carlos when providing care. Symptoms of trauma in the patient coupled with the biases of the medical staff can lead to an unproductive therapeutic relationship. VIAP staff bridge the divide between clients and clinicians by advocating on behalf of their clients, creating a trusting and safe environment for the patient to recover, and reminding medical staff to be empathetic and trauma-informed.

11.6   Conclusions and Future Directions

HVIPs have the ambitious mandate to break the cycle of community violence. The Boston VIAP aims to guide victims of violence through recovery from physical and emotional trauma, with the goal of empowering clients and families and facilitating recovery through services and opportunities to reduce retaliation, reinjury, and criminal involvement. These goals are supported by research documenting the enduring, positive effects that HVIPs have on their participants while saving money for hospitals and municipalities [2, 3, 7–9, 11]. A practical guide for launching and sustaining an HVIP was developed by the HAVI, with input from VIAP staff, and is recommended for any hospital treating at least 100 annual assaults, gunshot wounds, stab wounds, and other violence-related injuries [13].

This chapter integrates the procedures, partners, and standards of care for VIAP clients, with a detailed and complex case study of a pediatric gunshot victim, to provide an overall cohesive illustration of the model of care following pediatric firearm injury. The VIAP depends on the efforts of a diverse group of partners in the mental and physical recovery of their clients and those impacted by violence. VIAP staff also participate in community outreach in Boston middle and high schools to guide youths in neighborhoods most afflicted with violence, as well as in local and national trainings for peer advocacy and trauma-informed care. Cases involving pediatric victims can be particularly challenging and require additional support, as the violently injured youth is often inexperienced in decision-making regarding their own health care and well-being. Thus, parents, siblings, and other extended family members can become intimately involved in the pathway to recovery, both for the victim and for themselves.

In over 14 years of existence, the VIAP has celebrated many successes but has also met with substantial challenges. In partnership with the HAVI, the VIAP has made efforts to introduce new evidence-based care practices to better serve their clients. These practices include piloting new approaches to injury recovery and lifestyle intervention through a home visiting nurse program and through services offering more robust housing and employment options. However, the effectiveness of these initiatives has not yet been quantitatively assessed. While the data show great progress has been made in reducing the number of violently injured youths from 2006 to 2018 (Fig. 11.3b), there has been little to no reduction in the number of adult injuries. The VIAP continues to consider and evaluate new approaches to reach adults at high risk of violent injury or reinjury. Additionally, VIAP staff find there to be considerable challenges for clients in completing educational degrees and in establishing stable housing for clients who are homeless or experience chronically unstable housing. Nevertheless, VIAP Advocates can agree that the best marker of success is when a client has recovered from injury, is doing well, and no longer requires VIAP services. These past clients then ask how they can give back to their communities and help others.

Take Home Points
- The Boston Violence Intervention Advocacy Program (VIAP) is an ED-centered program, which takes advantage of the short window of time after a traumatic injury when the victim of violence is at a crossroads and may be more amenable to an intervention.
- VIAP partners with hospital and community groups to deliver a broad spectrum of care and offers local and national trainings in peer advocacy and trauma-informed care.
- Pediatric clients comprise 44% of the violent penetrating injuries presenting to the BMC ED over the history of VIAP, and 54% of these pediatric injuries were gunshot wounds.
- The 12-year downward trend in the overall number of violent penetrating injuries at BMC appears to exclusively be the result of a dramatic decrease in the number of pediatric injuries.
- When assisting young victims of firearm injury, VIAP stresses the importance of family support, trauma-informed care, patient advocacy, and addressing social determinants of health.

Acknowledgments The authors would like to thank Dr. Thea James of Boston Medical Center for her contributions to the founding of VIAP and the National Network of Hospital-Based Violence Intervention Programs (NNHVIP) and her continued efforts toward achieving health equity.

Conflict of Interest The authors have no conflicts of interest to disclose.

Authorship Statement All authors have approved the manuscript, made significant contributions, and have read and approved the final version of the manuscript.

References

1. Corbin TJ, Rich JA, Bloom SL, Delgado D, Rich LJ, Wilson AS. Developing a trauma-informed, emergency department–based intervention for victims of urban violence. J Trauma Dissociation. 2011;12(5):510–25.
2. Juillard C, Cooperman L, Allen I, Pirracchio R, Henderson T, Marquez R, et al. A decade of hospital-based violence intervention: benefits and shortcomings. J Trauma Acute Care Surg. 2016;81(6):1156–61.
3. James TL, Bibi S, Langlois BK, Dugan E, Mitchell PM. Boston violence intervention advocacy program: a qualitative study of client experiences and perceived effect. Acad Emerg Med. 2014;21(7):742–51.
4. Boston Police Department: Office of the Police Commissioner. City of Boston National Forum on youth violence prevention plan. Boston, MA; 2016.

5. Centers for Disease Control and Prevention. Web-based Injury Statistics Query and Reporting System (WISQARS) [Internet]. Available from: http://www.cdc.gov/injury/wisqars/index.html.
6. Boston Medical Center. Injury prevention center annual report 2014–2015; 2015.
7. Cooper C, Eslinger DM, Stolley PD. Hospital-based violence intervention programs work. J Trauma Acute Care Surg. 2006;61(3):534–40.
8. Purtle J, Dicker R, Cooper C, Corbin T, Greene MB, Marks A, et al. Hospital-based violence intervention programs save lives and money. J Trauma Acute Care Surg. 2013;75(2):331–3.
9. Bell TM, Gilyan D, Moore BA, Martin J, Ogbemudia B, McLaughlin BE, et al. Long-term evaluation of a hospital-based violence intervention program using a regional health information exchange. J Trauma Acute Care Surg. 2018;84(1):175–82.
10. Shibru D, Zahnd E, Becker M, Bekaert N, Calhoun D, Victorino GP. Benefits of a hospital-based peer intervention program for violently injured youth. J Am Coll Surg. 2007;205(5):684–9.
11. Purtle J, Rich JA, Fein JA, James T, Corbin TJ. Hospital-based violence prevention: progress and opportunities. Ann Intern Med. 2015;163(9):715–7.
12. Cunningham R, Knox L, Fein J, Harrison S, Frisch K, Walton M, et al. Before and after the trauma bay: the prevention of violent injury among youth. Ann Emerg Med. 2009;53(4):490–500.
13. Karraker N, Cunningham RM, Becker MG, Fein JA, Knox LM. Violence is preventable: a best practices guide for launching & sustaining a hospital-based program to break the cycle of violence. Washington, DC: Office of Victims of Crime, Office of Justice Programs, US Department of Justice; 2011.
14. Zimmerman MA, Stewart SE, Morrel-Samuels S, Franzen S, Reischl TM. Youth empowerment solutions for peaceful communities: combining theory and practice in a community-level violence prevention curriculum. Health Promot Pract. 2011;12(3):425–39.
15. Jennings A, National Center for Trauma Informed Care. Models for developing trauma-informed behavioral health systems and trauma-specific services [Internet]. Available from: http://www.theannainstitute.org/Models%20for%20Developing%20Traums-Report%201-09-09%20_FINAL_.pdf.
16. Mayor Menino, Boston Foundation join to launch youth anti-violence initiative, 'StreetSafe Boston' [press release, Internet]; 2008. Available from: https://www.tbf.org/news-andinsights/press-releases/2008/december/mayor-menino-boston-foundation-join-to-launch-youth-anti-violence-initiative-streetsafe-boston.
17. Decker SH, Bynum TS, McDevitt J, Farrell A, Varano S. Street outreach workers: best practices and lessons learned: innovative practices from the Charles E. Shannon Jr. Community safety initiative series. Institute on Race and Justice Publications. Paper 17; 2008.
18. Henderson SM, Peterson SS, Engel RS. Pulling levers to prevent violence: "the Boston miracle," its adaptations, and future directions for research. In: Teasdale B, Bradley MS, editors. Preventing crime and violence. Cham: Springer International Publishing; 2017. p. 281–96.
19. Zoubek R. Boston streetworker program [Internet]. Boston, MA; 2019. Available from: http://cultureandyouth.org/wp-content/uploads/2014/02/Boston-street-workers.pdf.
20. DeFreitas SC, Crone T, DeLeon M, Ajayi A. Perceived and personal mental health stigma in Latino and African American college students. Front Public Health. 2018;6:49.
21. Dobalian A, Rivers PA. Racial and ethnic disparities in the use of mental health services. J Behav Health Serv Res. 2008;35(2):128–41.
22. Jones MG, DeCherrie LV, Meah YS, Hernandez CR, Lee EJ, Skovran DM, et al. Using nurse practitioner co-management to reduce hospitalizations and readmissions within a homebased primary care program. J Healthc Qual. 2017;39(5):249–258.
23. Echeverry LM, Lamb KV, Miller J. Impact of APN home visits in reducing healthcare costs and improving function in homebound heart failure. Home Healthc Now. 2015;33(10):532–7.
24. Wu J, Dean KS, Rosen Z, Muennig PA. The cost-effectiveness analysis of nurse-family partnership in the United States. J Health Care Poor Underserved. 2017;28(4):1578–97.
25. Landy CK, Jack SM, Wahoush O, Sheehan D, MacMillan HL, Team NHR. Mothers' experiences in the nurse-family partnership program: a qualitative case study. BMC Nurs. 2012;11(1):15.

26. Briggs C. Nursing practice in community child health: developing the nurse–client relationship. Contemp Nurse. 2007;23(2):303–11.
27. Andrade AM, Silva KL, Seixas CT, Braga PP. Nursing practice in home care: an integrative literature review. Rev Bras Enferm. 2017;70(1):210–9.
28. Shaffer VO, Owi T, Kumarusamy MA, Sullivan PS, Srinivasan JK, Maithel SK, et al. Decreasing hospital readmission in ileostomy patients: results of novel pilot program. J Am Coll Surg. 2017;224(4):425–30.
29. Vehviläinen-Julkunen K. The characteristics of clients and public health nurses in child health services interactions. Scand J Caring Sci. 1993;7(1):11–6.
30. Health of Boston 2016-2017 [Internet]: Boston Public Health Commission Research and Evaluation Office Boston, Massachusetts 2016-2017. Available from: https://www.bphc.org/healthdata/health-of-boston-report/Pages/Health-of-Boston-Report.aspx.
31. Kalesan B, Vyliparambil MA, Bogue E, Villarreal MD, Vasan S, Fagan J, et al. Race and ethnicity, neighborhood poverty and pediatric firearm hospitalizations in the United States. Ann Epidemiol. 2016;26(1):1–6 e1–2.
32. Fowler KA, Dahlberg LL, Haileyesus T, Gutierrez C, Bacon S. Childhood firearm injuries in the United States. Pediatrics. 2017;140(1):e20163486.
33. Adler NE, Glymour MM, Fielding J. Addressing social determinants of health and health inequalities. JAMA. 2016;316(16):1641–2.
34. Artiga S, Hinton E. Beyond health care: the role of social determinants in promoting health and health equity [Internet]. Kaiser Family Foundation Issue brief. 2019;1-13. Available from: https://www.kff.org/racial-equity-and-health-policy/issue-brief/beyond-health-care-the-role-of-social-determinants-in-promoting-health-and-health-equity/.
35. Buitron de la Vega P, Losi S, Sprague Martinez L, Bovell-Ammon A, Garg A, James T, et al. Implementing an EHR-based screening and referral system to address social determinants of health in primary care. Med Care. 2019;57:S133–S9.
36. Rosenthal BS. Exposure to community violence in adolescence: trauma symptoms. Adolescence. 2000;35(138):271–84.
37. James TL, Bibi S, Langlois BK, Dugan E, Mitchell PM. Boston violence intervention advocacy program: a qualitative study of client experiences and perceived effect El Violence Intervention Advocacy Program de Boston: Estudio Cualitativo de las Experiencias y el Efecto Percibido del Usuario. Acad Emerg Med. 2014;21(7):742–51.
38. Fischer KR, Bakes KM, Corbin TJ, Fein JA, Harris EJ, James TL, et al. Trauma-informed care for violently injured patients in the emergency department. Ann Emerg Med. 2019;73(2):193–202.
39. Rich JA, Grey CM. Pathways to recurrent trauma among young black men: traumatic stress, substance use, and the "code of the street". Am J Public Health. 2005;95(5):816–24.
40. Oral R, Ramirez M, Coohey C, Nakada S, Walz A, Kuntz A, et al. Adverse childhood experiences and trauma informed care: the future of health care. Pediatr Res. 2016;79(1):227–33.
41. Maina IW, Belton TD, Ginzberg S, Singh A, Johnson TJ. A decade of studying implicit racial/ethnic bias in healthcare providers using the implicit association test. Soc Sci Med. 2018;199:219–29.
42. Park CY, Lee MA, Epstein AJ. Variation in emergency department wait times for children by race/ethnicity and payment source. Health Serv Res. 2009;44(6):2022–39.
43. James CA, Bourgeois FT, Shannon MW. Association of race/ethnicity with emergency department wait times. Pediatrics. 2005;115(3):e310–e5.
44. Bucknor-Ferron P, Zagaja L. Five strategies to combat unconscious bias. Nursing. 2016;46(11):61–2.

Chapter 12
Safety Devices for Firearms

James Dodington

> 'We need the iPhone of guns': Will smart guns transform the gun industry?
>
> By Michael S. Rosenwald
> February 17, 2014. *The Washington Post*

12.1 Introduction

Safe firearm storage is discussed throughout this book as a key element of pediatric firearm injury prevention. Importantly, in order to be able to counsel your patients on the practice of safe firearm storage, knowledge of firearm safety devices, their strengths and limitations, availability and costs, and some state and federal legislation and policy around these devices will be critical information to have on hand.

Multiple public health studies have demonstrated safe firearm storage is associated with decreased risk of pediatric firearm injury. This topic is reviewed in depth throughout this book as it relates to unintentional and intentional firearm injury prevention. In this chapter, we will review the specific types of firearm safety devices available and the limited research on community preferences for specific devices and implications for counseling and discuss the evolving area of "smart gun" technology. We will also briefly review policy and legislation around firearm safety devices and present a sample plan for a firearm safety device distribution community event.

12.2 Types of Firearm Safety Devices

There are multiple types of firearm safety devices, and it is critical to understand the options that patients and families have in counseling families on how to safely secure a firearm. In 2002, California established a law (California Penal Code

J. Dodington (✉)
Department of Pediatrics, Yale University School of Medicine, New Haven, CT, USA
e-mail: james.dodington@yale.edu

© Springer Nature Switzerland AG 2021 179
L. K. Lee, E. W. Fleegler (eds.), *Pediatric Firearm Injuries and Fatalities*,
https://doi.org/10.1007/978-3-030-62245-9_12

section 23620) requiring all firearm sales and transfers to be accompanied by a California Department of Justice-approved safety device. In addition, this law created a roster to catalogue all approved devices, which is maintained and accessible online (https://oag.ca.gov/firearms/fsdcertlist). You can use this roster to examine if the safety devices you plan to recommend or purchase for a community safety event are approved and its compatibility with a given firearm. We will now review the most common types of safety devices and their relative strengths and weaknesses.

12.2.1 Cable Lock or Trigger Lock

The cable lock (Fig. 12.1) is probably the most accessible and most widely known firearm safety device. The cable prevents the gun from firing as it obstructs the firing mechanism by running the cable through the barrel or "action" of the firearm or by preventing the use of ammunition by blocking the insertion of the magazine. The cable is usually secured by a traditional lock using either a key or combination. Many of these locks can be obtained for under $10.00 (USD), per device, but the least expensive ones have concerns related to their flimsiness. In contrast, a trigger lock is positioned over the trigger with a key or combination locking mechanism and obscures the trigger, so it can't be accessed. Importantly, however, cable locks and trigger locks can be compromised (i.e., broken off) more easily than other safety devices reviewed here. Thus, they should *always be used in conjunction with other safety strategies*. Most importantly for counseling, a cable lock or trigger lock should only secure *an unloaded firearm*. Although cable locks and trigger locks are affordable and allow a firearm to be transported and remain accessible, their weaknesses reduce their overall preference by firearm owners. A detailed guide with photographs of key steps on how to prepare a firearm for storage with a cable lock or trigger lock can be found at the National Crime Prevention Council, funded by the US Department of Justice (https://www.safefirearmsstorage.org/).

12.2.2 Lock Box

The firearm safe or lock box (Fig. 12.1) is another popular firearm safety device and comes in many forms. A safe or box may have a key or combination lock or an electronic interface, such as a biometric safe, allowing entry only for the "fingerprint" of the authorized user or users. They can also be anchored within a home or can be portable. These devices are popular in community-based studies, reviewed later in this chapter, because they allow for safe storage or transport and can allow for easy access to firearms without placement of a device over or around the firearm. The relative concerns related to these devices are the cost and ease of access. They are more expensive, over $100 to over $1000, for an electronic or biometric safe and,

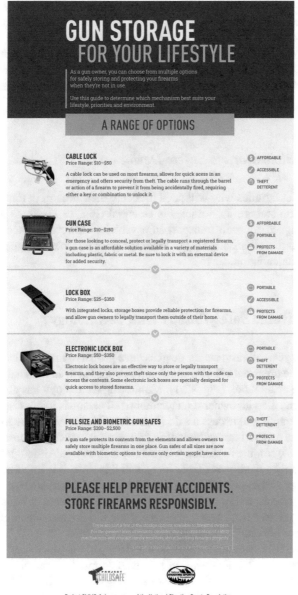

Fig. 12.1 Project ChildSafe – safe storage range of options infographics. (Reproduced with permission of Project ChildSafe, Newtown, CT)

according to some, may limit quick access to firearms, especially if keys or combination locks are used. There are multiple biometric safes in the $200–$300 range that provide quick access (2–3 seconds) to the firearms and can be used by multiple people if desired (i.e., multiple sets of fingerprints). Importantly, the American Academy of Pediatrics (AAP) recommends that even if a firearm is securely stored in a safe, the firearm should be *unloaded, and ammunition should be stored and locked separately.*

12.2.3 Vehicle Storage Safety Device

Importantly, for families who will need to secure their firearm in transport, reviewing safe firearm storage for vehicles is essential (Fig. 12.1). Some lock boxes or safes are designed for safe transport in a vehicle. However, if accessibility in a vehicle is required, an installed cargo area storage or console storage device may be the best recommendation.

12.3 Electronic Safety/Smart Gun Technology

In the past 10 years firearm safety devices have grown to include electronics incorporated into the firearm itself and/or holster, as opposed to an external safety device, such as a safe or lock box (Fig. 12.1). Monitoring technology has also been developed, which can alert an owner if an unauthorized person is in possession of a given firearm or attempting to access a safe (Fig. 12.1). Much in the way that cell phone technology has evolved to use biometric "fingerprint" readers almost ubiquitously, firearms are now coming to market with similar technology. Although many of these devices will not be readily available for sale at this time, it is important to know of this technology and its potential adoption in the future. These smart gun devices are of significant interest to law enforcement and others who want to limit the ability of an unauthorized user from being able to operate the firearm, when other forms of safe storage are not readily available.

In 2016, the US Government commissioned a report on "smart gun" technology in order to summarize developments in this field (https://obamawhitehouse.archives. gov/sites/default/files/docs/final_report-smart_gun_report.pdf). Smart gun technology has been in development since the 1990s, and these technologies are designed to contain *authorization systems,* which generally combine an "authentication mechanism that actuates a blocking mechanism in a seamless process that is designed to take less time than handling and firing a conventional gun." In 2016, when this report was published, there were no smart guns on the United States (US) market. This is due, in part, to the experience of New Jersey, which in 2002 passed "The New Jersey Childproof Handgun Law." This law mandated that 3 years after the first smart gun was sold ("came to market"), it would be illegal to sell any handgun unless that handgun is a personalized handgun. By 2014, viable smart guns became available, but gun stores willing to sell these guns were boycotted and threatened. The backlash, after passage of this law, was swift from the National Rifle Association and other organizations. This attempt to improve firearm safety may have inadvertently led to a slowdown of the development of personalized gun technology. By 2019, New Jersey repealed and amended the original law with a new version passed entitled, "AN ACT concerning personalized handguns and revising various parts of the statutory law." This 2019 law requires licensed firearm dealers in New Jersey to make available for purchase at least one personalized handgun within 60 days of the first personalized handgun being included on a roster of approved personalized handguns by a newly established commission.

In 2019, these technologies are still primarily in development, as the need for very high levels of reliability is critical to their market viability. According to the 2016 report, the "reliability of smart guns remains a topic of interest since early efforts at development in the mid-1990s, with reliability indicated as the most important concern by law enforcement practitioners regarding the potential use of this technology…Reliability can be defined as the probability that a device will perform its intended function for a specified period of time under stated conditions." The report notes what type of testing and certification would be appropriate, but that the US would not mandate this technology on sales. There is an irony that devices designed to inflict lethal injury have no safety standards. This is in part due to the framework used to establish the Consumer Product Safety Commission (CPSC) in 1972. Firearms were specifically excluded from the Consumer Product Safety Commission's jurisdiction, and this was passed into law in 1976. Firearms are essentially the only class of devices not regulated for safety in the US.

Importantly, recent smart gun technology has begun to meet standards of reliability stated by law enforcement and gun ownership groups, including a focus on smart gun technology not being "hacked" or compromised in some way, making the firearm inoperable. The authors of this text do not endorse any specific company/product in this review. One company making a device that contains this new technology is BioFire (Boston, MA, US), which has been highlighted as a firearm

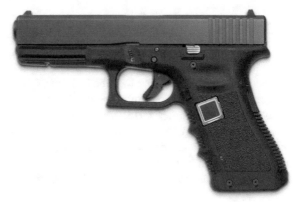

Fig. 12.2 Smart weapon from BioFire, Biometric "reader" indicated in blue box. (Reproduced with permission of BioFire)

safety device integrated into the handgun (Fig. 12.2). It only allows the authorized user to fire after a biometric "fingerprint" read. This gun has the critical additional feature of fast authorization in "less than 1 second" and a locking mechanism making the firearm fully inoperable without an authorized user in hand.

12.4   Safety Devices Are Critical to Safe Firearm Storage

The practice of safe firearm storage requires patients and families to choose from the above devices in order to secure their firearm, to prevent unintended use. It is important to keep in mind the *four* recommended practices of safe firearm storage include keeping a firearm:

- Locked
- Unloaded
- Storing ammunition in a separate location
- Storing ammunition in a locked container

These strategies have been shown to reduce firearm injuries in homes with children and teenagers where guns are stored. We will not review locking devices for ammunition, but it is important to review all four steps in your counseling when discussing firearm safety devices.

There are limited scientific studies on the effectiveness and use of specific firearm safety devices. Most studies examine the risk of injury for children and adolescents with and without a range of safe storage practices and report on preferences for safety devices. *The Journal of Trauma and Acute Care Surgery* did publish a 2018 evidence-based review, which concluded "(1) we conditionally recommend that gun locks be used to prevent unintentional firearm injury and (2) Because of the large effect size and the reasonable quality of available evidence with safe storage of firearms, we recommend safe storage to prevent firearm-related injuries."

12.5   Community Preferences for Firearm Safety Devices

Given the importance of clinician counseling on firearm safety devices in ensuring patients and families are able to effectively perform all four steps in safe firearm storage, we will review the limited research on overall community preferences for safety devices. In studies by Simonetti *et al.*, community-based "firearm safety device giveaway" events enrolled participants in surveys and asked their preferences for firearm safety devices. In two of these studies, a *preference for a firearm safe or lock box* as compared to a cable lock or trigger lock was reported. Although there are limitations to survey-based studies, community-based input is important to understand in clinician counseling or preparation for a firearm safety device give-away event. Of survey participants "residing with unlocked firearms, *84% reported they would consider using or definitely use a lock box*, whereas *11% reported they would never use a trigger lock*." Similarly, in a community-based survey evaluation, "9 of 10 participants preferred a lock box rather than a trigger lock." The authors point out that a clear-cut preference for a lock box is also misleading, given many gun safes or lock boxes are unable to support a long gun, and the cost is prohibitive for the storage of multiple firearms at times.

A study in rural Alaska examined if the installation of gun cabinets (installed gun safes) improved firearm storage practices. Grossman *et al.* performed a "waitlist" randomized trial of the installation of gun safes/cabinets and examined differences between those who received the immediate intervention and those who had to "wait" for the installation and accompanied safety instruction. In-person surveys were conducted at 12 and 18 months to determine the proportion of households reporting unlocked guns or ammunition. Direct observations of unlocked guns were also compared. The baseline level of having at least one unlocked gun in the home was *93% for both groups*. At 12 months, *35% of homes in the early group reported unlocked guns compared with 89% in the late group* ($P < 0.001$). The prevalence of these adopted safe storage practices was maintained at 18 months as well. The study authors concluded installed gun safes may be important to safe storage practices in communities with high levels of gun ownership and unlocked firearms in rural communities.

12.6 Community Acceptance of Smart Gun Technology

As discussed above, smart gun technology is yet to come into the mainstream in the US, and research is now being conducted on preferences and acceptance of this technology. A study by Crifasi *et al.* examined the preferences for smart guns or "personalized guns" through an online survey of gun owners in the US in 2016. Among gun owners surveyed, "48% had heard of personalized guns, and 79% thought licensed dealers should sell both traditional and personalized guns. Only 5% reported that they were very likely, and 13% were somewhat likely, to purchase a personalized gun that added $300 to the price." Similar concerns as those voiced in the 2016 US Government report arose, including concerns about the reliability of the technology and in this case the prices (56% of survey respondents were worried about price of technology). Importantly for counseling, those more interested in buying a personalized or smart gun were *already* more likely to perform safe firearm storage practices, and thus, the potential benefit overall to these new technologies may have limitations in its impact. Price points do not need to be a barrier to the sale of smart guns. As an analogy to electric vehicles and solar panels, federal and state rebates could cover the additional costs to induce early sales of smart gun technology.

12.7   Policy and Legislation Around Firearm Safety Devices

In 2005, Congress passed legislation making it unlawful for any licensed importer, manufacturer, or dealer to sell or transfer any handgun unless the transferee is provided with a secure gun storage or safety device. The legislation does not apply to transfers by private sellers and does not require transferees use the device.

Importantly, there are no US federal standards for firearm safety devices. Executive orders by President Obama called for the Consumer Product Safety Commission (CPSC) to review the effectiveness of gun locks and gun safes, including voluntary industry standards, and to take action to improve standards. It was noted in 2013 there had been safety recalls for "gun locks" through CPSC due to their failure to function properly. However, there is no clear federal guidance on approved safety devices, only state-based rosters and standards. Online resources can be used to examine specific state firearm laws around firearm safety devices (www.statefirearmlaws.org).

Only 11 states have laws around firearm safety devices, though 25 states have some form of child-access prevention (CAP) laws (9 states with recklessness laws and 16 states with negligence laws; see Chap. 13 for further details). As an example, Massachusetts requires all firearms be stored with a locking device in place. California, Connecticut, and New York also have this requirement, but only for certain situations. Recent state law changes have begun to focus on locking devices and access as key points for prevention of firearm injury. It is important for individuals to review their specific state's laws on firearm safety devices and child access prevention laws to provide the best counseling for which devices are approved and when they are mandated by state law. A few examples of state laws are as follows: (1) All firearms are required to be kept disabled with a locking device except when an authorized user is carrying it on his or her person or has the firearm under his or her immediate control (*Massachusetts, New York City*). (2) Locking devices are required on all firearms manufactured, sold, or transferred in the jurisdiction (*California*). (3) Standards are set for locking devices (*California, Connecticut, New York*). (4) Locking devices are tested and approved by a certified independent lab before they may be sold in the jurisdiction (*California*).

12.8   Key Points of Review for Counseling on Safety Devices from Professional Medical Societies

In order to counsel your patients and families on firearm safety devices, it may be helpful to review a list of key points on safety devices from the Massachusetts Medical Society and the Massachusetts Office of the Attorney General. These two organizations have developed two brochures: one for patients "Gun Safety and Your

Health (http://www.massmed.org/firearmguidanceforpatients/) and one for clinicians, "Talking to Patients About Gun Safety" (http://www.massmed.org/firearmguidanceforproviders/) (See Chap. 7). These can be downloaded and distributed for free. There is also information from the American College of Surgeons Committee on Trauma Brochure:

- The safest way to store a gun in your home is unloaded and securely locked, with the bullets locked in a separate [locked] container.
- Easy ways to store a gun safely include gun cases or safes, lock boxes, gun cabinets, and trigger and cable locks.
- Storage at a safe, remote location: As long as a gun is properly stored, a gun does not legally need to be kept in the owner's home. For instance, if a gun is mostly used for hunting, it could be stored in another location when not being used for that purpose. Examples of some remote locations might include in a bonded warehouse for gun storage or in a secure storage unit or in a garage or attic in a lock box or safe.
- Cars are *not* safe places to keep guns: Children can easily access guns left in cars, and cars are often targets for gun theft.

12.9   Creating a Community Safe Firearm Storage Giveaway Event

How to plan a firearm safety device distribution event with a focus on *safety device selection and purchase* and creation of a budget is the focus of the final section of this chapter. Multiple studies have shown the effectiveness of combining firearm safety information with distribution of a firearm safety device. A review of the literature in 2016 demonstrated firearm safety counseling with the distribution of a firearm safety device is the most effective way of ensuring increased safe firearm storage. The following is adapted and abbreviated from the "Safe Firearm Storage Giveaway Event Planning Toolkit," developed by Seattle Children's Hospital in 2017 (https:// www.seattlechildrens.org/pdf/safe-firearm-storage-giveaway-event-planning-toolkit.pdf). The sample event preparation steps below will give you the key steps to create an event, but we recommend reading the *full toolkit* for detailed information on each step and planning. The sample budget below outlines a distribution event for a firearm cable lock/trigger lock and firearm safe/lock box that can accommodate a handgun. The authors note that even with the known preference for gun safes or lock boxes (described in this chapter), they also distribute cable locks to attendees, fully aware that cable locks are often less preferable. Their experience and the evidence indicate if someone owns one firearm, they likely own multiple. Given funding often only allows distribution of one lock box or trigger lock per person, they also offer up to four additional cable locks, as they are a more affordable storage option that might bridge the gap and increase the safe storage of all firearms in the home.

12.9.1 Partnership with Community Organizations

Participation from local community organizations is critical to the success of any injury prevention event. In planning for your safety device giveaway, make sure to include health departments, sporting goods stores, first responders, firearm retailers, firearm range owners, firearm advocacy organizations, law enforcement, and community leaders.

12.9.2 Event Location

Make sure event locations are based on data related to firearm injuries and direct input from stakeholders including hospitals/systems, healthcare providers, and other potential community partners, perceived readiness of the community for the event, and availability of an event host (e.g., sporting goods store).[1] One must also ensure the venue has adequate parking for expected participants and space to accommodate a line of approximately 50–100 participants. If space permits, events are held inside the store and preferably near the firearm safe storage retail section of the store.

12.9.3 Event Host Responsibilities

Consider asking your event host to provide the following: indoor space to host the event. This often requires flexibility by the store manager to move store inventory and displays to create a cohesive and smooth flowing event. Depending on store hours, event attendees may have to form a line outside before the start of the event and allow event coordinators access to the space prior to store opening for setup. Provide a point person for pre-event planning and space/logistic questions. Preferably, the same person will serve as the day-of-event point person. If feasible, we ask the event host to provide a coupon or discount for safe storage devices sold in their store on the day of the event.

12.9.4 Event Promotion

A customized communication plan should be developed with input from local event partners and collaborators. Paid and earned promotion methods may include, but are not limited to, print and online ads (local newspaper, magazines/parent magazine,

---

[1] The authors of this guide indicated that through online polling, they were informed that holding events at a sporting goods location was of the highest interest to their population.

etc.), geo-targeted Facebook ads, social media posts from coordinating centers and community partners' social media platforms, and promotion on coordinating centers and partners' websites. When possible, promotional material should be translated into languages relevant to the local community.

12.9.5   Event Logistics and Considerations

Date selection: If possible, select a Saturday or Sunday to host the event. Weekends are generally the most available times for staff, volunteers, and potential event attendees. Be sure to examine any possible conflicting events that may impact event attendance, such as large firearms or outdoor shows, large community events, sporting events, holidays, etc.

Time of day: Event times may vary based on the event host's store/location hours. An event start time that allows for morning and early afternoon participation is recommended (e.g., 10 a.m.–1 p.m.). A maximum duration of 3–4 hours is recommended to ensure sufficient volunteer support.

12.9.6   Event Specifics

Consider implementing the following requirements for event attendees to receive a device: one item per person, two per household, must be 18 years old and present, and no ID required.

12.9.7   Safe Storage Device Selection

The lock box and trigger lock distributed in this toolkit were chosen based on their price, features, and approval on the *Roster of Firearm Safety Devices Certified for Sale by the State of California Department of Justice,* which provides standards for firearm safety devices (as mentioned in this chapter). Consider working with a local sporting goods wholesaler to purchase devices in bulk to receive discounted pricing. Please note, bulk ordering often requires a 2+ month lead time.

12.9.8   Firearm Safety Devices Chosen for Distribution

Lock box features include:
- Approval from California Department of Justice.
- Bulk pricing at or under $25 (approximate).

- Can be used to store most handguns.
- Cannot be used to store a long gun.
- Three-digit manual combination lock (preferred over a keyed device because children often know where keys are kept or can easily find keys. Combination locks avoid this problem.).
- Comes with cable to secure the lock box to heavy, immovable objects.
- Can be bolted to a hard surface by drilling holes through the bottom of the box.
- Foam in lock box does not have a petroleum smell.

   Trigger lock features include:

- Approval from California Department of Justice
- Bulk pricing at or under $10
- Fits most handguns and long guns
- Three-digit manual combination lock

   Cable lock features include:

- Approval from California Department of Justice
- Bulk pricing at or under $2
- Fits most handguns and long guns

12.9.9   Budget

An example budget can be found in the above link for a firearm safety event. The budget should be scaled to the likely number of attendees and with a focus on lock boxes which, for example, would be 350 lock boxes (350 @ $25 each) = $8750 (USD). Accounting for advertising and coordination assume that most events could run between $1200 and $20,000 (USD).

12.9.10   Event Sponsorship and Funding

Soliciting event sponsorships can help raise funds to host a large-scale event and help sustain an ongoing program.[2] Financial sponsors are given increased visibility through promotion. Community partners who agree to provide support with volunteers help with promotion, introductions to other community organizations. The ultimate goal of bringing on partners, both those who are able to sponsor and

---

[2]The authors note that a majority of their giveaway events have received financial support from local hospitals and/or healthcare systems and some smaller contributions have been made by additional community partners. However, they do not require a financial sponsorship to participate as a community partner for an event.

those that may not be able to, is to build community momentum around the event and important topic of safe firearm storage.

12.9.11   Event Evaluation

Attendees should complete a pre-event survey to assess current firearm storage practices, how they heard about the event, and the primary reason for attending. In addition, volunteers should conduct intercept surveys as people are leaving to ask what they learned, comfort level in using the storage device, what they liked, and what suggestions they have to improve the events.

12.10   Conclusions

In this chapter, we reviewed the most commonly used firearm safety devices on the market in the United States. We reviewed their relative strengths and weaknesses and the limited research on community preferences for devices, including an emphasis on firearm safes or lock boxes. We also reviewed some detail on smart gun technology that is likely to enter the US market in the future. We provided sample information to review with patients and provided an abbreviated safety device giveaway event plan. Clinician knowledge of firearm safety devices is important as part of firearm safety counseling with families. Engaging firearm-owning families in safety storing firearms is an integral part of increasing firearm safe storage to decrease firearm injuries and deaths to children and youth.

Take Home Points

- Gun safes are effective devices for firearm storage, and some studies have shown a preference for this device among community firearm owners.
- Electronic systems have been developed that directly secure a firearm without an external device. These are often referred to as "smart guns," and these technologies are likely to come to the market in the future.
- Educational materials for safety devices are readily available, and community events can effectively distribute safety devices and improve their use.
- Knowledge of firearm safety devices and effective counseling around their use is critical to preventing pediatric firearm injuries and deaths.

Suggested Readings

1. Azad HA, Monuteaux MC, Rees CA, Siegel M, Mannix R, Lee LK, Sheehan KM, Fleegler EW. Child access prevention firearm laws and firearm fatalities among children aged 0 to 14 years, 1991-2016. JAMA Pediatr. 2020;174(5):463–469.
2. Carbone PS, Clemens CJ, Ball TM. Effectiveness of gun-safety counseling and a gun lock giveaway in a Hispanic community. Arch Pediatr Adolesc Med. 2005;159(11):1049–54.
3. Coyne-Beasley T, Schoenbach VJ, Johnson RM. "Love our kids, lock your guns": a community-based firearm safety counseling and gun lock distribution program. Arch Pediatr Adolesc Med. 2001;155(6):659–64.
4. Crifasi CK, O'Dwyer JK, McGinty EE, Webster DW, Barry CL. Desirability of personalized guns among current gun owners. Am J Prev Med. 2019;57(2):191–6.
5. Grossman DC, Stafford HA, Koepsell TD, Hill R, Retzer KD, Jones W. Improving firearm storage in Alaska native villages: a randomized trial of household gun cabinets. Am J Public Health. 2012;102(SUPPL. 2):291–7.
6. Hoops K, Crifasi C. Pediatric resident firearm-related anticipatory guidance: Why are we still not talking about guns? Prev Med. 2019;124:29–32.
7. Rowhani-Rahbar A, Simonetti JA, Rivara FP. Effectiveness of interventions to promote safe firearm storage. Epidemiol Rev. 2016;38(1):111–24.
8. Siegel M, Pahn M, Xuan Z, Ross CS, Galea S, Kalesan B, Fleegler E, Goss KA. Firearm-Related Laws in All 50 US States, 1991-2016. Am J Public Health. 2017;107(7):1122–9.
9. Simonetti JA, Rowhani-Rahbar A, King C, Bennett E, Rivara FP. Evaluation of a community-based safe firearm and ammunition storage intervention. Inj Prev. 2018;24(3):218–23.
10. Simonetti J, Simeona C, Gallagher C, Bennett E, Rivara F, Rowhani-Rahbar A. Preferences for firearm locking devices and device features among participants in a firearm safety event. West J Emerg Med. 2019;20(4):552–6.
11. Teret SP, Culross PL. Product-oriented approaches to reducing youth gun violence. Future Child. 2002;12(2):119–31.
12. Violano P, Bonne S, Duncan T, Pappas P, Britton Christmas A, Dennis A, Crandall M. Prevention of firearm injuries with gun safety devices and safe storage: an Eastern Association for the Surgery of Trauma Systematic review. J Trauma Acute Care Surg. 2018;84(6):1003–11.

Chapter 13
Firearm Legislation and Advocacy

Jody Lyneé Madeira

> After Parkland, Indiana's 2018 gun bills tanked. A year later,
> it's an argument for them
>
> By Kaitlin Lange and Arika Herron
> February 12, 2019. *The Indianapolis Star*

13.1 Introduction

In contemporary America, there is little doubt that gun violence is a pervasive public health problem. There are over 80,000 firearm injuries annually, and over 39,000 fatalities—an average of over 100 people die by firearms per day, 9 of whom are children [1, 2]. Among fatal injuries in youth 15–19 years of age in 2018, more than 1 in 3 (34.4%) were firearm related. In youth under 20 years, almost 1 in 4 (24.0%) were firearm related [2]. The role of firearms in community and domestic violence endanger children's lives, create toxic stress, and increase risks of depression and mental health disorders [3]. Moreover, firearms in homes are associated with an increase in suicide in youth 10–19 years old. For every 10% increase in household gun ownership, youth suicide increased by 26.9% [4]. Public health research has also made important contributions to firearm injury prevention. For example, its methodologies, including epidemiological methods such as network analysis, have illustrated "how violence is transmitted by social interaction through networks of people" [5].

There is widespread consensus that firearm injury prevention is not the same as "gun control" [6]. "Gun control," or firearms regulation, includes the set of laws or policies regulating the manufacture, sale, transfer, possession, modification, or use of firearms by civilians. From a politicized perspective, people who advocate for

J. L. Madeira (✉)
Maurer School of Law, Center for Law, Society, & Culture, Indiana University,
Bloomington, IN, USA
e-mail: jmadeira@indiana.edu

© Springer Nature Switzerland AG 2021   193
L. K. Lee, E. W. Fleegler (eds.), *Pediatric Firearm Injuries and Fatalities*,
https://doi.org/10.1007/978-3-030-62245-9_13

gun control are frequently labeled as individuals who aim to broadly restrict or prohibit firearm use, motivated by opposition to the Second Amendment or the use of
firearms in general, though this may not be accurate. In contrast, public health
efforts to prevent or reduce firearm injury support narrowly tailored, evidence-based
measures (regulatory and non-regulatory) that can reduce the incidence of the most
common and preventable forms of firearm violence. These include efforts to
decrease firearm access to individuals at risk for harming others or themselves:
universal background checks and waiting periods; measures prohibiting felons,
individuals convicted of domestic violence misdemeanors, and those with certain
types of mental illness from gaining access to firearms; and child access prevention
laws to reduce pediatric fatalities. These injury prevention efforts also include
restrictions on the possession of military-style weapons and high-capacity magazines as well as other regulations.

This chapter will discuss pediatric clinician advocacy for firearm injury prevention legislation. It will first describe the sweeping changes the last 20 years have
wrought across legislative, commercial, and cultural landscapes. It will then explore
the evolution of medical professionals' advocacy efforts to reduce firearm violence.
Finally, it will explore particular ways in which pediatricians can advocate to reduce
firearm injuries from firearm violence.

13.2   Recent Changes in Firearm Markets, Laws, and Cultures

13.2.1   Changes in Firearm Markets

The annual "Firearms Commerce in the United States" report published by the
Bureau of Alcohol, Tobacco, and Firearms ("ATF") reveals a clear and compelling
pattern. Between 1986 and 2008, the number of firearms manufactured in the United
States (US) remained within a relatively limited range, from a high of 5.2 million in
1994 to a low of 2.9 million in 2001 [7]. From 2004 to 2013, however, this figure
steadily increased on average (with a sharp increase in 2009, the year after President
Obama was elected) until it reached a high of 11.5 M in 2016 (see Fig. 13.1) [7].
Approximately 165 million guns entered the US market between 2000 and 2017 [7].
At the same time, the total number of forms processed under the National Firearms
Act,[1] which are completed for items such as silencers, machine guns, and modified
shotguns, displayed the same upward trend, from 193,224 in 2004 to a high of
2,530,209 in 2016 [7]. Finally, firearm background checks have grown dramatically

---

[1] The National Firearms Act, passed in 1934, regulates certain firearms, requiring that purchasers
pay a $200 tax and register regulated firearms. These forms include applications to make NFA
firearms, tax exempt transfers between licensees, tax-paid transfers, tax-exempt transfers, and
exported NFA firearms.

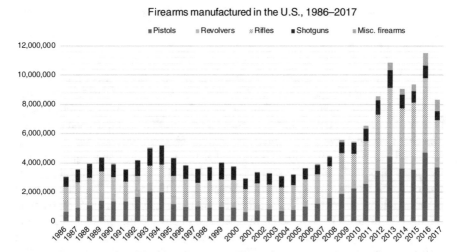

Fig. 13.1 Firearms manufactured in the US, 1986–2017; from the US Department of Justice, Bureau of Alcohol, Tobacco, Firearms, and Explosives, *Firearms Commerce in the United States, Annual Statistical Update*; 2019. https://www.atf.gov/firearms/docs/report/2019-firearms-commerce-report/download

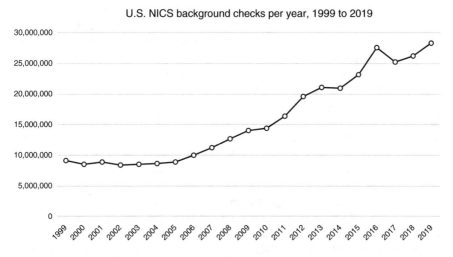

Fig. 13.2 US National Instant Criminal Background Check System (NICS) firearm background checks per year, 1999–2019; from the US Department of Justice, Federal Bureau of Investigation, NICS Firearm Checks (May 31, 2020). https://www.fbi.gov/file-repository/nics_firearm_checks_-_month_year.pdf/view

from 8.5 million in 2000 to an all-time high of 28,369,750 in 2019 (Fig. 13.2) [7]. By the end of 2020, background checks will have risen another 42% in a single year to just shy of a staggering 40 million. These trends indicate that more guns are being manufactured, purchased, and changing hands in the US.

13.2.2 Changes in Firearm Laws and Cultures

13.2.2.1 Federal Law

Federal law plays a limited role in firearm regulation, setting a floor rather than a ceiling for firearm regulation. *The National Firearms Act of 1934*, codified at 26 U.S.C. § 5801, includes taxes on the manufacture, sale, and transfer of some types of firearms, including machine guns, short-barreled shotguns, and silencers. *The Gun Control Act of 1968* (which repealed the *Federal Firearms Act of 1938* but reenacted many of its provisions) is codified at 18 U.S.C. § 921 and requires manufacturers, importers, and sellers to possess a federal license and maintain proper records, prohibits transfers to prohibited purchasers (those with "disabilities," such as prior felony conviction), establishes a minimum age for firearms purchases, requires all firearms to have serial numbers, and bans the importation of firearms with "no sporting purpose." *The Firearm Owners Protection Act of 1986* relaxed restrictions on firearm sellers and liberalized the definition of what it meant to "engage in the business" of selling firearms, allowing licensed dealers to sell at gun shows in the same state, and repealing requirements that ammunition sellers be licensed and that dealers track ammunition sales. It also explicitly banned a central federal database of dealer records. One of the best-known federal firearms regulations is the *Brady Handgun Violence Prevention Act of 1993*, which imposed a background check to determine whether a buyer is a prohibited purchaser. It also mandated if a check could not be completed quickly on the day of purchase, a buyer is entitled to take possession of the firearm in 3 days unless further information emerges. Contemporary background checks conducted by federally licensed firearms dealers involve submitting information to the National Instant Criminal Background Check System (NICS). The Brady Act's requirements were extended to shotguns and rifles in 1998. The *Federal Assault Weapons Ban*, passed in 1994, prohibited the manufacturer, transfer, and possession of semi-automatic assault weapons and the transfer and possession of large capacity magazines holding more than 10 rounds of ammunition, and outlawed 19 assault weapons by name along with any semi-automatic firearm with more than two military features and a detachable magazine (except for shotguns). This ban "sunsetted" or expired in 2004.

Two more federal laws have been passed after the turn of the century. The *Protection of Lawful Commerce in Arms Act and Child Safety Lock Act of 2005* enacted protections for the gun industry from torts suits, barring parties from suing for injuries resulting from the criminal or unlawful misuse of a firearm. There are exceptions for lawsuits alleging breach of contract or warranty, defective design or manufacturer, or negligence per se or negligent entrustment (supplying a firearm or ammunition to persons the seller reasonably should know or knows are likely to use them in ways creating unreasonable risk of physical injury) as well as lawsuits against transferors convicted of transferring a firearm knowing it would be used to commit a violent crime or who knowingly violated state or federal laws about the sale or marketing of firearms or ammunition. Finally, the *National Instant Criminal Background Check System Improvement Amendments Act of 2007* gave states financial incentives to report certain information to NICS (including disqualifying mental health records). It also authorized a grant program for states to establish and upgrade reporting capabilities. Participating states must create a program allowing eligible individuals to appeal and potentially remove disabilities from their records.

13.2.2.2   State Laws and Firearm Culture

For a comprehensive understanding of current state laws across the US, the interactive map at www.statefirearmlaws.org is a very useful resource and shows the evolution of state firearm laws from 1991 to the present. There is specific data available about each state and its laws. Figure 13.3 provides an overview of how many laws per state exist as of 2020 [8].

The unprecedented expansion in firearms markets that began in 2009 has been accompanied by state legislative reforms that relax or repeal "gun control" laws across the US regarding firearm sales, purchase, possession, and storage. State laws affect several types of conduct, including:

- Restricting or prohibiting possession by individuals because of mental health, substance use, or criminal histories (including domestic violence)
- Background checks
- Regulations on ammunition sales, firearm possession, concealed and open carry, "assault weapons," and large-capacity magazines (especially associated with the 2004 sunsetting of the Public Safety and Recreational Firearms Use Protection

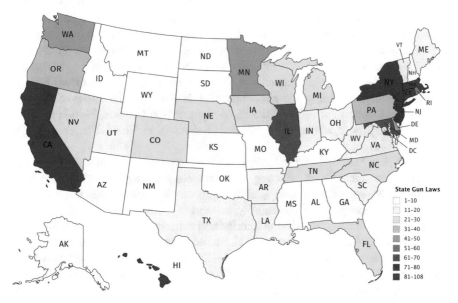

Fig. 13.3 Overview of gun laws per state as of 2020; from Dr. Michael Siegel, State Firearm Laws Database, www.statefirearmlaws.org/

Act, commonly called the Federal Assault Weapons Ban, which was a part of the Violent Crime Control and Law Enforcement Act of 1994)
- Safe gun storage and child access prevention
- Gun trafficking
- State preemption of local gun regulations
- State immunity statutes for gun manufacturers and sellers [8]

Recent trends in "gun rights" legislation include:

- Reforming state law to permit firearm concealed carry in traditionally sensitive areas such as schools, houses of worship, college campuses, and courthouses
- Repeal of license requirements for firearm purchases and concealed carry ("Constitutional Carry" laws)
- Preempting cities and municipalities from passing their own firearm regulations
- "Stand your ground" self-defense statutes
- Protective immunity legislation limiting or eliminating legal liability of gun manufacturers and sellers for violent acts committed with a firearm [8]

Since 2008, however, many states have also enacted "gun control" laws, including those regulating firearm possession for domestic violence offenders, background checks for concealed carry permits, and prohibitions on firearm possession for felons and those involuntarily committed for mental health treatment [8].

Attempting to identify whether the surges in firearm sales and state legislation were related to National Rifle Association (NRA) activities, Reich and Barth found that two variables contributed to these issues [9]. Conservative state legislatures were more likely to deregulate from 2009 to 2013 [9]. Moreover, NRA election spending (not lobbying) furthered deregulation in states where more residents flocked to buy firearms in the months before and after President Obama's election [9]. Reich and Barth have argued that preemptive firearm sales before the election opened the door for the NRA to influence state legislation in the direction of deregulation [9]. Many laws were passed in the wake of some of the largest mass killings in US history, including the shootings at Sandy Hook Elementary School in Newtown, Connecticut in 2012; the Pulse night club in Orlando, Florida in 2016; and the Marjory Stoneman Douglas High School in Parkland, Florida in 2018, among others.

These laws have both stemmed from and reinforced recent changes in US firearm culture, from recreational shooting to an emphasis on armed self-defense [10]. Carlson's research connects men's decisions to carry firearms as "citizen-protectors" to changing conceptions of masculinity, patterns of socioeconomic decline, perceptions of economic and physical insecurity, and concerns about perceived increases in crime and police ineffectiveness [11]. Stroud examines the cultural meanings of concealed carry for Texas permit holders [12]. In this article, respondents emphasized masculine goals such as protecting themselves and family members and compensating for lost physical strength due to age, or sex differences between women and male attackers.

13.2.2.3 State Laws That Could Reduce Gun Violence

The causal impact of state and federal laws on firearm violence and suicide remains controversial. Most studies use a panel regression method to "model differences in violent outcomes between states with and without a particular type of law over time" [8]. This methodology requires "data from a large number of states over a substantial period of time" to determine that the enactment or repeal of a law has a statistically significant association. However, until www.statefirearmlaws.org became available in 2017, no publicly available database allowed researchers to access "comprehensive information on a wide range of state firearm laws over an extended period of time," let alone an analysis of how the same firearm laws applied differently across states [8].

Research on gun violence was stymied after the Dickey Amendment in 1996 eliminated $2.6 million from the Centers for Disease Control and Prevention (CDC) budget. This occurred after the agency began to support firearms research, which demonstrated, among other findings, the increased risk of harm that firearms pose to members of a household. After passage of the Dickey Amendment, the role of the CDC was "relegated to monitoring firearm injuries by surveillance of firearm statistics," without making policy recommendations [13]. This restriction on firearm research funding quickly spread to the Nation Institute of Health (NIH) and Department of Health and Human Services (DHHS). Soon thereafter, databases related to firearm sales and ownership were eliminated, and data from background checks were destroyed within 24 hours [13]. Fortunately, since the Obama administration's action, the Institute of Medicine (now the National Academy of Medicine) has developed a research agenda aiming to reduce firearm-related violence, and funding for firearm research has finally been reinstated [14].

There are several types of laws that research suggests are effective and should be included in legislative advocacy efforts. Ultimately, these laws will be most effective if several of them are implemented across the country, for a robust interstate effect [15, 16].

- *Universal background checks*: This goal would be best achieved by requiring all firearm transfers and ammunition sales be completed through federally licensed dealers [17, 18]. It would ensure that all individuals who lawfully take possession of a firearm complete a background check and that records are kept for all sales and transfers. At a minimum, all firearm sales at gun shows, and all firearm sales between individuals, should include a background check and the requirement that transaction records are kept.
- *"Assault weapons" bans*: This could help prevent gun violence by restricting access to the types of weapons most frequently used in mass shootings. These weapons are capable of injuring or killing the most people at one time, without requiring the shooter to reload the weapon. Most current state bans on military-style rifles (predominantly enacted in the Northeast) list banned weapons by name or through listed features (banning weapons with one or two features).

They require assault weapon registration, prohibit transfers of previously owned qualifying weapons, and mandate owners have a location or license for previously owned qualifying weapons.

- *Limiting numbers of firearms that can be purchased within a certain time period*: One example includes laws limiting a firearm purchase to one per month [18]. These provisions help reduce illegal gun trafficking and deter dangerous individuals from building arsenals in a short period of time.
- *Buyer safety regulations*: These include laws require buyers to obtain a permit or license, require background checks, or mandate buyers undergo requisite safety training.
- *Child Access Prevention (CAP) laws*: These laws regulate the safe storage of guns from children by gun owners. Under strong CAP laws, prosecutors can charge owners who negligently store firearms and who know or reasonably should know that a minor could gain access, regardless of whether a minor actually accesses the firearm and/or harm occurs. A weaker version imposes criminal liability only when a child actually gains access, and the weakest version imposes criminal liability only if a child gains access and carries or uses the firearm. A less effective type of CAP law prohibits intentionally, knowingly, or recklessly allowing minors to access firearms, excluding negligence. Sometimes weak CAP laws only permit liability for parents or guardians if they provide a firearm to a minor knowing there is a substantial risk that the minor will use it to commit a crime.
- *Extreme risk protection order (ERPO) laws*: These laws help to remove access to firearms for a person who is at risk of harming themselves or others. Violence against one's self or others is often preceded by warning signs that family members or friends can detect. For this reason, as of 2020, 18 states and the District of Columbia allow family or household members, and in some cases law enforcement and health officials, to submit a petition for an ERPO. Other states allow others such as mental health professionals, coworkers, educators, or school administrators to petition. ERPOs can be ordered without notice (but may then last for a shorter time), or they can be issued after notice and a hearing. Final orders can last up to a year (depending on the state) and are subject to renewal, but individuals can request a hearing to prove that they are no longer a risk.

13.2.2.4 Notable Shifts Following Mass Shootings

The legislative "gun rights" tide is slowly ebbing, however. After the Sandy Hook Elementary School shooting in Newtown, CT, on December 14, 2012, some Northeastern states passed bans on "assault weapons" and high-capacity magazines, but federal reforms including a comprehensive background check requirement were not passed. On January 16, 2013, President Obama initiated 23 executive actions and 12 Congressional proposals mandating that federal agencies allow the *National Instant Criminal Background Check System (NICS)* access to relevant data, requiring traces of recovered crime guns, incentivizing states to share information with

NICS, providing guidance for federally licensed firearms dealers on how to conduct background checks for private sellers, training for armed attacks, reviewing current safety standards for gun locks and gun safes and gun safety technologies, developing model emergency response plans, and other measures. Connecticut revised its existing "assault weapons" ban prohibiting the sale of magazines holding more than ten ammunition rounds and requiring comprehensive background checks, which has been upheld as constitutional in federal court. New York's *SAFE act*, enacted on January 16, 2013, expanded the definition of "assault weapons" under state law, created a pistol permit database, implemented universal background checks, and prohibited all magazines holding over seven rounds. A federal court subsequently struck down the seven-round prohibition but upheld the "assault weapons" ban. Maryland enacted the *Firearm Safety Act of 2013*, which banned 45 types of firearms, required handgun licensing and fingerprinting for new owners, and restricted those who have been involuntarily committed to a mental health institution from possessing a firearm. This ban has also been upheld as constitutional by a federal court.

Finally, the Sandy Hook Elementary School and subsequent shootings have had a revolutionary effect on gun violence prevention advocacy. Moms Demand Action for Gun Sense in America (https://momsdemandaction.org/), founded the day after Sandy Hook, is a grassroots gun-violence prevention organization supporting measures to prevent gun violence, such as universal background checks. In April 2014, Moms Demand Action merged with Mayors Against Illegal Guns to form Everytown for Gun Safety (https://everytown.org), which has undertaken educational, policy, and lobbying activities, and spent more in the 2018 election cycle than the NRA and other gun rights organizations. Immediately after the shooting at Marjory Stoneman Douglas High School in Parkland, FL in 2018, student survivors founded March For Our Lives (https://marchforourlives.com), advocating student walkouts in schools across the country one month after the shooting. Thereafter, the organization dedicated itself to student-led activism to end gun violence and mass shootings.

13.3   Advocacy by Medical Professional Associations

Medical professionals have traditionally taken stands against public health issues such as tobacco use, unintentional poisoning, motor vehicle safety [19], and most recently, gun violence prevention. As Laine and Taichman emphasized in an *Annals of Internal Medicine* editorial:

> [w]hen public health crises arise, our powerful health care complex responds by doing what our scientific training and duty to help others require. We formulate questions that need answers, collect and analyze data to answer them, test hypotheses to discover remedies, study how to implement them, and monitor progress. . . . But it seems to stop when it comes to firearm injury. Why? [14]

This is especially true since safe storage has been shown to reduce the risk of suicide and unintentional injury for children and adolescents [20]. Research suggests that popular children's gun safety programs such as Eddie Eagle from the NRA are not effective, since when a child finds a gun, their behavior will likely not follow program guidelines [21]. Moreover, these programs place the burden of avoiding firearm injury on the child, instead of the adults around them. Child Access Prevention laws, specifically negligence laws promoting safe storage of firearms, are associated with reductions in pediatric firearm fatalities including homicides, suicides, and unintentional deaths [22]. In addition to addressing firearms in the child's home, parents and caregivers should also consider whether there are firearms in other homes visited by the child. The American Academy of Pediatrics (AAP) promotes the ASK (Asking Saves Kids) program [23], with the goal of increasing parents' willingness to ask about whether there are guns in the homes that their children visit [24].

As the gun violence prevention advocacy movement has grown, professional medical organizations such as the American Bar Association (ABA), American Medical Association (AMA), American Academy of Family Physicians (AAFP), American College of Emergency Physicians (ACEP), American Congress of Obstetricians and Gynecologists (ACOG), American College of Physicians (ACP), American College of Surgeons (ACS), American Psychiatric Association (APA), and the American Academy of Pediatrics (AAP) have joined together to "press… for increased research . . . to discover strategies to diminish firearm-related harms," supporting universal background checks and restrictions on "military-style weapons and high capacity magazines" [14, 24]. Individually, these organizations have created professional practice guidelines and policy recommendations and conducted member surveys. They have also published consensus statements that advocate approaching firearm violence as a medical or public health problem, encourage firearms counseling on safe storage and other initiatives, promote the development of research agendas, and support evidence-based violence prevention programs, federal research funding, and legislation such as that increasing funding and availability of mental health programs.

The AAP in particular has made firearm injury prevention a "high priority," including "advocating for better regulation of the use of and sale of firearms" [24]. Pediatricians have a unique opportunity to "play a critical role . . . in framing a message to convey to families in terms of child development and safety" [24]. The American College of Physicians, active in gun violence prevention for over 20 years, urges its members to "advocate for national, state, and local efforts to enact legislation to implement evidence-based policies . . . including, but not limited to universal background checks." They also support "appropriate regulation of the purchase of legal firearms to reduce firearms-related injuries and deaths," as well as completion of a firearms training program, domestic violence restraining orders and purchasing restrictions, bans on firearms undetectable through security screening, implementation of waiting periods following purchase, limiting concealed-carry expansion, and bans on future sales and possession of military-style firearms [25]. The AAP is openly supportive of child access prevention legislation as well as (1) mandatory waiting periods, (2) universal background checks, (3) mental health restrictions for gun purchases, and (4) restoration of the "assault weapons" ban [26]. It advises practitioners to connect with state AAP chapters, engage local media by sending letters to the editor (with speaking points), contact state and federal legislators to advocate for "improved gun safety legislation and funding for mental health services," and provide firearm safety anticipatory guidance [27].

Most recently, medical professionals have demonstrated a willingness to directly assert ownership over efforts to reduce gun violence and prevent firearm injury. In response to the publication of an American College of Physicians position paper in November 2018, the NRA tweeted that "self-important anti-gun doctors [should] stay in their lane." This spurred an avalanche of responses from medical professionals across the country, accelerated by another mass shooting that occurred less than 12 hours after the NRA tweet [6]. As Ranney *et al.* remarked, "the broad and rapid response to #ThisIsOurLane reflects not a new movement, but rather the convergence of multiple paths on which physicians had already embarked" [6].

13.4 Opportunities for Advocacy and Intervention for Pediatric Health Care Professionals

Like other successful health interventions requiring multi-pronged approaches, effectively addressing gun violence requires pediatric clinicians to engage in several activities, ranging from clinical practices to private expert testimony to initiating or joining professional associations' programming or participating in safety coalitions.

13.4.1 Counseling Patients

One of the most important advocacy opportunities is discussing firearms as a safety concern and providing anticipatory guidance to parents and patients, as one would for car seats, wood-burning stoves, or smoking in the home (See Chap. 7). This option, however, may not be easy, depending on caregiver attitudes toward firearms. Discussions on firearms, including firearm safety, between clinicians and families became highly controversial after state legislatures began to debate or enact laws restricting this conduct. The most infamous of these laws, Florida's *Firearm Owners' Protection Act of 2011* (FOPA) (also known as the Physician Gag Law), was passed on the heels of legislative testimony alleging that patients had been dismissed from practices, told that Medicaid would not cover visits if they refused to answer firearm-related questions, or otherwise were treated disparagingly. FOPA prohibited medical professionals from asking patients about firearms or intentionally entering disclosed information about firearm ownership into a patient's medical record unless it was relevant to the patient's or others' medical care or safety. In February of 2017, the US Court of Appeals for the Eleventh Circuit ruled that key FOPA provisions were unconstitutional for physicians on First Amendment grounds, because they impinged on medical professionals' First Amendment free speech rights. They held that patients had a right to learn such information and that no evidence suggested medical professionals had been inappropriately intrusive concerning patients' firearms ownership or been involved in firearms confiscation efforts [28]. The court did find that providers could not dismiss patients for refusing to discuss firearms. Other states have passed less draconian laws that still regulate some elements of physician-patient communication about firearms [29]. Minnesota, Missouri, and Montana all have restrictions on how firearm information can be collected and stored, but do not prohibit physician inquiries. However, these laws may still make health care workers wary about discussing guns.

Despite the outcome of this case, and assertions from the American Bar Association that firearm screening is compatible with the Second Amendment [19], researchers have found many practitioners are reluctant to screen for firearms or give anticipatory guidance, lest they seem "intrusive or offensive" [24]. Parents are receptive to physician counseling and most believe that pediatricians should provide safe storage advice [30]. In addition, 66% to 85% of physicians believe they have the right to counsel patients about firearm safety and a responsibility to prevent firearm-related injuries [31]. Yet, these beliefs are not carried over into practice, as few physicians counsel patients about firearms [32, 33]. This pattern has changed little over decades. In a 1997 study involving pediatric residents, firearms were not discussed in a single child-well visit out of 178 that were recorded [34]. A 2014 survey of 573 internists reported that 58% never asked whether patients had guns in the home, and 77% never discussed strategies for reducing the risk of gun-related injury [35].

This professional reluctance is unfortunate, because physician counseling can effectively promote safe storage [24]. During counseling, pediatricians can tailor advice to a child's developmental stage and discuss safety practices appropriate to those capacities, as well as describing "layers" of separation, such as both "gun safety" programs and physically separating the firearm from the child [24]. Screening for firearms is especially critical when there is an acute risk that a patient or parent will be violent to themselves or others (suicidal or homicidal ideation) and when certain individual factors are present (history of violence or substance abuse, serious mental illness, and conditions impairing cognition) [31]. Pediatricians are also readily able to debunk common myths about pediatric firearm injuries, such as that most firearm deaths are caused by mentally ill mass shooters, a gun in the home makes residents safer, and children don't know where parents' guns are kept in the home [36]. Critically, pediatric clinicians can also recommend emergency removal of firearms from a home where adolescents are depressed or have other indications of violence against self or others. Thus, it is paramount that clinicians know and understand their state laws regarding removal or prohibition of possessing or acquiring firearms for at-risk individuals.

For these reasons, several professional organizations, including the AAP and the AMA, are developing continuing education programs to educate physicians about how to discuss firearm safety with patients [37].

Clinicians who are reluctant to screen for firearms in the home can provide all patients with firearm safety information, but research has not yet demonstrated the efficacy of that approach [24]. Sanberg and Wang recommend a simple rubric, the "5 Ls": "If there is a gun in the home: (1) is it Locked, (2) is it Loaded, (3) are there Little children, (4) is anyone in the house feeling Low, and (5) is the owner Learned?" [36] As to the last point, even the most knowledgeable firearm owners can underestimate the risks associated with keeping loaded firearms in the home. It should also be noted regarding the presence of little children that adolescents are at significantly greater risk for death from firearms (i.e., suicide) than young children.

There are some potential barriers to firearm counseling. For example, patients could perceive that medical professionals are not trustworthy nor reliable sources of information because they "are not likely to be familiar with or accepting of firearms or firearm culture" [38]. To overcome this obstacle, firearms screening and counseling should be culturally sensitive, acknowledging both the protection of constitutional rights and protecting self and others from harm [39, 40]. To these ends, Betz *et al.* recommend that medical professionals educate themselves about federal and state laws (particularly Extreme Risk Protection Order "red-flag" laws applicable in high-risk situations passed in 18 states as of February 2020) to effectively discuss firearm safety and provide counsel [28, 36]. Physicians can also strive to learn about perceived risks and benefits of firearm ownership [28]. Physicians who own firearms could "provide leadership to their peers around developing competencies in firearm safety counseling" [38]. Researchers have also recommended that counseling include free gun locks, a step identified as "critical" in firearm safety promotion.

13.4.2   Collaborating with Community Organizations and Coalitions

Pediatric clinicians can also reach out to local community organizations, such as school districts and community mental health organizations, to offer their expertise with crisis planning. Such action increases public familiarity with a district's emergency plans and can make it easier to coordinate in case of a firearm-related incident. Community engagement can also allow pediatric clinicians to invite local officials or experts to visit professional settings or attend organizational events in turn to share expertise and stories.

Pediatric clinicians can participate in interdisciplinary coalitions to prevent firearm violence and injury. Some coalitions exist to achieve specific, pragmatic goals, such as the American College of Surgeons Committee on Trauma's "Stop the Bleed" program, a national public awareness campaign to train members of the public to help in a bleeding emergency (such as a significant trauma or a shooting) before professional medical help arrives. The program has excellent intentions, although it is unclear whether it has medical value. Nor do we know the unintended consequences of training people, including children and youth, to feel medically responsible during a mass shooting events, when this is something most people will never experience.

A second example is local partnerships that have developed between firearm ranges and public health professionals, with the purpose of providing suicide prevention education to gun shop customers and training employees how to identify at-risk customers. Of particular note, the National Shooting Sports Foundation has partnered with the American Foundation for Suicide Prevention to disseminate educational materials about suicide risk factors and warning signs to gun owners through firearms retailers and shooting ranges nationwide [6]. Finally, one residency program at Indiana University trains residents through Everytown's "Be Smart" program (https://besmartforkids.org/about), which raises awareness that storing guns locked, unloaded, and separate from locked ammunition can save children's lives. Residents are taught to perform bedside discussions with patients and chart these conversations. In addition, residents staff a table in support of the Be Smart program at community events while wearing their white coats.

Other collaborations are engaged in research and policy change. Health care leaders from several specialties formed the American Foundation for Firearm Injury Reduction in Medicine (AFFIRM), with the goal of producing research and collaborative action [6]. In more than 20 states, collaborations between firearm stakeholders and public health experts have been founded to "inform the development and implementation of effective, culturally-sensitive prevention and intervention efforts" [38]. For example, public health practitioners, firearm retailers, and local firearm instructors formed the New Hampshire Firearm Safety Coalition in 2009 following several suicides with recently purchased firearms, with the goal of preventing future instances [41]. This group is developing and sharing guidelines on how to identify potentially suicidal individuals. Part of their efforts also includes displaying and distributing suicide prevention materials tailored to firearm purchasers at firearm retailers. A similar group, the Colorado Firearm Safety Coalition, includes firearm instructors, Colorado Department of Public Health and Environment employees, and public health researchers. This group has also trained physicians and medical students on how to use and store firearms [38].

13.4.3   Engaging in Legislative Advocacy Through Letter-Writing or Expert Testimony

Legislative and legal advocacy to promote evidence-based policy measures can be efficacious in decreasing youth firearm injury and mortality [16]. These activities include both helping to pass certain types of legislation that can reduce firearm injury and actively opposing other legislation that could increase it. Recent years have witnessed a number of accomplishments for medical professional advocacy. It would be difficult to advocate for firearm screening and safety counseling if physicians had not challenged the constitutionality of FOPA on the grounds that such regulations may "interfere with medical practice [and quality of care] by substituting politics and legislative judgment for medical expertise" [42]. Moreover, physicians have successfully challenged similar laws in other states. In 2015, North Carolina physicians opposed House Bill 562, which barred any health care provider from asking a patient about their ownership or storage of firearms, except to prevent imminent deadly harm, or risk being fined. The medical community sent out press releases, called reporters, and had hallway conversations with legislators in a "White Coat Wednesday" event.

An excellent way to garner support for or against particular legislative initiatives is to publish a letter to the editor in a respected local or national publication. Individuals looking for assistance can consult the AAP website for speaking points on firearms, mental health, and school violence, and lists of media outlets and contacts by zip code. One area of regulation that needs to be addressed is the absence of safety regulations for firearms, over which the U.S. Consumer Product Safety Commission (CPSC) has elected not to exercise jurisdiction.

Engaging in legislative advocacy can require creative strategies depending on the context. The first question is what evidence legislators will find most persuasive. Peer-reviewed studies, the gold standard in evidence-based medical practice, are an excellent way to establish relationships between legislative actions and social trends. But they may not be useful in hearings where legislators attempt to debunk statistical conclusions or dismissively remark, "Correlation, not causation." Analyses using complex methodology such as the synthetic control technique can be difficult to explain in the few moments allotted for testimony [43]. In the age of "post-truth" politics, legislators may simply deem statistics and studies too abstract and elitist. Anecdotes, on the other hand, carry a great deal of emotional weight, but lack generalizability. Ideally, then, pediatricians who engage in legislative advocacy will equip themselves both with research evidence and anecdotes to both illustrate the consequences of legislative action or inaction and give their testimony the necessary sticking power. Effective advocates can also build relationships with news media and reporters, who cover legislative hearings and air interviews with experts.

Through letter-writing, speaking to legislators, and providing legislative testimony, pediatric clinicians can advocate for several specific state-level regulations to reduce gun violence.

- Comprehensive background checks for all firearm purchases (including private sales between individuals). These laws could prevent some firearms from reaching prohibited purchasers; currently, 40% of transfers (an estimated 6.6 million) take place outside a federally licensed dealer [19].
- Paired waiting periods of 3 days to pick up a firearm after purchase. These laws have also been associated with reducing fatalities.
- Increasing funding for and access to mental health care. Most mental illness by itself is not a disqualifying factor for firearm ownership [19].
- Extreme Risk Protective Order (ERPO) "red flag" laws. These laws allow families and law enforcement to report patients at risk of harming themselves or others. They could be advantageous so long as they balance rights with public safety,

promote confidentiality, and do not deter patients from seeking treatment [19]. Most ERPO laws do not allow health care clinicians (including psychiatrists) to petition the courts, but they can still be an effective tool in times of crisis. Expanding current ERPO laws to allow health care clinicians to petition is another way to help patients.

- Releasing the facilitation of temporary transfer of firearms during times of crisis. These laws are needed to protect recipients of firearms from liability [44, 45].
- Regulating or prohibiting private ownership of "military-style" weapons and high-capacity magazines. These laws could reduce the risk of shooting casualties [19].

13.5 Conclusions

For nigh on three decades, the majority of medical professional associations, including the American Academy of Pediatrics, have incorporated firearm injury prevention advocacy into their policy statements, standards of care, and organizational calls to action. Years ago, it was easier to understand why medical professionals might initially be uncomfortable with advocating to reduce firearm injury and violence. Not only were firearms highly politicized, but also it was easier to construe "advocacy" to mean promoting subjective viewpoints over evidence-based practices and forsaking the role of trusted professional for that of biased pundit. Now, in the face of irrefutable evidence that firearm injuries are a public health crisis, staying silent runs counter to a healing ethos. It is no longer ethical [46] to passively confront the impact that firearm injuries and deaths have upon the families and youth; advocacy and local action are prime weapons against this epidemic [47, 48].

Take Home Points
- Most laws regulating the sale, purchase, and ownership of firearms are instituted on the state, not the federal, level.
- Pediatric clinicians should be aware of the certain types of laws in their state, including child access prevention (CAP) and extreme risk protection order (ERPO) laws, that are directly related to child safety.
- Anticipatory guidance by pediatrician clinicians to their patients is important to decrease firearm injuries and deaths to children and youth. Recent attempts by state legislatures to limit physicians' ability to provide firearm safety anticipatory guidance to patients and families have not been upheld in higher courts.
- Advocacy on the state level for effective firearm injury prevention legislation can be done in various ways by pediatric clinicians and public health advocates.

References

1. Baackes J, Seidman R. Why we should be treating gun violence like every other epidemic [Internet]. California health report 2018; 2020 [cited Mar 24]. Available from: https://www.calhealthreport.org/2018/04/26/treating-gun-violence-like-every-epidemic/. Accessed 29 Aug 2019.
2. Centers for Disease Control and Prevention. Data and statistics (WISQARS) [Internet]; 2020 [cited Mar 24]. Available from: https://www.cdc.gov/injury/wisqars/index.html
3. American Academy of Pediatrics (AAP), Council on Injury, Violence, and Poison Prevention Executive Committee. Firearm-related injuries affecting the pediatric population. Pediatrics. 2012;130(5):e1416–23.
4. Knopov A, Sherman RJ, Raifman JR, Larson EL. Household gun ownership and youth suicide rates at the state level, 2005–2015. Am J Prev Med. 2019;56(3):335–42.
5. Green B, Horel T, Papchristos AV. Modeling contagion through social networks to explain and predict gunshot violence in Chicago, 2006 to 2014. JAMA Intern Med. 2017;177(3):326–33.
6. Ranney ML, Betz ME, Dark C. #ThisIsOurLane - Firearm safety as health care's highway. N Engl J Med. 2019;380(5):405–7.
7. United States Department of Justice, Bureau of Alcohol, Tobacco, Firearms, & Explosives. Firearms commerce in the United States: annual statistical update 2019 [Internet]; 2020 [cited Mar 24]. Available from: https://www.atf.gov/firearms/docs/report/2019-firearms-commerce-report/download
8. Siegel M, Pahn M, Ziming X, Ross CS, Galea S, Kalesan B, Fleegler E, Goss KA. Firearm-related laws in all 50 US states, 1991–2016. Am J Public Health. 2017;107(7):1122–9.
9. Reich G, Barth J. Planting in fertile soil: the National Rifle Association and state firearms legislation. Soc Sci Q. 2019;98(2):485–99.
10. Yamane D. The sociology of U.S. gun culture. Soc Compass. 2017;11(7):e12497.
11. Carlson J. Citizen-protectors: the everyday politics of guns in an age of decline. New York: Oxford University Press; 2015.
12. Stroud A. Good guys with guns: the appeal and consequences of concealed carry. Chapel Hill: University of North Carolina Press; 2016.
13. Cagle MC, Martinez JM. Have gun, will travel: the dispute between the CDC and the NRA on firearm violence as a public health problem. Politics Policy. 2004;32(2):278–310.
14. Laine C, Taichman DB. Reducing firearm-related harms. Ann Intern Med. 2015;163(4):325–6.
15. Santaella-Tenorio J, Cerdá M, Villaveces A, Galea S. What do we know about the association between firearm legislation and firearm-related injuries? Epidemiol Rev. 2016;38(1):140–57.
16. Kaufman EJ, Morrison CN, Brana CC, Wiebe DJ. State firearm laws and interstate firearm deaths from homicide and suicide in the United States: a cross-sectional analysis of data by county. JAMA Intern Med. 2018;178(5):692–700.
17. Fleegler EW, Lee LK, Monuteaux MC, Hemenway D, Mannix R. Firearm legislation and firearm-related fatalities in the United States. JAMA Intern Med. 2013;173(9):732–40.
18. Lee LK, Fleegler EW, Farrell C, Avakame E, Srinivasan S, Hemenway D, Monuteaux MC. Firearm laws and firearm homicides: a systematic review. JAMA Intern Med. 2017;177(1):106–19.
19. Weinberger SE, Hoyt DB, Lawrence HC 3rd, Levin S, Henley DE, Alden ER, et al. Firearm-related injury and death in the United States: a call to action from 8 health professional organizations and the American Bar Association. Ann Intern Med. 2015;162(7):513–6.
20. Grossman DC, Mueller BA, Riedy C, Dowd MD, Villaveces A, Prodzinski J, et al. Gun storage practices and risk of youth suicide and unintentional firearm injuries. JAMA. 2005;293(6):707–14.
21. Himle MB, Miltenberger RG, Gatheridge BJM, Flessner CA. An evaluation of two procedures for training skills to prevent gun play in children. Pediatrics. 2004;113(1 Pt 1):70–7.

22. Azad HA, Monteaux MC, Rees CA, Siegel M, Mannix R, Lee LK, et al. Child access prevention firearm laws and firearm fatalities among children aged 0 to 14 years, 1991–2016. JAMA Pediatr. 2020;174(5):463–9.
23. American Academy of Pediatrics (AAP). 8 things you can do to support ASK (Asking Saves Kids) day [Internet]; 2020 [cited Mar 24]. Available from: https://www.aap.org/en-us/about-the-aap/aap-press-room/news-features-and-safety-tips/Pages/8-Things-You-Can-Do-to-Support-ASK-(Asking-Saves-Kids)-Day.aspx
24. Dowd MD. Firearm injury prevention: the role of the clinician. Pediatr Ann. 2017;46(4):e127–30.
25. Butkus R, Doherty R, Bornstein SS. Reducing firearm injuries and deaths in the United States: a position paper from the American College of Physicians. Ann Intern Med. 2018;169(10):704–7.
26. American Academy of Pediatrics (AAP). Addressing gun violence [Internet]. https://www.aap.org/en-us/advocacy-and-policy/aap-health-initiatives/Pages/Gun-Violence-Matrix%2D%2DIntentional-(Federal).aspx. Accessed 29 Aug 2019.
27. American Academy of Pediatrics (AAP). How pediatricians can advocate for children's safety in their communities [Internet]. https://www.aap.org/en-us/advocacy-and-policy/Pages/How-Pediatricians-Can-Advocate-for-Childrens-Safety-in-Their-Communities.aspx. Accessed 29 Aug 2019.
28. Betz ME, Ranney ML, Wintemute GJ. Physicians, patients, and firearms: the courts say "yes". Ann Intern Med. 2017;166(10):745–6.
29. McCourt AD, Vernick JS. Law, ethics, and conversations between physicians and patients about firearms in the home. AMA J Ethics. 2018;20(1):69–76.
30. Garbutt JM, Bobenhouse N, Dodd S, Sterkel R, Strunk RC. What are parents willing to discuss with their pediatricians about firearm safety? A parental survey. J Pediatr. 2016;179:166–71.
31. Wintemute GJ, Betz ME, Ranney ML. Yes, you can: physicians, patients, and firearms. Ann Intern Med. 2016;165(3):205–13.
32. Grossman DC, Mang K, Rivara FP. Firearm injury prevention counseling by pediatricians and family physicians: practices and beliefs. Arch Pediatr Adolesc Med. 1995;149(9):973–7.
33. Hoops K, Crifasi C. Pediatric resident firearm-related anticipatory guidance: why are we still not talking about guns? Prev Med. 2019;124:29–32.
34. Roszko PJD, Ameli J, Carter PM, Cunningham RM, Ranney ML. Clinician attitudes, screening practices, and interventions to reduce firearm-related injury. Epidemiol Rev. 2016;38(1):87–110.
35. Butkus R, Weissman A. Internists' attitudes toward prevention of firearm injury. Ann Intern Med. 2014;160(12):821–7.
36. Sandberg M, Wang NE. Pragmatic firearm advocacy for pediatricians. Hosp Pediatr. 2017;7(6):361–3.
37. Massachusetts Medical Society. Talking to patients about gun safety [Internet]; 2020 [cited Mar 24]. Available from: http://www.massmed.org/Continuing-Education-and-Events/Online-CME/Courses/Patient-Conversations-About-Firearms/Talking-to-Patients%2D%2DAbout-Gun-Safety/
38. Jager-Hyman S, Wolk CB, Ahmedani BK, Zeber JE, Fein JA, Brown GK, et al. Perspectives from firearm stakeholders on firearm safety promotion in pediatric primary care as a suicide prevention study: a qualitative study. J Behav Med. 2019;42(4):691–701.
39. Marino E, Wolsko C, Keys S, Wilcox H. Addressing the cultural challenges of firearm restriction in suicide prevention: a test of public health messaging to protect those at risk. Arch Suicide Res. 2018;22(3):394–404.
40. Betz ME, Wintemute GJ. Physician counseling on firearm safety: a new kind of cultural competence. JAMA. 2015;314(5):449–50.
41. Barber C, Frank E, Demicco R. Reducing suicides through partnerships between health professionals and gun owner groups—beyond docs vs. Glocks. JAMA Intern Med. 2017;177(1):5–6.
42. Lee TT, Curfman GD. Physician speech and firearm safety, *Wollschlaeger v. Governor of Florida*. JAMA Intern Med. 2017;177(8):1189–92.

43. Donohue JJ, Aneja A, Weber KD. Right-to-carry laws and violent crime: a comprehensive assessment using panel data and a state-level synthetic control analysis [Internet]. National Bureau of Economic research working paper; 2020 [Cited Mar 24]. Available from: https://www.nber.org/papers/w23510

44. Gibbons MJ, Fan MD, Rowhani-Rahbar A, Rivara FP. Legal liability for returning firearms to suicidal persons who voluntarily surrender them in 50 US States. Am J Public Health. 2020;110(5):685–8.

45. Fleegler EW, Madeira JL. First, prevent harm: Eliminate firearm transfer liability as a lethal means reduction strategy. Am J Public Health. 2020;110(5):619–20.

46. Masiakos PT, Warshaw AL. Stopping the bleeding is not enough. Ann Surg. 2017;265:37–8.

47. American Foundation of Suicide Prevention. American Foundation for Suicide Prevention and the National Shooting Sports Foundation partner to help prevent suicide [Internet]; 2016. https://afsp.org/american-foundation-suicide-prevention-national-shooting-sports-foundation-partner-help-prevent-suicide/. Accessed 29 Aug 2019.

48. Vriniotis M, Barber C, Frank E, Demicco R, New Hampshire firearm safety coalition. A suicide prevention campaign for firearm dealers in New Hampshire. Suicide Life Threat Behav. 2014;45:157–63.

Chapter 14
How to be a Firearm Legislative Advocate

Naveen F. Sangji and Peter T. Masiakos

The government spending bill includes a major victory for gun safety advocates

By The Editorial Board
December 19, 2019. *The Washington Post*

Physicians have a long history of advocating for their patients and for the American public. From 1776, when four physicians signed the United States (US) Declaration of Independence, to the 116th US Congress, which included 15 physicians, doctors have served in federal, state, and local government. They have served as heads of regulatory agencies, as advocates through professional organizations and hospital systems, and as individuals for issues impacting patient care and physician practice [1, 2]. The American Medical Association's (AMA) Declaration of Professional Responsibility states that physicians should "advocate for social, economic, educational, and political changes that ameliorate suffering and contribute to human well-being" [3].

In addition to the AMA, physician societies and medical associations such as the American College of Surgeons (ACS), the American College of Physicians (ACP), the American Academy of Pediatrics (AAP), the American College of Cardiology (ACC), and the American Academy of Family Physicians (AAFP) have advocacy arms focused on individual and public health. Some of the areas of engagement include expanding population access to and affordability of health care, improving delivery of health care, decreasing physician regulatory burden, improving undergraduate and graduate medical education, and addressing public health crises—including injuries [4–7]. These organizations rely on the engagement of physician

N. F. Sangji
Department of Acute Care Surgery, University of Michigan, Ann Arbor, MI, USA
e-mail: nsangji@med.umich.edu

P. T. Masiakos (✉)
Department of Pediatric Surgery, Massachusetts General Hospital, Harvard Medical School, Boston, MA, USA
e-mail: pmasiakos@partners.org

© Springer Nature Switzerland AG 2021
L. K. Lee, E. W. Fleegler (eds.), *Pediatric Firearm Injuries and Fatalities*,
https://doi.org/10.1007/978-3-030-62245-9_14

members to bring forward their concerns and the concerns of their patients to our elected representations at the state, local, and federal levels, and to proffer practical solutions.

Firearm injury is a public health crisis in the US. It is the second leading cause of death in people 10–24 years old [8]. Yet, for the past two decades, federal funding for firearm injury prevention research has been restricted due to the 1996 Omnibus Consolidated Appropriations Act [9]. In response to the Centers for Disease Control and Prevention (CDC)-funded studies demonstrating that firearm ownership was a risk factor for homicide in the home, the National Rifle Association (NRA) lobbied Congress to eliminate $2.6 million from the 1996 CDC budget. This was the exact amount the CDC had allocated to gun violence research the previous year [10]. The 1996 appropriations bill included a rider proposed by Rep. Jay Dickey (R-AR) stating "none of the funds made available for injury prevention and control at the Centers for Disease Control and Prevention may be used to advocate or promote gun control." [11]. The CDC subsequently ceased all firearm-related research, as did the National Institute for Health (NIH) and the Department of Health and Human Services (DHHS). Given the politically divisive nature of any discussion on firearm legislation, addressing this public health crisis will require active engagement and advocacy from all stakeholders, including physicians, who care for the victims of firearm injury. Finally, in 2020, after multiple well-publicized mass shootings and shifts in public opinion on firearm deaths as a public health crisis, $25 million in federal funding was appropriated to the CDC and NIH for firearm-related research for the first time since 1996.

Although this funding is an important step for firearm research, a multi-pronged strategy is necessary to decrease firearm injuries and deaths to US children. This includes clinician-led advocacy focused on stronger legislation and increased public health and research funding. A number of recent physician-led efforts at the federal and state levels highlight key mechanisms by which clinicians can get involved in and be successful at legislative advocacy. These strategies are applicable to efforts on firearm injury legislation at the state and federal levels as well. We propose the following three steps as essential for successful physician advocacy:

1. Establish relationships with legislators
2. Develop coalitions
3. Persist, despite repeated failures

14.1 Federal-Level Advocacy

Physicians have a strong history of legislative advocacy on the federal level. We illustrate here one example, with principles, which potentially could be applied to future firearm legislation. One of the greatest challenges to the physician practice of medicine during this past decade was the impending payment cuts of 21% for physician services under the Medicare Sustainable Growth Rate (SGR) formula. This threat was averted with the passage of the Medicare Access and CHIP (Children's Health Insurance Program) Reauthorization Act (MACRA) of 2015 [12]. Repeal of the SGR took a concerted, decade-long effort by physicians who worked with their medical professional societies to meet with legislators and highlight the impact of payment cuts to their practices and to the patients they serve. Medical associations such as the AMA, the ACS, and the ACC coordinated their strategies and worked in concert to lobby for repeal and replacement legislation. Physicians sent thousands of letters, made phone calls to their representatives in the US House and Senate, had in-person meetings, participated in medical association "lobby days," and testified in front of congressional committees to advocate for repeal and replacement. The repeal efforts failed year after year as "patches" were enacted to avert payment cuts at the last minute each year, until 2015 with the passage of MACRA [13]. Successful repeal of the SGR required years of coordinated efforts in the face of repeated failures, spearheaded by medical associations with the support of physicians delivering care in clinics, hospitals, rural communities, and academic medical centers alike.

14.2 State-Level Advocacy

In an era of gridlocked national politics, state-level legislation can be highly impactful for healthcare access and delivery, patient safety, and physician practice. This includes firearm safety legislation. Working relationships between physicians and their state representatives are crucial to these efforts. We include two examples in this chapter to illustrate the importance of relationships, coalition-building, and persistence in the face of great odds for successful advocacy [14, 15]. First is the passage of Sean's Law in Massachusetts in 2010, which prohibits children less than 14 years old from riding an all-terrain vehicle (ATV) on public lands. The second is the defeat of Proposition 46 in California in 2014, which would have raised the cap on non-economic damages in medical liability lawsuits. Then finally we include an example of physician advocacy with the AAP, which resulted in overturning the Firearm Owners' Privacy Act, "physician gag law," in Florida.

14.3 Passage of Sean's Law

In 2006, 8-year-old Sean Kearney suffered severe head injuries from an all-terrain vehicle (ATV) crash while at a friend's house. He died 5 days later from these injuries. Sean's parents questioned how this could have happened to their child, and they wanted to prevent something like this from happening to another child in the future. Their grief motivated Sean's trauma surgeon to be a physician advocate for the Kearney family to help pass state legislation prohibiting ATV riding in children.

Initial meetings with Massachusetts state Senator Stephen Baddour (D-Methuen) established a strong working relationship. This ultimately led to submitting a formidable bill prohibiting children less than 14 years old from riding an ATV on public lands and moving it through the legislative process. A coalition of medical clinicians joined an unlikely "out of the box" coalition consisting of environmental advocates. This multidisciplinary coalition led the 4-year-long effort spanning two legislative sessions. In the first legislative session, the bill did not even come to a vote. The medical and environmental coalitions increased their efforts in the second legislative session, and "Sean's Law" was eventually enacted in 2010 [14]. This law mandated a minimum age of 14 years for ATV use by children, the first law of its kind in the US [16]. A study assessing ATV injury data up to 3 years after the enactment of Sean's Law revealed a 40% decrease in pediatric ATV-related injuries in Massachusetts [17]. An unlikely partnership between a trauma surgeon and a state Senator, coalition building among other medical clinicians and environmental advocates, along with persistence in the legislative process is a demonstration of how physician advocacy can lead to legislative change. This ultimately decreased injuries and deaths from ATVs in Massachusetts. Similarly, as more restrictive state-level firearm laws are associated with decreased firearm deaths and injuries, these principles can be applied by clinicians to advocate for stronger state-level firearm legislation.

14.4   Defeat of Proposition 46

John Maa, MD, FACS, a trauma surgeon in San Francisco, CA, led a collaboration between the California chapters of the ACS and the California Medical Association (CMA), which ultimately helped to defeat a statewide ballot measure in 2014 (Proposition 46). This ballot measure would have raised the cap on noneconomic damages in medical liability lawsuits, with detrimental effects on patient access to care [15]. Under Dr. Maa's leadership, these medical associations joined a broader collaboration with government, advocacy, and labor organizations such as the California Chamber of Commerce, American Civil Liberties Union (ACLU), and Service Employees International Union (SEIU) to defeat this ballot measure. Physicians organized lobby days at the California statehouse, offered testimony, and wrote letters to editors of newspapers to raise awareness of the impact of this ballot measure on healthcare access. The efforts of the coalition were rewarded at the ballot, where Proposition 46 was soundly defeated. The broad coalition was a key factor ensuring defeat of this ballot measure. This is another example of the effectiveness of clinician advocacy on the state-level with multi-disciplinary coalition building on affecting state-level change.

14.5   Overturning the Physician Gag Law

In 2011, the state of Florida enacted the Firearm Owners' Privacy Act (FOPA), also known as the "physician gag law," which prohibited health care practitioners from asking about firearm ownership by a patient or family member unless this information was relevant to the patient's medical care or safety. In addition, this law prohibited including any information about firearm ownership in the medical record and prohibited the clinician from harassing or discriminating against patients based on firearm ownership. Shortly after this law passed, several physicians and physician professional organizations, including the AAP, sued on the basis that this law violated a physician's First Amendment rights to freedom of speech. After concerted efforts by physicians working with the AAP and others, the inquiry, record-keeping, and anti-harassment provisions of the law were finally overturned in 2017 in an *en banc* decision by the US Court of Appeals for the Eleventh Circuit in *Wollschlaeger v. Governor, Florida*. Pediatricians working with the AAP were crucial to moving this case through the appeals process and eventually having this law overturned. Although this Florida law was successfully overturned, there are continued state-level efforts at limiting physicians' inquiry of firearms in the home. It is important for clinicians to be knowledgeable about laws as well as impending legislation in their state to become engaged in state-level legislative advocacy for harm prevention against firearm injuries and deaths [18].

14.6 Physician-Led Advocacy Efforts on Firearm Violence

Recently, the American College of Physicians (ACP) released a position paper on reducing injury and deaths from firearms [19]. In response, the NRA asked for "self-important, anti-gun doctors to stay in their lane" on the social media platform Twitter [20]. Joseph Sakran, MD, MPP, FACS, a trauma surgeon and survivor of a firearm injury as a teenager, challenged the NRA and created a Twitter account @ ThisIsOurLane, which incited a maelstrom of support from physicians and allied healthcare professionals who care for the victims of firearm-related injuries [20]. Trauma surgeons, emergency medicine physicians, pediatricians, medical students, and nurses, among many others, responded with heartfelt and graphic testimony on the impact of firearm injuries on their patients and the families of the victims. Dr. Sakran's efforts made national headlines and helped bring advocacy related to firearms to the forefront of physician consciousness. In eight short months, physicians who were told they had no role in this public health discussion are now helping to lead it.

Given the complex intertwining of issues such as Second Amendment rights, political convictions, unintentional injuries, intentional violence, and mental health, efforts to decrease firearm-related injuries in the US must occur on many fronts. Physicians, being on the frontlines of those who care for victims of firearm injuries, can make important contributions. Individuals like Dr. Sakran can have a tremendous impact just by sharing their stories, as can any physician who cares for patients who are victims of firearm injuries. Medical associations and professional organizations can serve as vehicles for lobbying state and federal governments. For example, in 2018, the AMA House of Delegates passed a number of new policies in response to tragedies such as the Orlando massacre of 2016 in response to activism from AMA members [21]. The ACS has convened a task force, including members who own firearms and practice trauma surgery, to reach common sense consensus to reduce firearm injuries. They hosted discussions on firearm injury prevention at national forums such as their annual Clinical Congress and Leadership and Advocacy Summit [22]. Other physician organizations, including the AAP, have also organized similar efforts.

In addition, there are now also a number of physician-led organizations dedicated solely to firearm injury research and education. The American Foundation for Firearm Injury Reduction in Medicine (AFFIRM) and Firearm Safety Among Children and Teens (FACTS) are two recently founded organizations. They are both focused on funding research, disseminating best practices, and organizing education on firearm injury prevention. They both have useful resources for medical professionals interested in firearm-related advocacy and research [23, 24].

14.7   Resources for the Engaged Clinician

There are numerous resources for interested clinicians to engage in advocacy around firearm injury, or any other public health-related topic of interest, through their state and professional organizations [4–7]. Advocacy can be, but does not have to be, time consuming. Many medical professional associations, state societies, and healthcare institutions support platforms that can send form letters outlining policy positions electronically with as few as two clicks to their members' representatives. Legislators pay attention to these letters from you, their constituent. They take the views of their constituents into account when adopting positions on specific issues or bills.

For those who are willing and able to engage further, a number of professional associations such as the ACS and the AAP organize federal lobby days in Washington, D.C. In addition, the state chapters of these professional associations organize annual state lobby days, which provide a great opportunity for physicians to meet with their US and state representatives, respectively. During these meetings, clinicians can share patient stories and experiences and start developing the relationships that can lead to two-way exchanges of information and collaboration between clinicians and legislators. Physicians and other healthcare professionals can make themselves available for providing testimony on important issues such as firearm injury when bills addressing those are debated in their state legislature or in the US Congress. US Representatives and Senators also have in-district office hours open to constituents, which are listed and readily available on their web pages. Interested clinicians can make appointments to meet with their US Representatives or Senators within their own district, when legislators are likely to have less harried schedules and are hence able to dedicate time to constituent concerns.

Here are some specific steps to engage in state-level legislative advocacy:

1. Meet with your institution's government relations office, if you work in an institution that has such an office.

    (a) They can assist with developing relationships with state and federal legislators.

   (b) They can help develop and introduce state-level legislation to decrease firearm injuries and deaths.

2. Understand the current firearm-related laws and any impending legislation in your state.
3. Identify and arrange a meeting with your state representative and state senator. Start to develop a relationship with your legislator and/or his/her staff person.

   (a) Express your support of legislation to decrease firearm injuries and deaths to US residents. This can also be accomplished through e-mail, written letter, and/or phone call in addition to an in-person meeting.

4. Use resources from the ACS, AAP, and ACP for talking points.
5. Engage with your medical professional organization (e.g., ACS and AAP) to participate in their advocacy efforts in your state. This could include providing written or oral expert testimony.
6. Publish an Op-Ed in your local or national newspaper or other news source advocating for stronger firearm legislation to decrease firearm injuries and deaths to children. Universal background checks, Child Access Prevention (CAP), and Extreme Risk Protection Order (ERPO) laws are three laws with some pediatric specific implications.
7. Participate in state lobby days through your institution and/or medical professional organization.

Each day in the US, 109 people are killed as a result of firearm violence [25]. It has become clear that combating this public health crisis will require active and sustained engagement from physicians and other medical professionals who are on the frontlines and deal with the toll of firearm injuries and the social consequences of these injuries. As a closing note, in 2015, Ex-Representative Jay Dickey voiced his deep regret about the amendment bearing his name, which stymied firearm research for a generation [26]. After decades of lobbying by clinician groups and others, in 2020, Congress finally authorized $25 million for firearm violence. It is a relatively small start, but an important key to moving forward as we strive to decrease firearm-related deaths and injuries to US children and youth.

Take Home Points
- Clinicians have an important role in legislative advocacy for harm prevention to improve the health and well-being of children and youth, including against firearm injuries and deaths.
- Medical professional organizations can guide interested clinicians in advocacy.
- Advocacy can occur at the state and federal levels.
- Similar to other successful advocacy efforts, firearm injury legislation requires engagement of clinicians, building of coalitions, and persistence in the face of failure.

References

1. Editorial. Four physicians who signed the declaration of Independence. N Engl J Med. 1961;265:1318–9.
2. Dyrda L. Becker's Healthcare; 2017 Jan 9. Meet the 15 physician members of the 115th US Congress [Internet]. Available from: https://www.beckershospitalreview.com/hospital-management-administration/meet-the-15-physician-members-of-the-115th-us-congress.html. Accessed 11 June 2019.
3. American Medical Association. Declaration of professional responsibility: medicine's social contract with humanity [Internet]. Available from: www.ama-assn.org/ama/upload/mm/369/decofprofessional.pdf. Accessed 11 June 2019.
4. American College of Surgeons (ACS), Advocacy [Internet]. Available from: https://www.facs.org/advocacy. Accessed 11 June 2019.
5. American Academy of Pediatrics (AAP), Advocacy and Policy [Internet]. Available from: https://www.aap.org/en-us/advocacy-and-policy/Pages/Advocacy-and-Policy.aspx. Accessed 11 June 2019.
6. American College of Cardiology (ACC), Advocacy at the ACC [Internet]. Available from: https://www.acc.org/tools-and-practice-support/advocacy-at-the-acc. Accessed 11 June 2019.
7. American Academy of Family Physicians (AAFP), Advocacy [Internet]. Available from: https://www.aafp.org/advocacy.html. Accessed 11 June 2019.
8. Murphy SL, Xu J, Kochanek KD, Curtin SC. Deaths: Final data for 2015. Natl Vital Stat Rep. 2017;66(6):1–75.
9. Rubin R. Tale of 2 agencies: CDC avoids gun violence research but NIH funds it. JAMA. 2016;315(16):1689–91.
10. Kellerman AL, Rivara FP. Silencing the science on gun research. JAMA. 2013;309(6):549–50.
11. Dzau VJ, Rosenberg M. Congress hasn't banned research on gun violence. It just won't fund it [Internet]. The Washington Post; 2018 Mar 21. Available from: www.washingtonpost.com/opinions/how-research-canhelp-us-address-gun-violence/2018/03/21/ecde2128–2c4d-11e8–8ad6-fbc50284fce8_story.html?utm_term=.ad7c443b6193. Accessed 25 May 2018.
12. Public Law 114–10, 114th Congress. Medicare access and CHIP reauthorization act of 2015 [Internet]. 2015 Apr 16. Available from: https://www.congress.gov/114/plaws/publ10/PLAW-114publ10.pdf. Accessed 11 June 2019.
13. American College of Surgeons. ACS declares victory with passage of law repealing the SGR [Internet]. 2015 June. Available from: bulletin.facs.org/2016/08/the-acs-andadvocacy-a-tradition/. Accessed 11 June 2019.
14. Ackerman T, Rosen J. Surgeons as state advocates: success stories [Internet]. Bull Am Coll Surg. 2014;99:9. Available from: http://bulletin.facs.org/2014/09/surgeons-as-advocates-success-stories/. Accessed 11 June 2019.
15. Maa J, Sutton J. The defeat of proposition 46 in California: a case study of successful surgeon advocacy [Internet]. Bull Am Coll Surg. 2016;101:1. Available from: http://bulletin.facs.org/2016/01/the-defeat-of-proposition-46-in-california-a-case-study-of-successful-surgeon-advocacy/. Accessed 11 June 2019.
16. Commonwealth of Massachusetts, General Laws, Part I, Title XIV, Chapter 90B, Section 26. Prohibited or limited operation by underage persons; restrictions [Internet]. Available from: https://malegislature.gov/Laws/GeneralLaws/PartI/TitleXIV/Chapter90B/Section26. Accessed 11 June 2019.
17. Flaherty MR, Raybould T, Kelleher CM, Seethala R, Lee J, Kaafarani HMA, Masiakos PT. Age legislation and off-road vehicle injuries in children. Pediatrics. 2017:e20171164.
18. Lee TT, Curfman GD. Physician speech and firearm safety: Wollschlaeger V. Governor, Florida. JAMA Intern Med. 2017;177(8):1189–92.
19. Butkus R, Doherty R, Bornstein SS. Health and public policy committee of the American College of Physicians. Reducing firearm injuries and deaths in the United States: a position paper from the American College of Physicians. Ann Intern Med. 2018;169(10):704–7.

20. Warmsley L. After NRA mocks doctors, physicians reply: 'this is our lane' [Internet]. National Public Radio; 2018 Nov 11. Available from: https://www.npr.org/2018/11/11/666762890/after-nra-mocks-doctors-physicians-reply-this-is-our-lane. Accessed 13 June 2019.
21. AMA Staff. AMA recommends new common sense policies to prevent gun violence [Internet]. Press Release; 2018 June 12. Available from: https://www.ama-assn.org/press-center/press-releases/ama-recommends-new-common-sense-policies-prevent-gun-violence. Accessed 13 June 2019.
22. ACS Staff. ACS takes a public health approach to firearms [Internet]. Clinical Congress Daily Highlights; 2018 Oct 22. Available from: https://www.facs.org/clincon2018/resources/highlights/mon/ps124. Accessed 13 June 2019.
23. American Foundation for Firearm Injury Reduction in Medicine (AFFIRM) [Internet]. Available from: https://affirmresearch.org/what-we-do/. Accessed 30 Mar 2020.
24. Firearm-safety Among Children and Teens (FACTS) [Internet]. Available from: https://www.icpsr.umich.edu/icpsrweb/content/facts/about/consortium.html. Accessed 30 Mar 2020.
25. Centers for Disease Control and Prevention, Web-Based Injury Statistics Query & Reporting System (WISQARS) fatal injury reports, national, regional and state (Restricted), 1999–2017 [Internet]. Available from: https://webappa.cdc.gov/cgi-bin/broker.exe. Accessed 13 Aug 2019.
26. Ex-Rep. Dickey Regrets Restrictive Law On Gun Violence Research [Internet]. National Public Radio (NPR), Morning Edition. 2015 Oct 9. Available from: https://www.npr.org/2015/10/09/447098666/ex-rep-dickey-regrets-restrictive-law-on-gun-violence-research. Accessed 30 Mar 2020.

Chapter 15
Future Directions for Firearm Injury Intervention, Policy, and Research

David Hemenway and Michael C. Monuteaux

The gun rights debate in Georgia intensifies with 2020 nearing

By Greg Bluestein and Tamar Hallerman
August, 9, 2019. *The Atlanta Journal-Constitution*

15.1 Introduction

As documented elsewhere in this volume, pediatric firearm injury is a national, clinical, and public health concern in the United States (US). Firearms are the second leading cause of death among US youth of ages 1–17 years [1]. From 2009 through 2014, there were over 20,000 firearm-related emergency department visits by pediatric patients [2]. In 2014, there were 10 emergency department visits for firearm-related injuries per 100,000 persons who were 0–18 years old [3]. Addressing this growing public health crisis requires a comprehensive approach integrating efforts from clinicians, public health professionals, policy makers, educators, researchers, community leaders, law enforcement, and others. In this chapter, we will discuss the future directions of pediatric firearm injury prevention from three perspectives: interventions, public policy, and research.

When considering the prevention of future pediatric firearm injury, the following points should be considered. First, interventions and policy proposals should be evidence-based whenever possible. We can maximize effectiveness by leveraging existing data and capitalizing on previous experiences to craft and implement future efforts. That is not to say, however, that our responses need be delayed while we

D. Hemenway
Department of Health Policy and Management, Harvard T.H. Chan School of Public Health, Boston, MA, USA
e-mail: hemenway@hsph.harvard.edu

M. C. Monuteaux (✉)
Department of Pediatrics, Division of Emergency Medicine, Boston Children's Hospital, Boston, MA, USA
e-mail: Michael.monuteaux@childrens.harvard.edu

© Springer Nature Switzerland AG 2021   223
L. K. Lee, E. W. Fleegler (eds.), *Pediatric Firearm Injuries and Fatalities*,
https://doi.org/10.1007/978-3-030-62245-9_15

wait for definitive data as dozens of children suffer firearm injuries each day. Action is needed now, informed by the best evidence available, with each iteration building on the lessons learned from earlier efforts.

Second, our future efforts should integrate the support and involvement of all relevant stakeholders – clinicians, public health professionals, policy makers, law enforcement, survivor organizations, firearm owners, and others in the firearm community (such as gun retail outlets/range owners and firearm trainers). The involvement of the latter groups can be especially informative and important when crafting and delivering injury prevention messages to firearm owners [4, 5].

Third, intervention programs, public policy, and research are inter-related efforts, each informing and influencing the others. For instance, a new public policy permitting law enforcement or family members to request the temporary removal of firearms from a person who may present a danger to themselves or others (i.e., Extreme Risk Protective Order or "red flag laws") might motivate a research study to measure the impact of the law on firearm violence rates. Likewise, a research study demonstrating that the provision of lock boxes during routine well visits to a pediatrician office increases safe firearm storage among gun-owning parents might lead to support for the initiation of similar interventions at other health care delivery settings. For ease of disposition, we will consider each of these three perspectives in turn, but we will remain cognizant that these efforts are not operating in a vacuum. Progress in one area can and often will be a springboard to meaningful progress in another. Thus, the recommendations that follow should not be restricted to the area within which they are presented.

15.2   Intervention

Few pediatric firearm injury prevention programs have strong empirical evidence of success. A recent comprehensive review included 46 studies implemented across several settings (i.e., school, healthcare, community) evaluating a variety of interventions, such as safe storage encouragement, screening programs, and education programs on firearm use and carriage. The authors did not find consistent results supporting an evidence-based approach to prevention and noted that methodological shortcomings were common in the reviewed literature [6]. However, another review by Rowhani-Rahbar et al. of interventions to encourage safe storage of firearms concluded that counseling coupled with the provision of a safe storage device can significantly improve the firearm storage practices of parents with young children, although there were not enough studies ($n = 3$) to support a formal meta-analysis [7]. There are also community-based programs with some evidence demonstrating reductions in violence, although these are not firearm- nor pediatric-specific [8].

We can make the following recommendations to help guide future intervention and prevention programs. First, interventions should be tailored to a specific mechanism and intent of firearm injury. Evidence shows that the epidemiology [9] and risk factors for self-inflicted, violent, and unintentional firearm injury differ considerably [10]. These differences should translate into mechanism-specific intervention features and designs. Successful approaches to preventing youth suicide by firearm may differ from those having an impact on firearm-related interpersonal violence. Even within the context of interpersonal violent firearm injury prevention, it is likely that gang-related violence, intimate partner violence and other forms of interpersonal violence may each require distinctive approaches. Second, where possible, outcome evaluation should be included as a vital element of future interventions, regardless of whether the program is expected to be the subject of a research study. Interval evaluations of success using *a priori* defined metrics are essential to make continual improvements in effectiveness. Third, when planning intervention evaluations, practitioners and researchers alike should utilize randomized and controlled designs whenever feasible. As demonstrated by our colleagues in criminology, it is often possible to create interventions using randomized, controlled trials [11, 12].

There are several intervention modalities that can be highlighted as promising avenues for future efforts. As noted above, safe storage interventions, including the provision of a safe storage device, have been shown to improve storage practices among firearm owners. Since there is strong evidence that safe storage is protective against self-inflicted and unintentional firearm injury among youth [13], these behavioral changes can ultimately result in fewer injuries and deaths [14]. Healthcare settings (e.g., emergency departments and primary care clinics) represent a prime opportunity to implement intervention programs (including anticipatory guidance with or without the provision of safe storage devices) that can reach large numbers of children and their parents. However, many clinicians have reported feeling inadequately trained to counsel patients about firearm safety and did not believe such guidance to be efficacious [15]. In response, educational interventions for clinicians should be developed and evaluated [16]. Interventions for children exposed to firearm violence, either as an injured victim or as a witness, are warranted, as these experiences are harmful to children's development and well-being [17]. Finally, public health messaging and information campaigns about the risks of firearm ownership (especially regarding suicide and intimate partner violence), the benefits of safe firearm storage, and the importance of adequate firearm training should be developed and tested in partnership with stakeholders from the firearm community.

Health care organizations (including its accreditation bodies) are not the only non-governmental organizations that can play a role in reducing firearm injuries, and whose policies and programs call for evaluation. Corporations, for example, can actively try to reduce firearm violence [18]. Walmart has written strict procedures for the selling of firearms to reduce the likelihood of straw purchasing [19]. Dick's Sporting Goods Stores have stopped selling assault-style weapons, and in 2020, they stopped selling firearms altogether in 575 of their 857 stores [20]. In local areas, the faith community has been important in engendering cooperation between the police and the community [21]. Imagine the possible effect on gun trafficking if there was a concerted national effort across all faiths to make gun sales to strangers without a background check the equivalent of a mortal sin, whether or not local authorities said it was illegal [22].

15.3   Policy

Recent reviews have summarized the literature on the association between public policy and firearm injury among children. Briefly, Zeoli and colleagues reviewed twenty studies and found evidence that child access protection (CAP) laws were associated with reductions in unintentional firearm death among youth, although the findings varied by the severity of the criminal liability imposed by the law and the ages of the children under study [23]. No association was found for laws regulating minimum age restrictions for purchase or possession of a firearm and pediatric firearm injury outcomes. There were too few studies focused on other laws (e.g., background checks, stand your ground laws) to draw substantive conclusions about the protective effect of these types of laws and pediatric firearm injuries and deaths [23]. A 2020 study by Azad and colleagues looked at CAP laws by type – recklessness laws and negligence laws – across 25 years and found that negligence laws were associated with lower child fatality rates for homicide, suicide, and unintentional firearm deaths [24]. A RAND Corporation review found supportive evidence (the strongest strength of evidence designation employed by the review) that CAP laws were protective against both self-inflicted and unintentional firearm injuries and deaths among youth [25].

We can propose several recommendations to inform future policy initiatives. First, although limited, the empirical evidence evaluating existing policies should inform the development of new policy efforts, which when implemented should include a funded mechanism for methodologically sound evaluation. As novel policies take effect at the state or municipal levels, they can be evaluated, and the results disseminated widely in a timely fashion. Policies proven effective should be adopted by other locales, which then in turn contribute data to the shared body of evidence. Of course, because states and municipalities differ widely in the strength and breadth of their firearm regulation, policies enacted in one locale can be compromised by the more permissive firearm statutes of neighboring locales through the trafficking of firearms [26]. One way to mitigate this problem is to nationalize the most effective polices through federal legislation. A challenge exists of course in that it may take years of data to show true effectiveness.

Second, efforts should be made to optimize the implementation, enforcement, and dissemination (in terms of raising public awareness) of new laws/policies, in order to maximize their effect and facilitate valid evaluations. For example, CAP laws are only effective to the extent that parents are both aware of the passage of the law and change their behavior vis-à-vis the use and storage of their firearms in response to this awareness. As another example, some state-level ERPO "red flag" policies allow family members to petition a court to remove firearms from a person deemed in crisis [27], but the extent to which the public is cognizant of this preventive measure is unknown. Most states do not allow physicians, psychologists, or other health care providers to petition. Across states, the use of ERPO laws varies significantly. In the first year after passage in Massachusetts, only 20 petitions to remove a gun in a dangerous situation were filed [28]. In the year prior to implementation, there were 262 firearm fatalities including 152 suicides. Thus, passage of CAP and red flag policies should be accompanied by wide-reaching multimedia public messaging campaigns targeting firearm owners and their families to maximize awareness. In other instances, local law enforcement officials have made known their refusal to enforce duly approved state-level statues intended to reduce firearm violence [29]. Political measures to ensure the uniform enforcement of new policies are advised.

Third, policy makers should recognize the myriad manifestations of firearm violence among children (e.g., unintentional, gang activity, suicides, mass shootings, domestic violence, homicide) and understand how a novel policy might impact these various types of violent events differently. Policies could also exert a differential effect on children by age, whereby a policy may be protective against unintentional firearm injuries among school-aged children but have less impact on older youth where firearm injuries are more likely to be intentional (i.e., homicide or suicide). Policies might also impact children differently by race, ethnicity, urban-rural residence, or socioeconomic status. It is important when designing policy to be precise in considering what type of firearm violence it is intended to prevent and who is expected to see the benefit.

There are several policy ideas, some already part of the public conversation, that may be considered more broadly by policy makers and other stakeholders moving forward. For instance, only two states have thus far attempted to regulate the production and distribution of the so-called "ghost guns," which use legal loopholes to allow users to easily assemble untraceable guns. Recently, plans have been distributed for the printing of guns using 3D printers; these firearms are untraceable and do not trigger metal detectors [30].

There are no policies preventing the manufacture of replica-style toy guns, which are designed explicitly to look and feel like real firearms. In fact, firearm manufacturers allow toy companies to produce replicas of their products. A recent investigation found there have been over 150 persons brandishing these replica-style toys who were shot by law enforcement since 2015 [31].

Some political figures have endorsed the arming of teachers and/or other school personnel as a safeguard against active shooter events. In 2019, Florida passed a law allowing teachers to carry guns in school. Given the non-zero probability that an accessible, loaded firearm will inflict an inappropriate injury (i.e., unintentional injuries, self-inflicted injuries, or interpersonal violence that is not perpetrated in self-defense), policy makers should consider carefully whether placing a loaded firearm in every classroom during each and every school day would cause more morbidity than it might prevent.

Finally, it is imperative to recognize that government at all levels has many policy levers that can help prevent firearm injuries. For example, job programs for adolescents and young adults, nurse visits for families, and after-school activities for children and adolescents can buffer vulnerable youth from harmful influences, provide coping skills to children and caregivers, and help identify high-risk youth for clinical intervention. Government policies directed specifically at firearms include taxing or prohibiting large capacity magazines and imposing strict liability for gun owners whose firearms are stolen and used in crime. Government can also advance promotion of safety standards for firearms and use its purchasing power through law enforcement and the military to purchase the so-called "smart guns" (see Chap. 12). Local governments can use their zoning and other powers to regulate sub-standard gun shops. The public health problems associated with firearms are broad, requiring broad policies on the local, state, and federal levels [32].

15.4   Research

A 2019 special issue of the *Journal of Behavioral Medicine* [33] contained five comprehensive reviews of the scientific literature related to pediatric firearm injury, covering the following topics: youth firearm carriage [34], risk and protective factors [35], primary prevention efforts [6], long-term outcomes of exposure to firearm violence [36], and the effects of laws on pediatric firearm injury outcomes [23]. We refer the reader to these excellent works to review and understand the contemporary landscape of scientific work in this area at the time of this writing.

When summarizing these reviews, Cunningham et al. noted that the failure of federal agencies to fund firearm injury research has resulted in a paucity of published studies in the area [33]. Indeed between 2004 and 2015, gun violence research was considerably underfunded and understudied compared to other leading causes of death in the US [37]. This funding draught is also reflected in the strength of the evidence (or lack thereof) found in currently available studies. Thus, the evidence base describing pediatric firearm injury available to the clinical, policy, and public health communities has been lacking [33].

Beyond these excellent points, we can make a few additional recommendations to help guide future research efforts. Most of the policy research examining pediatric firearm injury (and firearm outcomes in general) to date has relied on ecological study designs, which suffer from well-known methodological limitations including the so-called ecologic bias (i.e., an inconsistency between a given ecological association and the individual-level effect) [38]. Where possible, future assessments of policy effects should take advantage of methodologically stronger study designs.

1. For example, individual-level behavior changes (e.g., a change in firearm storage practices) made in response to polices could be are linked to subsequent firearm-related outcomes.
2. Or, studies could examine variations in the characteristics of specific injuries (e.g., whether the firearm used was purchased legally or operated by a person under the minimum age cutoff) before and after the implementation of the relevant policy within a jurisdiction and/or between jurisdictions with and without the policy.

In general, future studies would benefit from longer, prospective follow-up periods and examination of both intermediate (e.g., changes in firearm storage practices and replacement of conventional firearms with "smart guns") and distal (i.e., pediatric firearm injuries and mortality) outcomes to fully characterize the chain of causation. Lastly, it is imperative that we develop more accurate, detailed, and nationally comprehensive firearm injury surveillance systems, surveys of firearm-related behaviors across age (e.g., gun ownership and carriage), and data warehouses of firearm-related administrative and forensic data (e.g., gun-tracing and concealed-carry permit data) [39]. Thankfully, the National Violent Death Reporting System finally has funding for all 50 states; better circumstantial data on non-fatal firearm injuries are sorely needed.

A recent publication provided a comprehensive research agenda to guide scientific efforts toward the prevention of firearm injuries among children and adolescents. The Firearm Safety Among Children and Teens (FACTS) Consortium, a multidisciplinary organization, used a modified nominal group technique to identify five broad research areas: epidemiology and risk and protective factors, primary prevention, secondary prevention and sequelae, policy, and data enhancement. Within these areas, 26 specific agenda items with examples of specific research questions were identified [40].

Beyond the thorough and thoughtful research agenda described above, we can highlight further potential directions for future research efforts. First, machine learning methods and related sophisticated statistical techniques can be utilized to develop and refine prediction models for firearm-related outcomes among high-risk individuals (e.g., suicide attempts among patients with depression and violent retaliation by victims of assault). Such methods are being developed to predict clinical outcomes in emergency department samples [41], including pediatric patients [42, 43], which could ultimately be used to inform and guide clinical practice. Separate prediction models could be developed for suicide risk and interpersonal violence (both as perpetrator and as victim). Such tools, if validated, could be used to focus limited prevention resources.

Second, the ubiquitous presence of social media and other online activities among Generation Z (i.e., the demographic cohort born from the mid-1990s through the early 2000s, aka, the "smartphone generation") should be investigated. Several questions about the impact of this technology on these youth warrant careful study. For example, little is known about their attitudes toward firearms, their intake of firearm-related online content (and the nature of this content), their awareness of firearm violence within their community and across the country, the impact of this awareness on psychological and attitudinal outcomes, or the role of social media and other online platforms in transmitting inflammatory communications that can instigate a firearm-related incident (be it suicide or interpersonal violence), just to name a few.

Third, the development of wide-ranging research networks and committed funding mechanisms is crucially important to advancing the science in this area. As is well known, there was a prolonged moratorium on support for firearm-related research from the National Institutes of Health (NIH) and Centers for Disease Control and Prevention (CDC). As a result, the field of firearm violence prevention (and pediatric firearm violence in particular) is still struggling to meet the challenge of providing evidence-based solutions and guidance to policy makers and clinicians. Thankfully, there are signs of improvement. The aforementioned FACTS Consortium, which is funded by NIH, is a network of scientists and stakeholders focused on cultivating research resources in this area [44]. The American Foundation for Firearm Injury Reduction in Medicine (AFFIRM) is a group of healthcare professionals and researchers working together to find lasting solutions to curb firearm violence. Firearm-focused conferences sponsored by multidisciplinary teams have taken place, where researchers had the opportunity to share their work, network, and cultivate new collaborations [45]. Following the lead of the Wellness Foundation and the Joyce Foundation, the National Collaborative on Gun Violence, a philanthropic fund launched with Arnold Foundation support, recently funded its first round of firearm research projects [46]. Health care organizations such as Kaiser Permanente and Massachusetts General Hospital are currently providing funds for firearms research as are three state governments (California, New Jersey, and Washington). There are online repositories for firearm researchers, where datasets, publications, reports, and other resources are available [47–49]. Research leaders, philanthropists, health care organizations and state and federal funding agencies should continue this momentum and commit to expanding these resources.

15.5   Conclusions

The statistics on firearm violence among youth are grim. Firearms are the second leading cause of death among individuals less than 19 years old in the US. In 2018, there were more school shootings than in any other year since 1970 [50]. The popular media provide us with daily reminders of our national firearm violence epidemic. It has been estimated that there are more than 350 million firearms currently in circulation in the US [51, 52], with more and deadlier weapons sold every day.

Facing these facts, one might acquiesce to the notion that firearm violence is woven into our national DNA, an embedded cultural tumor beyond excision. However, our firearm problem need not be intractable. As evidence, there have been substantial, culture-shifting public health successes in the past. Smoking rates among US adults dropped from 42% in 1965 to 14% in 2017 [53]. Would today's cultural attitudes toward smoking in public spaces such as bars and restaurants have seemed plausible to persons living in the 1970s or 1980s? Yet these changes were realized. Similar national behavioral shifts toward healthier practices have occurred in other areas (e.g., seatbelt usage, drinking and driving).

Policy, research, intervention, informing, supporting, and reinforcing each other can advance reciprocally and exert a meaningful reduction on the burden of pediatric firearm injury and mortality. Understanding the scope of the problem of firearm injuries and deaths, examining potential solutions for decreasing these injuries and deaths, and advocating for effective policies are critical for starting to work on addressing this important health problem. We must no longer sit on the sidelines and watch as more children and youth are injured or killed by firearms, while potential solutions languish. Only by healthcare professionals, child advocates, policy makers, gun owners, and citizens working together can we turn the tide on firearm deaths and injuries for children and youth in the US.

Take Home Points
- Addressing the crisis of pediatric firearm injury requires a comprehensive approach, integrating efforts from clinicians, public health professionals, policy makers, educators, researchers, community leaders, law enforcement, and others.
- Toward addressing pediatric firearm injury, there are important opportunities across the policy, research, and intervention domains that should be explored.
- Interventions should be tailored for specific mechanisms of injury (i.e., unintentional, intentional, self-harm). Priority areas for intervention include safe storage interventions, healthcare setting-based intervention programs, and interventions focused on children who are victims of or are exposed to violence.
- Effective policies should be optimized in terms of implementation, enforcement, and dissemination to maximize their effect and facilitate their evaluations.
- The development of wide-ranging research networks and committed funding mechanisms are essential for conducting high-quality research needed to decrease firearm injuries and deaths.
- Policy, research, interventions, informing, supporting, and reinforcing each other can advance reciprocally and exert a meaningful reduction on the burden of pediatric firearm injury and mortality.

References

1. Cunningham RM, Walton MA, Carter PM. The Major Causes of Death in Children and Adolescents in the United States. N Engl J Med. 2018;379(25):2468–2475.
2. Cutler GJ, Zagel AL, Spaulding AB, Linabery AM, Kharbanda AB. Emergency Department Visits for Pediatric Firearm Injuries by Trauma Center Type. Pediatr Emerg Care. 2019 May 22. Online ahead of print.
3. Gani F, Canner JK. Trends in the Incidence of and Charges Associated With Firearm-Related Injuries Among Pediatric Patients, 2006-2014. JAMA Pediatr. 2018;172(12):1195–1196.
4. Henn M, Barber C, Hemenway D. Involving firearm stakeholders in community-based suicide prevention efforts. Curr Epidemiol Reports. 2019;6(2):231–7.

5. Jager-Hyman S, Benjamin Wolk C, Ahmedani B, et al. Perspectives from firearm stakehold-ers on firearm safety promotion in pediatric primary care as a suicide prevention strategy: a qualitative study. J Behav Med. 2019;42(4):691–701.
6. Ngo Q, Sigel E, Moon A, et al. State of the science: a scoping review of primary prevention of firearm injuries among children and adolescents. J Behav Med. 2019;42:811–29.
7. Rowhani-Rahbar A, Simonetti JA, Rivara FP. Effectiveness of interventions to promote safe firearm storage. Epidemiol Rev. 2016;38(1):111–24.
8. Cure violence: scientific evaluations [Internet]. Avaiable from: http://cureviolence.org/results/scientific-evaluations/.
9. Centers for Disease Control and Prevention. Web-based Injury Statistics Query and Reporting System (WISQARS) [Internet]. Available from: http://webappa.cdc.gov/sasweb/ncipc/nfi-rates2001.html. Published 2019.
10. Monuteaux MC, Mannix R, Fleegler EW, Lee LK. Predictors and Outcomes of Pediatric Firearm Injuries Treated in the Emergency Department: Differences by Mechanism of Intent. Acad Emerg Med. 2016;23(7):790–5.
11. Farrington DP, Welsh BC. Randomized experiments in criminology: what have we learned in the last two decades? J Exp Criminol. 2005;1:9–38.
12. Braga AA, Welsh BC, Papachristos AV, Schnell C, Grossman L. The growth of random-ized experiments in policing: the vital few and the salience of mentoring. J Exp Criminol. 2014;10(1):1–28.
13. Grossman DC, Mueller BA, Riedy C, et al. Gun storage practices and risk of youth suicide and unintentional firearm injuries. J Am Med Assoc. 2005;293(6):707–14.
14. Monuteaux MC, Azrael D, Miller M. Association of Increased Safe Household Firearm Storage With Firearm Suicide and Unintentional Death Among US Youths. JAMA Pediatr. 2019;173(7):657–662.
15. Price JH, Thompson A, Khubchandani J, Wiblishauser M, Dowling J, Teeple K. Perceived roles of Emergency Department physicians regarding anticipatory guidance on firearm safety. J Emerg Med. 2013;44(5):1007–16.
16. Kwong JZ, Gray JM, Rein L, Liu Y, Melzer-Lange MD. An educational intervention for medi-cal students to improve self-efficacy in firearm injury prevention counseling. Inj Epidemiol. 2019;6(Suppl 1):27.
17. Rajan S, Branas CC, Myers D, Agrawal N. Youth exposure to violence involving a gun: evi-dence for adverse childhood experience classification. J Behav Med. 2019;42:646–57.
18. Hemenway D. Gun safety is a business issue [Internet]. Harvard Business Review. Available from: https://hbr.org/2012/12/gun-safety-is-a-business-issue. Published 2012.
19. Walmart. Walmart statement on firearms policy [Internet]. Available from: https://corporate.walmart.com/newsroom/2018/02/28/walmart-statement-on-firearms-policy. Published 2018. Accessed 24 Feb 2020.
20. Zhang H. Dick's Sporting Goods will stop selling guns at 440 more stores [Internet] Available from: https://www.cnn.com/2019/03/14/investing/dicks-sporting-goods-guns/index.html. Published March 10, 2020. Accessed 28 Dec 2020.
21. Winship C, Berrien J, McRoberts O. Religion and the Boston miracle: the effect of black min-istry on youth violence. In: Bane M, Coffin B, Thiemann R, editors. Who will provide?: the changing role of religion in American social welfare. Boulder: Westview Press; 2000. p. 336.
22. Hemenway D, Azrael D, Miller M. Selling a gun to a stranger without a background check: acceptable behaviour? Inj Prev. 2018;24(3):213–217.
23. Zeoli AM, Goldstick J, Mauri A, Wallin M, Goyal M, Cunningham R; FACTS Consortium. The association of firearm laws with firearm outcomes among children and adolescents: a scoping review. J Behav Med. 2019;42(4):741–762.
24. Azad HA, Monuteaux MC, Rees CA, Siegel M, Mannix R, Lee LK, Sheehan KM, Fleegler EW. Child access prevention firearm laws and firearm fatalities among children aged 0 to 14 Years, 1991–2016. JAMA Pediatr. 2020;174(5):463–69.
25. RAND Corporation. Gun policy in America [Internet]. Available from: https://www.rand.org/research/gun-policy.html. Accessed 15 Aug 2019.

26. Giffords Law Center to Prevent Gun Violence. Statistics on gun trafficking & private sales [Internet]. Available from: https://lawcenter.giffords.org/gun-traffickingprivate-sales-statistics/.

27. Giffords Law Center to Prevent Gun Violence. Extreme risk protection orders [Internet]. Available from: https://lawcenter.giffords.org/gun-laws/policy-areas/who-can-have-a-gun/extreme-risk-protection-orders/.

28. Rosmarin D. Massachusetts' 'red flag' gun law needs an update [Internet]. WBUR. Available from: https://www.wbur.org/cognoscenti/2019/08/21/massachusetts-extreme-risk-protection-order-red-flag-gun-law-david-rosmarin. Published 2019. Accessed 25 Feb 2020.

29. National Public Radio. When Sheriffs won't enforce the law [Internet]. Available from: https://www.npr.org/2019/02/21/696400737/when-sheriffs-wont-enforce-the-law.

30. Giffords Law Center to Prevent Gun Violence. Ghost guns [Internet]. Available from: https://lawcenter.giffords.org/gun-laws/policy-areas/hardware-ammunition/ghost-guns/#federal.

31. The Trace. Gunmakers are profiting from toy replicas that can get kids killed [Internet]. Available from: https://www.thetrace.org/2019/05/replica-gun-licensing-deals/.

32. Hemenway D. Injury prevention class exercise: three-pronged list making. Inj Prev. 2019;25(6):565–569.

33. Cunningham RM, Carter PM, Zimmerman M. The Firearm Safety Among Children and Teens (FACTS) Consortium: defining the current state of the science on pediatric firearm injury prevention. J Behav Med. 2019;42(4):702–705.

34. Oliphant SN, Mouch CA, Rowhani-Rahbar A, Hargarten S, Jay J, Hemenway D, Zimmerman M, Carter PM; FACTS Consortium. A scoping review of patterns, motives, and risk and protective factors for adolescent firearm carriage. J Behav Med. 2019;42(4):763–810.

35. Schmidt CJ, Rupp L, Pizarro JM, Lee DB, Branas CC, Zimmerman MA. Risk and protective factors related to youth firearm violence: a scoping review and directions for future research. J Behav Med. 2019;42(4):706–723.

36. Ranney M, Karb R, Ehrlich P, Bromwich K, Cunningham R, Beidas RS; FACTS Consortium. What are the long-term consequences of youth exposure to firearm injury, and how do we prevent them? A scoping review. J Behav Med. 2019;42(4):724–740.

37. Stark DE, Shah NH. Funding and Publication of Research on Gun Violence and Other Leading Causes of Death. JAMA. 2017;317(1):84–85.

38. Morgenstern H. Ecological studies. In: Rothman KJ, Greenland S, Lash TL, editors. Modern epidemiology. 3rd ed. Philadelphia: Lippincott Williams & Wilkins; 2008. p. 511–31.

39. Hemenway D. Firearms data, and an ode to data systems [Internet]. Chance. 2018; Available from: https://doi.org/10.1080/09332480.2018.1438703.

40. Cunningham RM, Carter PM, Ranney ML, et al. Prevention of firearm injuries among children and adolescents: consensus-driven research agenda from the firearm safety among children and teens (FACTS) consortium. JAMA Pediatr. 2019; Online ahead of print.

41. Raita Y, Goto T, Faridi MK, Brown DFM, Camargo CA Jr, Hasegawa K. Emergency department triage prediction of clinical outcomes using machine learning models. Crit Care. 2019;23(1):64.

42. Bertsimas D, Dunn J, Steele DW, Trikalinos TA, Wang Y. Comparison of Machine Learning Optimal Classification Trees With the Pediatric Emergency Care Applied Research Network Head Trauma Decision Rules. JAMA Pediatr. 2019;173(7):648–656.

43. Goto T, Camargo CA, Faridi MK, Freishtat RJ, Hasegawa K. Machine learning-based prediction of clinical outcomes for children during emergency department triage. JAMA Netw Open. 2019;2(1):e186937

44. FACTS Consortium. FACTS: firearm safety among children and teens [Internet]. Available from: https://www.icpsr.umich.edu/icpsrweb/content/facts/index.html. Published 2019.

45. University of Connecticut. Correlates, causes, and solutions for firearm violence in America [Internet]. Available from: https://dpp.uconn.edu/preventfirearmviolence.

46. RAND Corporation. National collaborative on gun violence research [Internet]. Available from: https://www.ncgvr.org/.

47. Gun Violence Archive [Internet]. Available from: https://www.gunviolencearchive.org/. Published 2019.

48. GVPedia. Gun Violence Research [Internet]. Available from: https://www.gvpedia.org/. Published 2017.
49. McClenathan J, Pahn M, Siegel M. The Changing Landscape of U.S. Gun Policy: State firearm laws [Internet]. Available from: http://www.statefirearmlaws.org/.
50. Zimmerman MA, Carter P, Cunningham R. The facts on the US children and teens killed by firearms [Internet]. The Conversation. Available from: https://theconversation.com/the-facts-on-the-us-children-and-teens-killed-by-firearms-118318. Published Aug. 6, 2019.
51. Azrael D, Hepburn L, Hemenway D, Miller M. The stock and flow of U.S. firearms: results from the 2015 National Firearms Survey. Russell Sage Found J Soc Sci. 2017;3(5):38–57.
52. Levine PB, McKnight R. Three million more guns: The Spring 2020 spike in firearm sales [Internet] Brookings. Available from: https://www.brookings.edu/blog/up-front/2020/07/13/three-million-more-guns-the-spring-2020-spike-in-firearm-sales/. Published July 13, 2020.
53. LaVito A. CDC says smoking rates fall to record low in US [Internet]. CNBC. Available from: https://www.cnbc.com/2018/11/08/cdc-says-smoking-rates-fall-to-record-low-in-us.html. Published 2018.

Index

© Springer Nature Switzerland AG 2021
L. K. Lee, E. W. Fleegler (eds.), *Pediatric Firearm Injuries and Fatalities*,
https://doi.org/10.1007/978-3-030-62245-9

Printed in the United States
by Baker & Taylor Publisher Services